INTERNATIONAL
FIRST RESPONDER

UK Edition

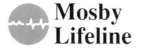

Mosby
Lifeline

INTERNATIONAL
FIRST RESPONDER

UK Edition

Walt A Stoy

Medical Adviser and Editor: **Dr Juergen Klein**

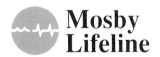

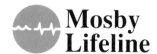
Mosby Lifeline

Publisher:	Terry Robinson
Editor:	Claire Hooper
Design and layout:	Mark Howard
Photography:	Tim Fisher
	Henry Sung
	Carlos Dominguez
Illustration:	Jenni Miller
	Marion Tasker
Tables:	Lee Riches
Copyediting:	Robert Whittle
Proofreading:	John Ormiston
Index:	Laurence Errington
Production:	Melanie Vandevelde

Published in 1998 by Mosby Consumer Health and Safety, a division of Mosby International Ltd, Lynton House, 7–12 Tavistock Square, London WC1H 9LB, UK.
© Copyright 1998 Mosby International Ltd.

ISBN: 0 7234 3130 2

Designed by Twenty-Five Educational,
25 Marylebone Road, London NW1 5JR
Printed and bound by Grafos S.A. Arte sobre papel, 1998.

Picture Credits

Figures 5.30, 6.5, 8.3, 8.4, 8.6, 8.7, 9.9, 9.14, 9.17, 10.4, and 10.5 from Mills, Morton & Page: *Color Atlas and Text of Emergencies*, 2nd Edition. London: Mosby International Ltd, 1995.

Figure 11.9 from Al-Azzawi: *Color Atlas of Childbirth and Obstetric Techniques*. London: Mosby International Ltd, 1990.

Figure 9.12 courtesy of Peter Driscoll, Consultant, Accident and Emergency Department, Hope Hospital, Salford.

Figures 2.3, 6.1, 8.5 and section openers for sections 1, 7 and 8 provided by John Callan, SHOUT Picture Library, 58–59 Great Marlborough Street, London W1V 1DD.

Figures 12.5, C.8 and C.10 by Mark Howard, Twenty-Five Educational.

Every effort has been made to contact holders of copyright to obtain permission to reproduce copyrighted material. If any have been inadvertently overlooked, however, the publishers will be pleased to make the necessary arrangements at the first opportunity.

Foreword

I T IS INDEED WITH ENTHUSIASM and a sense of pride that I write the Foreword for this textbook. The authors of the original textbook were honoured to be asked to share their materials for the development of a textbook to be used in the United Kingdom. Many talented individuals have been actively involved in the design and development of this textbook. The goal of this textbook is to give you information that will empower you with knowledge and skills to help you in care for patients.

The original textbook was based upon the 1995 'U.S. Department of Transportation National Highway Traffic Safety Administration, National Standard Curriculum for First Responders'. We designed this curriculum to meet the needs of those individuals who arrive on the scene of a medical or traumatic emergency first, before additional personnel with more knowledge and skills to care for the patient. We know that this textbook will meet that need in the United Kingdom as well.

Speaking for the authors of the original text, and the individuals who have taken this text to the next level, we hope that you enjoy it. Our sincere desire is for you to be better prepared to help in the care of the patients you encounter. Your willingness to learn this material will benefit mankind. For that, we thank you.

Walt A. Stoy PhD EMT-P
Director of Education
Center for Emergency Medicine
of Western Pennsylvania
Pittsburgh
USA
1998

Preface

I N THIS DECADE before the millennium, unprecedented changes have been seen in the concepts and strategies underlying the provision of pre-hospital immediate care. The concepts of 'chain of survival' and 'chain of trauma care' have arisen to provide state-of-the-art emergency care from the pre-hospital phase right through to the rehabilitation phase after hospitalisation. These new EMS strategies, which are a result of international co-operation and joint efforts on both sides of the Atlantic, are geared towards improving response times and providing a greater chance of survival for medical patients and trauma victims alike.

International First Responder (UK Edition) has been initiated in the current spirit of international exchange of pre-hospital care research and education. It is unique in that its contents reflect current British pre-hospital immediate care practice, while at the same time providing a basic curriculum for an adult-learner orientated First Responder Provider Course.

International First Responder (UK Edition) is a complete revision of *Mosby's First Responder Textbook*, written by Dr Walt A. Stoy and the Center for Emergency Medicine, Pittsburgh, Pennsylvania, and published in the USA in 1997. The project of anglicisation and adaptation of the American textbook to produce the first comprehensive textbook for First Responders in the UK was endorsed by the Chief and Assistant Chief Fire Officers Association (CACFOA) in June 1997. Representatives from eight fire brigades across the United Kingdom of Great Britain and Northern Ireland, and the National Fire Service College in Moreton-in-Marsh, shared their enthusiasm and their pre-hospital expertise to rewrite and review each chapter, and to re-illustrate the text.

The objectives of the *International First Responder* (**UK Edition**) are:

1) To disseminate the concept of the 'First Responder' and the knowledge required for fire-fighters to contribute effectively to an integrated and comprehensive Emergency Medical System;
2) To provide a core textbook for every fire-fighter in the UK who is involved in pre-hospital patient care as part of their statutory fire and rescue responsibilities;
3) To emphasise the importance of and to equip the reader with the relevant knowledge concerning patient assessment, basic airway care and oxygen therapy, Basic Life Support and Automated External Defibrillation;
4) To serve as the textbook for the 'First Responder Provider Course', leading to a Certified First Responder qualification after successful completion;
5) To establish the Certified First Responder qualification as an entry-level foundation in order to encourage the further establishment of UK course programmes and qualifications.

The *International First Responder* (**UK Edition**) would never have been completed in the allocated time frame without the team spirit and hard work of the individuals seconded to the CACFOA Editorial Working Group by their respective fire brigades and the National Fire Service College. On behalf of CACFOA and the Publishers, I would like to thank them for their invaluable input, enthusiasm and stimulating discussion around the table. Finally, special thanks must go to Andrew Kent, RGN, for his major contribution to the completion of this textbook.

Dr Juergen Klein Dip IMC RCSEd DA (UK)
Specialist Registrar in
Anaesthesia and Intensive Care,
Leicester Royal Infirmary NHS Trust,
Leicester
UK
1998

Contributors

CACFOA Editorial Working Group

It is important to note that *International First Responder* (**UK edition**) is essentially the end result of the work of Fire Service Personnel within the UK. Members of the CACFOA Editorial Working Group (listed below) conducted the mammoth task of identifying the key issues, writing their assigned sections and carrying out spirited peer review. Without them, this project could not have come to fruition.

Malcolm Alcock FIFireE MISM, County Fire Officer, Suffolk County Council Fire Service

Ian S. Black GIFireE CertEd, ALS Provider, Station Officer, London Fire Brigade

William Clark GIFireE, Brigade Emergency Planning Staff Officer, Northern Ireland Fire Brigade

William Denny EMT, Sub Officer, Personnel and Training Department, Strathclyde Fire Service

Kevin Ford, Acting Station Officer, Cleveland Fire Brigade

John Harding GCGI GIFireE, Divisional Officer, Greater Manchester County Fire Service

David Hutchinson LICG, Deputy Commandant, Strathclyde Fire Brigade Training Centre

Andrew Kent, MA RCN ENB 199, Clinical Nurse Manager, Accident & Emergency Department, Cumberland Infirmary, Carlisle

Mazen Khuri, Divisional Officer, Cleveland Fire Brigade

Dr Juergen Klein Dip IMC RCSEd DA (UK), Specialist Registrar in Anaesthesia and Intensive Care, Leicester Royal Infirmary NHS Trust, Leicester

Michael Lambell OStJ JP MIFireE, Group Commander, London Fire Brigade

Michael McCarthy, Assistant Divisional Officer and Senior RTA Instructor, Fire Service College, Moreton-in-Marsh

Gerry O'Neill BA (Hons) MIFireE, Acting Assistant Chief Fire Officer, Lancashire Fire and Rescue Service

Alan Wilson GIFireE AIMgt, Divisional Officer (Training Manager), North Wales Fire Service

Acknowledgements

The CACFOA Editorial Working Group and the Publisher would like to give special thanks to the following individuals and organisations:

CACFOA (Chief and Assistant Chief Fire Officers Association); Richard Bull, CACFOA Personnel and Training Committee, for nominating and facilitating the Editorial Working Group; All those individuals who gave up their time to organise and take part in photographic sessions; John Callan, SHOUT Picture Library; Tim Fisher, Photographer; Carlos Dominguez, Photographer; Henry Sung, Brigade Photographer, Lancashire Fire and Rescue Service; Mark Skelton, Station Officer, Strathclyde Fire Brigade; Cameron Black, Sub-Officer, Strathclyde Fire Brigade; John Taylor, Media and Public Relations Officer, Lancashire Fire and Rescue Service; Ian Williams, Sub Officer, North Wales Fire Service; Her Majesty's Coastguard, MRSC, Belfast; Her Majesty's Coastguard, Holyhead, North Wales; Professor Graham Page, Accident and Emergency Department, Aberdeen Royal Infirmary; Barry Hart, Circuit Paramedic, Snetterton Circuit, Norwich; London Ambulance Service Training Directorate. Equipment was kindly supplied by: Laerdal Medical Ltd, Orpington, Kent; Physio Control UK Ltd, Basingstoke, Hants; Ferno UK, Cleckheaton, W. Yorkshire; and Response Medical Equipment Ltd, Chipping Campden, Gloucestershire.

About this book

WELCOME to ***International First Responder* (UK Edition)**. The goal of the authors and reviewers involved in this project is to provide you with a basic textbook for easy and quick reference to the information necessary to succeed in becoming a First Responder. The text has been carefully planned to meet the needs of both instructors and students, using abundant illustrations to provide a visually appealing book complete with easy-to-read text and accessible diagrammatic information.

The Approach

This textbook focuses, quite simply, on what First Responders *need-to-know*. One of the problems in providing too much information is that students are forced to determine what content is really important – where to focus their attention. Therefore, the topics covered in this text are more concise and focused than that of similar texts. Nonetheless, all the information that First Responders must know in order to provide quality emergency care is covered here, with as much background information and explanation as necessary for students to become excellent pre-hospital care providers. **Principle boxes** highlight essential information and procedures. Additional in-depth information that some First Responders may need to know is covered in the **Appendices** at the back of the book.

Organisation of Content

This textbook is divided into eight divisions. Division One, **Preparatory**, is designed to help the student understand the emergency medical services and how the First Responder fits into this system. It also includes material on the well-being of the First Responder, the relevant core information on human anatomy and physiology, and techniques for lifting and moving patients. Division Two, **The Airway**, focuses on basic and advanced airway and ventilation techniques and oxygen delivery. Division Three, **Patient Assessment**, describes scene assessment and the patient assessment process, including triage, primary assessment, First Responder physical examination, and secondary assessment. Division Four, **Circulation**, covers circulation and the steps of cardiopulmonary resuscitation for adults, infants and children. Division Five, **Illness and Injury**, provides an overview of medical emergencies, including near-drowning, bleeding and soft tissue injuries with emphasis on the pathophysiology of shock and burns. Division Six, **Childbirth and Children**, contains information about childbirth and caring for infants and children. Division Seven focuses on **EMS operations**, including general

aspects of air medical transport, hazardous materials incidents and the principles of extrication. Finally, Division Eight contains the **Appendices**, which provide additional information that is not covered in the main text. Appendices A and B cover information on oxygen delivery and other ventilation devices. Appendix C includes information on assessing vital signs. Appendix D contains the information First Responders will need to know to use an automated external defibrillator. Appendix E has the information needed to apply simple splints. At the end of the text is a **Glossary** which defines the key terms used throughout the book. A **Further Reading** section provides a list of important books and other publications that you should refer to for additional background information. Finally, a detailed **Index** is also provided to ensure ease of access to the information contained within this book.

Structure of Chapters

Each chapter has a specific, carefully planned structure that will help you to read and learn the material more easily.

Chapter Outline

Each chapter begins with an outline of the material included within, allowing you to see how the information fits together at a glance.

Key Terms

Each chapter starts with a list of key terms, providing brief definitions for important terms used within the chapter.

First Responder Objectives

The objectives provided at the start of each chapter mirror those of the curriculum of the UK First Responder Qualification. **Cognitive** objectives include what you should know after reading and studying the chapter. **Affective** objectives focus on attitude – what you should understand and feel about patients and family members in relation to the chapter content. **Psychomotor** objectives list what you should be able to do after studying the chapter and practising the skills in your course.

First Response 'Scenario'

Each chapter opens with a short account of First Responder patient care in a realistic pre-hospital situation. The patient's problem relates to the chapter topic. These scenarios will help you to focus on the material covered in the chapter, and will help you to put the First Responder skills you learn from the chapter into real-life context.

Text

The text of each chapter is broken into small sections of information to allow you to proceed with your reading and learning in a flexible but organised manner.

Information Boxes and Tables

Information boxes and tables are placed throughout the text to highlight special information, making it easier to learn and review. These special displays include **First Responder Alerts**, which call attention to critical information or safety warnings.

Review Questions

Review Questions are featured throughout the chapters to test your comprehension of the material covered thus far. If you have difficulty answering any of these questions, you should go back and review the material before proceeding to the next section.

Illustrations

The textbook is heavily illustrated throughout with full-colour photographs and diagrams. The important aspects of First Responder skills are illustrated in a step-by-step format to help you learn the correct procedures before you begin practising them.

Chapter Summary

At the end of each chapter is a summary organised around the key topics in the chapter. This will allow you to integrate all of the key information in the chapter, as well as to return to the chapter later for a quick content review.

International First Responder

Contents

DIVISION ONE: PREPARATORY

Chapter 1: Introduction to the Emergency Medical Services System   3

The Emergency Medical Services System   5
Access to the Emergency Medical Services system   6
Levels of Education   6
The Health-Care System   6
Roles and Responsibilities of the First Responder 7
Personal Safety   7
Scene Safety   7
Patient Assessment and Care   7
Handover to a Higher Level of Care   8
Professional Attributes   8
Medical Direction   8
Strategic Medical Direction   10
Medical Direction   10

Chapter 2: Well-Being of the First Responder   11

Emotional Aspects of Emergency Care   13
Dying and Death   13
Stressful Situations   14
Stress   14
Critical Incident Stress Debriefing   15
Comprehensive Critical Incident Stress Management   16
Safety   17
Scene Safety   17
Personal Safety   19

Chapter 3: The Human Body   23

The Respiratory System   24
The Airway   24
The Lungs   25
The Respiratory System of Infants and Children   26
The Circulatory System   26
The Heart   27
Blood Vessels   27
The Blood   28
The Circulation of Blood   28

The Musculoskeletal System   29
The Skeletal System   29
The Muscular System   30
The Nervous System   33
The Skin   33
The Digestive System   33
The Endocrine System   34

Chapter 4: Lifting and Moving Patients   35

Role of the First Responder   37
Body Mechanics and Lifting Techniques   37
Guidelines for Lifting   37
Guidelines for Carrying   37
Guidelines for Reaching   40
Rescue Board Technique   40
Helmet Removal   42
Guidelines for Pushing and Pulling   42
Principles of Moving Patients   42
General Considerations   42
Emergency Moves   43
Non-urgent Moves   44
Patient Positioning   44
Equipment   45
Wheeled Stretcher   45
Scoop Stretcher   45
Carrying Chair   46
Spinal Boards   46
Immobilisation Extrication Devices   46
Cervical Collar   47

DIVISION TWO: THE AIRWAY

Chapter 5: The Airway   51

The Respiratory System   54
Components and Function of the Respiratory System   54
Considerations for Infants and Children   55
Opening the Airway   55
Manual Positioning   56
Inspecting the Airway   56
Airway Adjuncts   57

Clearing the Compromised Airway and
Maintaining an Open Airway   **60**
The Recovery Position   60
Finger Sweeps   60
Suctioning   60
Assessing Breathing   **64**
Determine the Presence of Breathing   64
Determine the Adequacy of Breathing   64
Artificial Ventilation   **65**
Mouth to Mask Ventilation Technique   65
Mouth-to-Barrier Device Ventilation Technique   67
Mouth-to-Mouth Ventilation Technique   67
Special Considerations for Trauma Patients   68
Assessing the Effectiveness of Artificial Ventilation 68
Special Situations in Airway Management   **69**
Patients with Laryngectomies   69
Ventilating Infants and Children   70
Gastric Distension   70
Facial Trauma   70
Dental Appliances   70
Foreign Body Airway Obstruction (FBAO)   **70**
FBAO in the Responsive Patient   71
FBAO in the Adult Patient   71
FBAO in Infants and Children   73

DIVISION THREE: PATIENT ASSESSMENT

Chapter 6: Patient Assessment   79

Scene Assessment   **82**
Universal Precautions   82
Scene Safety   82
Nature of Illness and Mechanism of Injury   83
High-Speed Deceleration Injuries   85
Number of Patients and Need for Additional Help   86
Triage   **86**
Triage 'Sieve'   86
Primary Assessment   **88**
General Impression of the Patient   88
Assess Responsiveness   88
Assess the Airway   89
Assess Breathing   89
Assess Circulation   90
Reporting to Responding Ambulance Crews   91
First Responder Physical Examination   **91**
Performing a Physical Examination   92
Medical Patients and Patients with
No Significant Injury or Mechanism of Injury   94
Patient History   **94**
Medical Condition Identification Insignia   94
The AMPLE History   94
Secondary assessment   **95**

DIVISION FOUR: CIRCULATION

Chapter 7: Circulation   101

Review of the Circulatory System   **103**
Function   103
Anatomy   103
Physiology   104
Cardiopulmonary Resuscitation   **105**
Definition   105
Chain of Survival   105
Techniques of Adult CPR   **105**
Steps of Adult CPR   106
Hand Position for Chest Compression in the Adult 108
Two-Rescuer CPR   109
Techniques of Infant and Child CPR   **110**
Steps of Infant and Child CPR   110
Hand Position for Chest Compression in the Infant 112
Hand Position for Chest Compression in the Child 112
Interacting with the Patient's
Family and Friends   **114**

DIVISION FIVE: ILLNESS AND INJURY

Chapter 8: Medical Emergencies   117

General Medical Complaints   **119**
Specific Medical Complaints   **120**
Altered Mental Status   120
Fitting   121
Exposure to Cold   122
Near-Drowning   125
Exposure to Heat   126
Behavioural Emergencies   **127**
Behavioural Changes   128

Chapter 9: Bleeding and Soft Tissue Injuries   131

Shock   **133**
Signs and Symptoms of Shock   134
Role of the First Responder   134
Treatment of Shock   135
Bleeding   **135**
External Bleeding   136
Internal Bleeding   138
Role of the First Responder   138
Specific Injuries   **138**
Types of Injuries   139
Role of the First Responder   139
Special Considerations   140

Burns 143
Depth of Burns 143
Role of the First Responder 144
Special Considerations 145
Dressing and Bandaging 146

Chapter 10: Injuries to Muscles and Bones 151

Review of the Musculoskeletal System 153
The Skeletal System 153
The Muscular System 153
Injuries to Bones and Joints 154
Mechanism of Injury 154
Bone and Joint Injuries 154
Role of the First Responder 156
Injuries to the Spine 157
Mechanism of Injury 157
Assessment of a Casualty with
Suspected Spinal Injury 157
Signs and Symptoms of Potential Trauma 157
Management of Spinal Injuries 158
Role of the First Responder 158
Injuries to the Brain and Skull 159
Head Injuries 159
Role of the First Responder 159

DIVISION SIX: CHILDBIRTH AND CHILDREN

Chapter 11: Childbirth 165

Reproductive Anatomy and Physiology 167
Labour 168
First Stage of Labour 168
Second Stage of Labour 169
Third Stage of Labour 169
Pre-delivery Emergencies 169
Delivery 170
Role of the First Responder 171
Initial Care of the Newborn Baby 171
Post-Delivery Care of the Mother 172

Chapter 12: Infants and Children 175

The Airway 177
Anatomical and Physiological Concerns 177
Opening the Airway 177
Suctioning 178
Using Airway Adjuncts 178
Assessment 179

**Common Medical Problems in Infants
and Children** 180
Airway Obstruction 180
Respiratory Emergencies 180
Circulatory Failure 182
Fits 182
Altered Mental Status **182**
Sudden Infant Death Syndrome (SIDS) 183
Trauma **183**
Head Injury 183
Chest Injury 184
Abdominal Injury 184
Injury to an Extremity 184
**Reactions to Ill and Injured Infants
and Children** **184**

DIVISION SEVEN: EMS OPERATIONS

Chapter 13: EMS Operations 189

Phases of an EMS Response **191**
Preparation for the Call 191
Mobilisation 192
On the Way to the Scene 192
Arrival at the Scene 192
Transferring the Patient to the Ambulance 193
Post-run 193
Air Medical Transport **193**
Selection of Landing Sites 193
Landing Site Preparation 194
Safety 195
Fundamentals of Extrication **196**
Principles of Extrication 196
Team Approach System 197
Extrication Techniques 199
Supplementary Restraint Systems (SRS) 200
Hazardous Materials **202**
Safety 202
Radiation 203
Mass Casualty Situations **204**
Basic Triage 204
Procedures 205

DIVISION EIGHT: APPENDICES

Appendix A: Supplementary Oxygen Therapy 209

Oxygen **210**
Oxygen Delivery Equipment **211**
Oxygen Regulators 211
Oxygen Delivery Devices 211

Appendix B: Advanced First Responder Ventilation Techniques   215

Advanced First Responder Ventilation Techniques   **216**
Mouth-to-Mask with Supplementary Oxygen Technique   216
Two-Person Bag–Valve–Mask Technique   217
Flow-Restricted, Oxygen-Powered Ventilation Device Technique   218
One-Person Bag–Valve–Mask Technique   218
Assessing the Adequacy of Artificial Ventilation   **219**

Appendix C: Vital Signs   221

Vital Signs   **222**
Breathing   223
Pulse   224
Skin   225
Pupils   226
Blood Pressure   227
Vital Sign Reassessment   **228**

Appendix D: Automated External Defibrillation   231

The Automated External Defibrillator   **233**
Overview of the Automated External Defibrillator   233
Advantages of the Automated External defibrillator   234
Operation of the Automated External Defibrillator   234
Post-Resuscitation Care   238
Maintenance of the Automated External Defibrillator   **238**
Automated External Defibrillator Skills   **238**

Appendix E: Principles and Techniques of Splinting   241

Injuries to Bones and Joints   **242**
Signs and Symptoms of Bone and Joint Injury   242
Emergency Care for Casualties with Bone and Joint Injuries   242
Splinting   **243**
Reasons for Splinting   243
Principles of Splinting   243
Splinting Equipment and Techniques   244
Risks of Splinting   246

Glossary   249

Further Reading   254

Index   255

Division One:
Preparatory

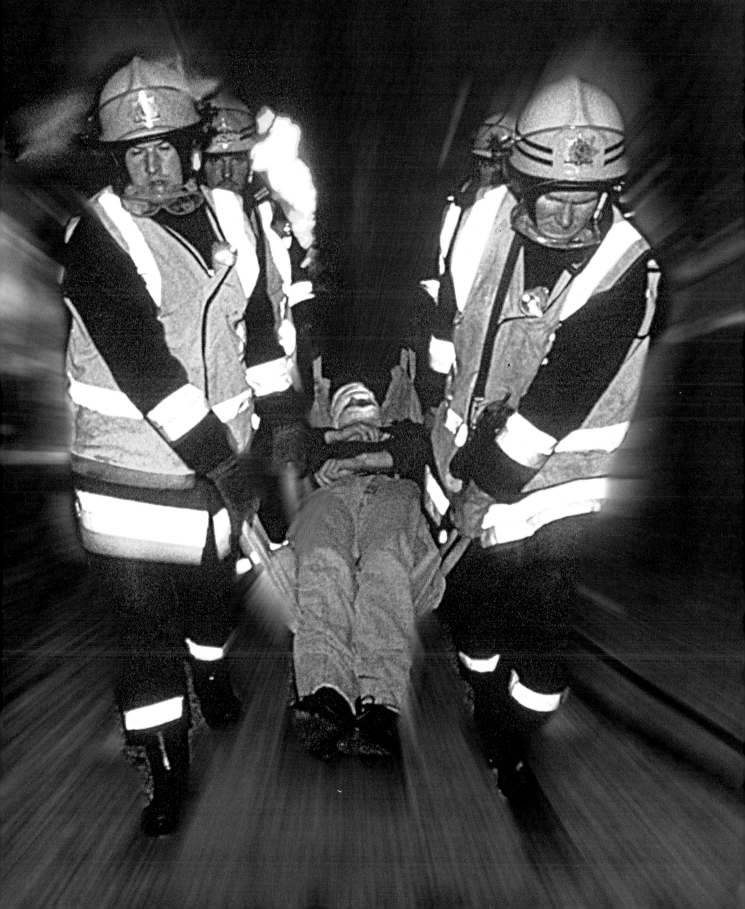

Chapter One

Introduction to the emergency medical services system

I. **The Emergency Medical Services system**
   A. Access to the emergency medical services system
   B. Levels of education
   C. The health-care system

II. **Roles and responsibilities of the First Responder**
   A. Personal safety

   B. Scene safety
   C. Patient assessment and care
   D. Handover to a higher level of care
   E. Professional attributes

III. **Medical direction**
   A. Strategic medical direction
   B. Medical direction

Key terms

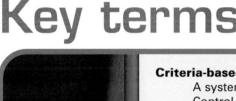

Criteria-based dispatch
A system by which an Ambulance Control Operator, who has received special training, uses a computerised dispatch program or cardex system to prioritise calls according to information received, and may provide pre-arrival instructions to emergency callers or others over the telephone before arrival of the EMS.

Emergency Medical Services (EMS) System
A system of many agencies, personnel and institutions involved in planning, providing and monitoring emergency care.

Ambulance Technician
An emergency care provider, cardiac trained, who may administer low risk drugs and gases and may carry out defibrillation.

Ambulance Paramedic
An emergency provider with training above the level of Ambulance Technician to include advanced airway management, intravenous (IV) cannulation, drug therapy and defibrillation.

First Responder
An EMS provider who utilises a minimum amount of equipment to perform initial assessment and intervention and who is trained to assist other EMS providers, e.g. a suitably trained fire-fighter, First Aider or member of the public.

Strategic Medical Direction
Any direction provided by medically qualified personnel that does not involve speaking with providers in the field, including but not limited to, systems design, protocol development, education and quality improvement.

Medical Direction
The process (usually by medically trained personnel) of ensuring that the care given to casualties is medically appropriate, also called medical control ('MEDCON'). This may include direct communication between medically trained personnel and care providers in the field.

Quality Improvement
A system for continually evaluating and making necessary adjustments to the care provided within an EMS system.

Objectives

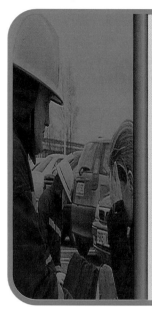

On completion of this chapter you will be able to meet the following objectives:

Cognitive Objectives

1. Define the components of the Emergency Medical Service (EMS) System.
2. Differentiate the roles and responsibilities of the First Responder from other pre-hospital care providers.
3. Define medical direction and discuss the First Responder's role in the process.
4. Discuss the types of strategic medical direction that may affect the medical care provided by the First Responder.

Affective Objectives

5. Accept and uphold the responsibilities of a First Responder within the standards of an EMS system.
6. Explain the rationale for maintaining an appropriate 'professional' approach when carrying out the role of the First Responder.
7. Describe why it is appropriate to treat a patient in a non-judgemental manner and to offer equal standards of care to all.

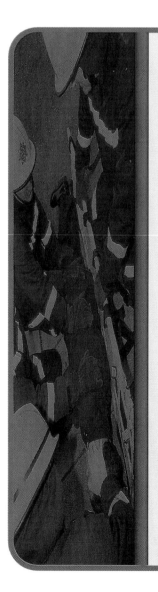

First response

FOLLOWING THE COMPLETION of his probationary period, Gary had been nominated to attend a First Responder course which was being organised by the brigade. He knew that ambulance personnel were there to offer this type of assistance, but he had chosen to become a fire-fighter not an ambulance paramedic or a doctor. During a lunch break he decided to discuss the matter with Adam, a veteran First Responder on his watch. Adam explained to him that being a First Responder was nothing like being a doctor. He explained the Emergency Medical Services (EMS) system to Gary and told him what an integral part of that system the First Responders were. Adam explained to Gary that, as a fire-fighter, his First Responder training would be extremely valuable. It was certain that during his career Gary would respond to many incidents where casualties would need medical assistance. The people that he would provide care for would be members of his community, other brigade personnel and possibly members of his family.

Adam further explained that fire-fighters were not the only ones serving in this vital capacity. He told Gary about police officers who became First Responders as part of their training. He also talked about some industrial response teams in which business and industry use First Responders to provide emergency care in their facilities before the arrival of the EMS. He also provided some examples of other people who serve as First Responders as part of their jobs, such as helicopter crews, mountain rescue teams and life boat personnel.

Adam recalled the time that he responded to a road traffic accident (RTA) and found an unresponsive patient. He opened the woman's airway, monitored her breathing and controlled severe bleeding. The ambulance crew told Adam that his actions probably saved the woman's life. Adam told Gary that his initial training as a First Responder, and the continuation courses and refresher training he completed whilst in the brigade, made him feel much more comfortable in performing his job as a fire-fighter. Gary left the discussion with a new outlook on becoming a First Responder and fire-fighter.

First Responders are an integral component of any Emergency Medical Services (EMS) System. First Responders initiate care until the ambulance service arrives or provide care for casualties in situations that cannot be reached by ambulance personnel immediately. They therefore require a solid foundation of knowledge in basic emergency procedures. This textbook will provide you with a pathway for learning how to become a First Responder.

This chapter marks the beginning of your education in becoming a First Responder. The chapter outlines the roles, responsibilities and attributes of a First Responder. It also describes the **Emergency Medical Services (EMS) system** and the role of First Responders within the system. The EMS system is the system of volunteers and professionals who provide emergency medical care, beginning when someone initially realises an injured or ill person requires such care and continues through to the patient's admission to the hospital (**Fig. 1.1**)

THE EMERGENCY MEDICAL SERVICES SYSTEM

Working or volunteering as a First Responder is an important role which can be both demanding and rewarding. Few other activities have such an impact on people's lives on a daily basis.

Every day, people's lives are touched by EMS. From an elderly patient who must reach the doctor's surgery for an appointment, to a child with a life-threatening airway emergency, all of the casualties you will encounter have one thing in common – they need help. They require the assistance of a competent, qualified, caring individual. The EMS system is a network of resources that provides emergency care and transport to victims of sudden illness and/or injury.

The EMS system increasingly has a role to play in injury and illness prevention. Just as fire-fighters and police officers spend much of their time on fire- or crime prevention, some EMS personnel are beginning to make efforts directed at reducing preventable injury and illness. First Responders can impact upon lives by teaching people how to lead a healthy life and how to prevent injury where possible.

The initial component of the EMS system is the response to emergencies. The public must recognise that there has been an emergency and must inform the emergency services, who can give telephone advice to assist in any early life-saving intervention.

First Responders may be part of a designated EMS response or they may be members of the public, work as fire-fighters, police officers or other form of rescue team. First Responders are often sent to the scene of an emergency to initiate emergency medical pre-hospital care until the ambulance and additional EMS help arrives. In this role the First Responders have an important job: scene safety, the initial assessment and treatment of the injured.

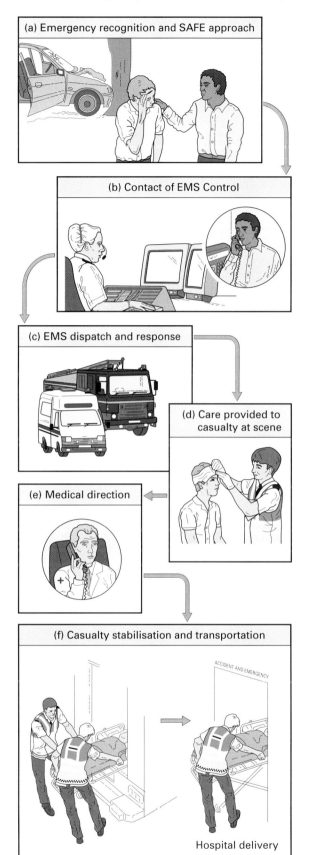

Fig. 1.1 The EMS system encompasses **(a)** emergency recognition and SAFE approach (**S**hout for help, **A**pproach with care, **F**ree from danger, **E**valuate AcBCs – airway/cervical spine, breathing, circulation), **(b)** contact of EMS Control, **(c)** EMS personnel dispatch and response, **(d)** care provided to the casualty at the scene, **(e)** medical direction when necessary, and **(f)** casualty stabilisation, transportation and delivery to the hospital.

Once additional help arrives, First Responders may continue to provide care by helping the ambulance personnel as they arrive at the scene. In some cases, this may require First Responders to help Ambulance personnel during transport of casualties to the hospital (e.g. assisting with resuscitation).

The following sections will help you better understand the role of the EMS system.

Access to the emergency medical services system

The manner in which the public contacts the EMS system is extremely important. The commonest access number in the United Kingdom is the **999** system. However, **112** is also used and is the recognised European version. Telephone exchanges are equipped to identify the location of the caller using these emergency service numbers, and all calls are taped onto computer recording systems.

Public information campaigns at local and national level give the public the type of information they require to access the system and also inform them of the information required by the emergency service controller who will take their call (**Fig. 1.2**).

Levels of education

There are several recognised levels of pre-hospital care provider. The five main levels are: Certificated First Aider, First Responder, Ambulance Technician, Ambulance Paramedic and Emergency Doctor.

A ***Certificated First Aider*** is a person who has received approved first aid training.

A ***First Responder*** is a person who will assess and commence initial care of the patient. The focus of this role is to provide initial stabilisation until additional EMS resources arrive.

The ***Ambulance Technician*** provides primary medical care before the patient reaches hospital. Ambulance Technicians are cardiac trained and may also administer some low risk drugs. They may also carry out defibrillation. The level of training is dependent on each local ambulance authority protocol.

An ***Ambulance Paramedic*** has a higher skill level than an Ambulance Technician. Their training includes more complex techniques such as advanced airway management, intravenous access and drug therapy and defibrillation. As with the Ambulance Technicians, the levels of training are dependent on each ambulance authority.

An ***Emergency Doctor*** is a doctor who, ideally, is trained to the Diploma in Immediate Medical Care standard, and provides additional advanced skills and expertise in the pre-hospital field.

The health-care system

The EMS system is an integral component of the overall health-care system in the United Kingdom. This health-care system has many components. Most important to the First Responders is the pre-hospital setting. Certificated First Aiders, First Responders, Ambulance Technicians, Ambulance Paramedics and Emergency Doctors are the primary pre-hospital care providers.

The sequence of an EMS event begins when someone notices or discovers a patient's illness or patient's injury and calls the EMS system through the emergency number. First Responders may already be at the scene and will provide initial care until more advanced EMS personnel arrive. Also involved are professional emergency-service controllers who, as part of the system know as 'Criteria Based Dispatch', not only forward the emergency call to the responding crews, but may also give pre-arrival medical care instructions by telephone or via mobile radio (**Fig. 1.3**).

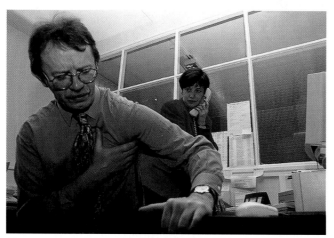

Fig. 1.2 In the United Kingdom, '999' is the universal number for access to police, fire and ambulance services.

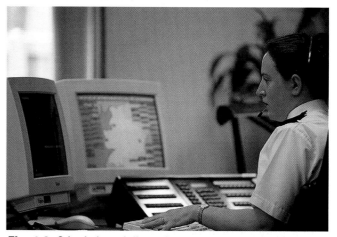

Fig. 1.3 Criteria-based dispatch operators are trained to give medical care instructions to emergency callers, First Responders and others on the scene, and to EMS crews before they arrive at the scene.

The next step in the health-care system is the hospital. Typically, this begins with arrival at the Accident and Emergency department. Health-care workers in the Accident and Emergency Unit include doctors, nurse practitioners, nurses and health-care assistants. Over and above immediate emergency care, the Unit can also provide services such as blood investigations, electrocardiograms (ECGs) and X-rays.

Some casualties may need the attention of a specialised unit such as a trauma unit, a burns unit, a children's unit or a poisons centre. These units can provide EMS personnel with additional specialist information as required.

ROLES AND RESPONSIBILITIES OF THE FIRST RESPONDER

The roles and responsibilities of First Responders are continually evolving. First Responders must understand these roles and responsibilities to be competent members of the health-care system (**Box 1.1**).

Personal safety

As a First Responder you have an initial responsibility for your personal safety and to be physically and mentally fit. This is discussed in depth in Chapter 2, 'The well being of the First Responder'. Personal safety at the scene includes using universal precautions and surveying the emergency scene for hazards or potential hazards before entering. Chapter 6, 'Patient Assessment', describes the appropriate measures to be taken in this important procedure.

Scene safety

First Responders are initially responsible for the safety of crew members, patients and bystanders. As discussed in the following chapters, this includes maintaining scene safety and coping with stress. You are responsible for providing the best possible care for patients whilst carrying out safety precautions that will prevent injury to patients or yourself from any hazards at the scene. The safety of bystanders must also be considered. By securing a safe scene and communicating effectively with bystanders, you protect everyone's safety.

Patient assessment and care

Patient assessment is a primary responsibility of the First Responder (**Fig 1.4**). In some cases, you may have to gain access to the patient before you can begin care. Special tools and equipment may be necessary to gain access to some casualties who may be trapped in vehicle wreckage, etc.

First Responders assess the patient's needs and provide the basic medical care established by that assessment. Chapter 6, 'Patient Assessment', describes how to assess a patient. As a First Responder you should practice and master these skills. The emergency care you provide is based on assessment findings. This approach allows for rapid management of life-threatening injuries and helps to relieve the patient's discomfort quickly.

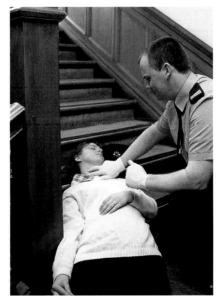

Fig. 1.4 First Responders assess patients to determine needs and provide appropriate care.

Box 1.1	**Roles and Responsibilities of the First Responder**

• Personal safety
• Scene safety
• Casualty assessment and care
• Handover to a higher level of care

Handover to a higher level of care

First Responders must confirm that EMS personnel with a higher level of training and the means to transport the patient to the hospital are en route. They must also ensure that care is continued for the patient. As additional EMS providers arrive, First Responders may assist them in providing continued care for the patient, as required.

When the patient has been evaluated and treated, he or she will be prepared for transport. First Responders must be able to assist in lifting and moving the patient safely. You should ensure the environment is safe for lifting, for example, by moving debris off the roadway before moving a patient over it. You must also use safe lifting and moving techniques as described in Chapter 4, 'Lifting and Moving patients'.

First Responders may have to complete a pre-hospital care handover report that includes information about the scene, the patient's injuries and care provided. This report will become part of the patient's record and may be used in quality improvement systems (**Fig. 1.5**).

Professional Attributes

First Responders must behave 'professionally'. In the context of this chapter, the term 'professional' refers to a level of competence rather than whether the First Responder is voluntary or paid.

Professional attributes include smart appearance, a positive attitude, the ability to communicate effectively with other personnel, up-to-date knowledge and skills, and making the patient's needs a top priority without endangering yourself or others.

First Responders are health-care practitioners and are an important component of the health-care team. You should strive, therefore, to project a smart appearance. A patient and his or her family may derive their first impressions of health-care personnel from their initial contact with you. An unkempt First Responder may imply sloppy patient care.

Maintaining calm and composure in emergency situations, and a caring, confident manner towards the patient and family while waiting for additional EMS personnel to arrive, will help relieve their anxiety.

An additional role of the First Responder is liaison with other health-care system professionals. It is important that the First Responder communicates effectively and develops a professional working relationship with such personnel.

As a First Responder you should keep abreast of changes and advances in medical care. Continuation training is an important aspect of your role. You should attend continuation training courses whenever possible and should practice skills that are not often used. You should also attend refresher courses to update your skills and knowledge on a regular basis. There are many journals that can help keep First Responders informed about trends in pre-hospital care. Journals targeted to specific professions that utilise First Responders also provide excellent information regarding trends in emergency medical services.

First Responders should be patient advocates, i.e. they should represent the interests of the patient when he or she is incapable of doing so. With the exception of their own safety and that of the crew, First Responders must put the needs of the patient first. Serving as a patient advocate requires good judgement, which will develop further with clinical experience.

MEDICAL DIRECTION

Medical Direction is the process through which medically trained personnel monitor the care given to casualties by First Responders. Your local EMS service will be able to give you information about medical direction and First Responders. Every EMS system must have medical direction.

Care provided can be monitored through the two components of medical direction: **Strategic Medical Direction** and **Medical Direction**, sometimes called Medical Control (MEDCON).

Review Questions

Roles and responsibilities of the First Responder

1. Which of the following is a role or responsibility of a First Responder?
   A. Vehicle extrication
   B. Fire suppression
   C. Patient assessment
   D. Crime prevention

2. A First Responder's professional appearance and confidence help reduce a patient's _____?
   A. Blood pressure
   B. Length of stay
   C. Level of consciousness
   D. Anxiety

3. Continuation training courses help maintain the First Responder's _____?
   A. Knowledge and skills
   B. Professionalism
   C. Certification and registration
   D. All of the above

4. After ensuring the safety of the First Responder, the crew, the patient and bystanders, which of the following is the most important?
   A. Obtaining insurance information
   B. Initial assessment of patient
   C. Teaching the new First Responders
   D. Vehicle maintenance

1. C; 2. D; 3. D; 4. B

Date: ☐☐☐☐☐ **Time:** ☐☐☐☐

One form to go with patient, one form to be retained

PATIENT REPORT FORM

Patient details: _____

Name: _____
Address: _____

Age: _____ D.O.B: _____ Sex: M ☐ F ☐
Contact: _____ Tel: _____

Comments: _____

_____
_____
_____
_____
_____

Chief complaint:

Trauma ☐   Burn ☐

Smoke inhalation ☐   Fall   >6ft ☐   <6ft ☐

Cardiac arrest ☐   Other _____

Mark apparent injuries	Mark apparent burns
FRONT BACK	FRONT BACK

RTA

✕ Position of patient
→ Point of impact
▨ Damaged area
† Fatality

Estimated time of accident: _____

Vehicle occupant ☐   Seat belt ☐

Trapped ☐   Ejected ☐

Extrication   Immediate ☐   Controlled ☐
                               Time _____

Motor cyclist ☐   Helmet worn ☐

Cyclist ☐   Pedestrian ☐

Estimated speed of impact _____

Airway	Open	Partial obstruction	Obstructed	Chin lift	Jaw thrust
Adjunct	None	Finger sweep Suction	Oral airway	Nasal airway	Finger sweep
Cervical spine	Manual hold	Collar	Board	All	
Breathing (per min)	Absent | <10	10–20	20–30	Regular	Irregular
Oxygen therapy	Yes	No	Amount given	Litres =	Time =
Circulation (pulse rate)	<50	50–70	70–100	>100	
Pulse location	Radial	Femoral	Carotid	Absent	
Skin colour	Pale	Normal	Cyanosed		
Responsiveness	Alert	Verbal	Painful	Unresponsive	
CPR	One person 15:2	Two person 5:1	Time =	AED | Yes	No

Form completed by: _____

Fig. 1.5 The pre-hospital care handover report forms part of the patient's record. This form, completed in duplicate by the First Responder, should include information about the scene, the patient's injuries and the care provided.

Strategic medical direction

Strategic Medical Direction consists of the organisational overview through which medically trained personnel influence care. These is achieved by elements such as designing the EMS system, developing protocols and standing orders, providing initial and continuation training, as well as other aspects such as reviewing pre-hospital care reports and managing data collection. EMS systems should also participate in **quality improvement**, a system for continuously evaluating and improving the care provided within the EMS system.

Medical direction

Medical Direction involves direct communication between the medically trained personnel and the provider in the field. This communication may occur via mobile phone, radio or telephone (land line). In some cases, the medically trained personnel may be present at the scene, allowing pre-hospital providers to speak directly with them. The role of a medically trained person at the emergency scene may vary. Local protocol dictates the proper procedure for following the orders and advice of this person at the emergency scene.

CHAPTER SUMMARY

The emergency medical services system

The EMS is a system of many agencies and institutions involved in planning and monitoring emergency medical care.

The five main levels of pre-hospital care providers are: Certificated First Aider, First Responder, Ambulance Technician, Ambulance Paramedic and Emergency Doctor. All EMS personnel interact with other health-care system professionals. First Responders should establish a strong working relationship with these other personnel.

Roles and Responsibilities of the First Responder

The First Responder has many roles and responsibilities, including personal safety; the safety of the crews, casualties and bystanders; patient assessment; patient care based on assessment findings; patient handover; and patient advocacy.

The First Responder is a health-care practitioner with certain professional attributes including projecting a smart appearance, maintaining knowledge and skills at a competent level, attending continuation training courses and serving as a patient advocate.

Medical direction

Quality care and medical direction go hand in hand. Medical direction establishes that all care given to a patient is medically appropriate. Strategic Medical Direction includes other activities such as system planning, protocol development, education, training and quality improvement. Medical direction involves direct contact between the medically trained personnel and the providers in the field.

Chapter TWO

The well-being of the First Responder

I. **Emotional aspects of emergency care**
    A. Dying and death
    B. Stressful situations
    C. Stress
    D. Critical incident stress debriefing
    E. Comprehensive critical incident stress management

II. **Safety**
    A. Scene safety
    B. Personal safety

Key terms

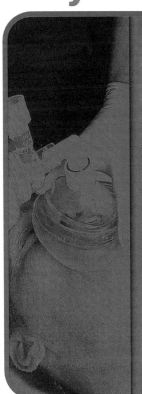

Universal precautions
Measures taken to prevent First Responders from coming into contact with a patient's blood, body fluids, or airborne pathogens via secretions.

Burnout
A condition characterised by physical and emotional exhaustion resulting in chronic, unrelieved job-related stress and ill health.

Critical incident
Any situation that causes emergency workers to experience strong emotional reactions and that interferes with their ability to function, either immediately or at sometime in the future.

Critical incident stress debriefing (CISD)
A debriefing process conducted by either a team of peer counsellors or specially trained health professionals, in order to help emergency workers deal with their emotions and feelings after a critical incident.

Hazardous material
A substance that poses a threat or unreasonable risk to life, health or property if not properly controlled during manufacture, processing, packaging, handling, storage, transportation, use or disposal.

Stress
Bodily or mental tension caused by physical or emotional factors; can also involve a person's response to events that are threatening or challenging.

Objectives

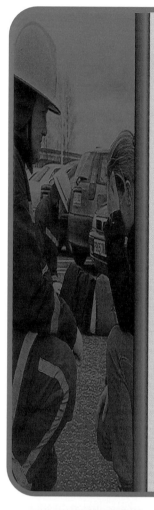

On completion of this chapter you will be able to meet the following objectives:

Cognitive objectives

1. List possible emotional reactions that the First Responder may experience when faced with trauma, illness, dying and death.
2. Discuss the possible reactions that a family member may exhibit when confronted with dying and death.
3. State the steps in the First Responder's approach to the family confronted with dying and death.
4. State the possible reactions that the family of the First Responder may exhibit owing to their outside involvement with EMS.
5. Recognise the signs and symptoms of critical incident stress.
6. State possible steps that the First Responder may take to help reduce or alleviate stress.
7. Explain the need to determine scene safety.
8. Discuss the importance of universal precautions.
9. Describe the steps the First Responder should take for personal protection from airborne and blood-borne pathogens or pathogens transmitted via other body fluids.
10. List the personal protective equipment necessary for each of the following situations: hazardous materials, rescue operations, crime scenes, exposure to blood, exposure to airborne pathogens and exposure to blood-borne pathogens.

Affective objectives

11. Explain the rationale for serving as an advocate for the use of appropriate protective equipment.

Psychomotor objectives

12. Given a scenario with potential infectious exposure, the First Responder will use appropriate protective equipment. At the completion of the scenario, the First Responder will properly remove and clean or discard the protective garments.
13. Given the above scenario, the First Responder will complete disinfection and cleaning, and all reporting documentation.

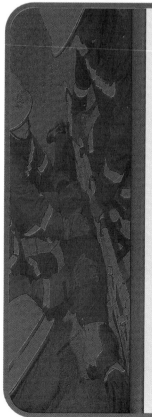

First response

A WEEK AFTER THE FATAL PLANE CRASH, Debbie again awoke from a nightmare of the crash scene. She still couldn't accept that a crash with no survivors had happened in her town. She remembered getting the initial call to an aircraft down and hurrying to the scene in the fire appliance as a First Responder. Dozens of ambulances responded within minutes of Debbie's arrival, but there were no survivors to receive medical care. The First Responders, EMS personnel, paramedics, nurses and doctors had felt helpless. Debbie had thought about the incident every day since it happened. She had lost her appetite and couldn't concentrate on work. Everyone involved in the response had been supposed to talk to the critical incident stress debriefing (CISD) team, but Debbie didn't feel that talking would help.

When Debbie arrived for work, her supervisor, Alan, met her at the door. "I think we need to talk," Alan said. In the last few days, he had noticed a change in attitude and had tried to approach her, but she didn't want to talk. He discussed the problem with Debbie and asked her to see the CISD team.

Now, having talked to the team and other First Responders who had attended the incident, Debbie still thinks about the crash, but without the negative emotions and tension she felt a week ago. The CISD team helped Debbie work through her frustration at being unable to care for the victims of the crash and to remember the value of the work she does every day.

EMS is a stressful profession. First Responders and other emergency professionals are regularly called on to help the injured and dying. First Responders must deal with physical injuries and dying, as well as with the emotions of the patient, the patient's family and themselves (**Fig. 2.1**). First Responders must be prepared to deal with these stresses effectively.

First Responders also face personal risk in the form of scene hazards, exposure to disease and stress. Knowing the warning signs of stress and how to protect yourself can help you have a long and healthy career as a First Responder.

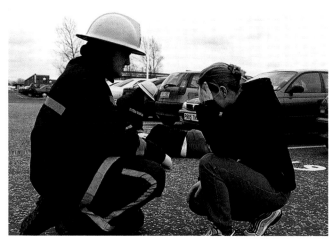

Fig. 2.1 First Responders must handle the emotions of patients and their family members, as well as their own emotions.

EMOTIONAL ASPECTS OF EMERGENCY CARE

Dying and death

Death is the natural end to all living things. At some time in our lives, we will all face death – the death of a family member or friend, a patient and eventually our own death. Different people have different ways of coping with death, but there are some similarities in general coping mechanisms. Familiarity with the normal grieving process provides insight to the reactions of patients, their family members and yourself. People generally go through five stages: denial, anger, bargaining, depression and acceptance.

Denial – "Not me." "It can't be true." These are defence mechanisms that allow people to feel there must be a mistake when they learn that they or someone they care about is dying. 'The medical tests were wrong.' 'The results were misinterpreted.' 'Something else went wrong.' People often deny the facts even in the face of overwhelming evidence. This can make them very difficult to deal with. It is important to be straightforward and honest with both the patient and the family regarding questions you are asked about your knowledge of the patient's condition.

Anger – "Why me?" Once a patient begins to accept the fact he or she is dying, a common response is anger. Patients may vent their anger at those nearby who are in good health, at the doctor who informs them of their condition, at their family or at the First Responders who try to help them. Remember that the patient is not actually angry with you and do not take any insults or anger personally. Be tolerant and patient, and do not become defensive. Listen empathically to what the patient has to say, and answer all questions truthfully. Do not give false reassurance such as, "Of course you will be all right", or "Don't worry, everything is fine."

Bargaining – "OK, but first let me …" Once patients begin to accept their imminent death, they may try to postpone the inevitable event by bargaining. "OK, I know I'm going to die, but let me live a while longer to see my first grandchild." Patients may try to bargain with doctors, themselves or God.

Depression – "OK, but I haven't …" Once patients realise that bargaining won't work, sadness and despair may set in. They think of all the happy things in their lives that they will miss and all of the things that they will never get to do. These patients are often silent and retreat into their own world. They are preparing and grieving for their own death.

Acceptance – "OK, I'm not afraid." At this stage, people have made peace with themselves and are willing to accept that they are dying. Acceptance does not imply that the patient is happy about dying, only that he or she realises his or her fate. Some family members still may not accept death and may require more emotional support than the patient. Be supportive of the wishes of family members and the patient.

Not everyone moves through these stages in the same way in the same time frame. Some patients may experience the stages in a different order or skip stages, or they may return to a previous stage. The response to death is as varied as people are. The patient's progression through these stages is influenced by age, duration of any illness and family support.

Dealing with a dying patient and comforting the family members is not an easy task. Kindness, compassion and understanding may help the patient or family members cope with their emotions. Listen empathically and speak with a gentle tone of voice. Allow the patient and family members to express their emotions, including rage, anger and despair.

Patients should always be treated with respect, and their privacy should be protected. Patients may feel the need to have some control over their treatment and their wishes should be honoured when possible. Always explain your actions to the patient and family members and treat the patient with dignity, even when the patient is unresponsive. Often a gentle touch is remembered more than the most expert care. Let the patient and family know that everything that can be done for the patient will be done, but do not falsely reassure them about the situation.

The well-being of the First Responder

Stressful situations

Stress and working as a First Responder often go hand in hand. First Responders feel stress in many different situations. Although different people find different situations stressful, some situations cause almost all emergency service workers to feel stress (**Box 2.1**).

First Responders not only have their own stress to deal with, but often also have to manage bystanders or patients who are experiencing stressful reactions.

Stressful situations may cause the First Responder to feel stress long after the incident. After caring for an injured child, for example, First Responders may be more protective of their own children in the days and weeks that follow. Stress can also be caused by a slow build up of smaller stressful situations. You must know the warning signs of severe stress and be able to recognise them in yourself and co-workers to help manage stress.

Stress

Stress is a bodily or mental tension caused by physical or emotional factors. It involves the person's response to events that are threatening or challenging. Not all stress is negative. If we didn't feel the stress of knowing there is an exam at the end of this course, we might not read the book for class. If not for the stress of being late for work, we might never get out of bed. Stress becomes a problem when it is felt so strongly that it begins to hinder our ability to function. Emergency workers are not immune to the stress of emergency situations. You must be aware of the signs of stress in yourself and in co-workers so you know when to take steps to manage stress.

Burnout is a condition resulting from chronic job-related stress. It is characterised by physical and emotional exhaustion.

Warning signs of stress

There are warning signs of stress to be recognised in order to manage stress appropriately. The warning signs of stress are listed in **Box 2.2**.

Stress management

The ways in which we handle stress are as different as people's reactions to stress. Too much stress can unquestionably affect your health and ability to perform your job. The following are some proven guidelines that help many people deal with their stress and avoid burnout (**Fig. 2.2**).

Change your diet – A healthy diet keeps your body in good condition and prepared to respond to an emergency. Consume only small amounts of sugar, caffeine and alcohol. Avoid fatty foods but increase carbohydrates. Also avoid excessive salt, which may increase your blood pressure. It is easy to miss meals during a busy day; don't forget to take care of yourself and eat meals regularly.

Stop smoking – Cigarette smoking increases your blood pressure and heart rate, and doubles your chances of a fatal heart attack. Cigarettes contain hundreds of toxins that increase your chances of lung disease and cancer, and cigarettes contribute to thousands of deaths every year. Although it is difficult to quit smoking, most people can do it once they are committed to their decision. The benefits of quitting smoking are unquestionable: cigarette smoking is the number one changeable risk factor for heart disease.

Get regular exercise – Regular exercise improves cardiovascular fitness, strength and flexibility and lowers your chances of becoming ill or injured. Exercise contributes to psychological and physical well-being.

Balance your work, recreation and family – Plan time away from duty and emergency work, and don't lose interest in your family and outside activities.

Change your work schedule – If you find that you are feeling severe effects of stress, request a change of duty assignment to a less busy area or a change of shift which allows you to spend some time on less arduous tasks, or even take time off to spend with

Box 2.1	**Situations That Cause Stress**

- Mass casualties
- Paediatric casualties
- Death
- Infant and child trauma
- Amputations
- Violence
- Infant and child abuse
- Elder abuse, spouse abuse
- Death or injury of a co-worker or other EMS personnel

Box 2.2	**Stress Warning Signs**

- Irritability with co-workers, family or friends
- Inability to concentrate
- Difficulty sleeping or nightmares
- Anxiety
- Indecisiveness
- Guilt
- Loss of appetite
- Loss of interest in sexual activities
- Isolation
- Loss of interest in work

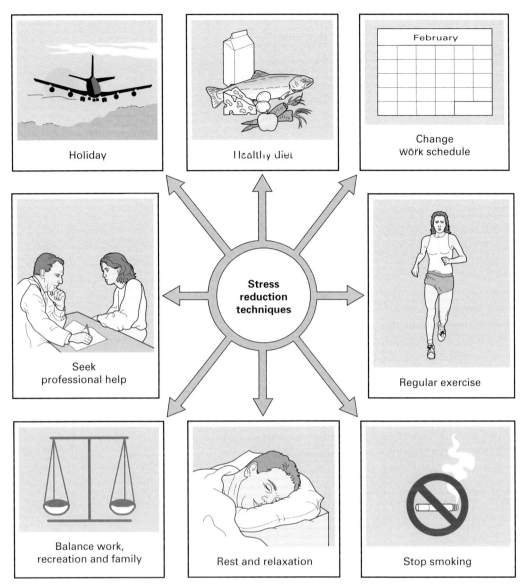

Fig. 2.2 Stress reduction techniques.

Holiday

Healthy diet

February

Change work schedule

Stress reduction techniques

Seek professional help

Regular exercise

Balance work, recreation and family

Rest and relaxation

Stop smoking

your friends and family. No one expects emergency workers to be immune to stress. It is not a weakness to need time to recover from stressful situations.

Seek professional help – You can benefit from professional help if the symptoms of stress are severe. Occupational health workers, social workers and clergy can all provide assistance with these sorts of issues.

First Responders and other emergency service personnel are not the only ones who experience job-related stress. Family and friends of these workers also experience stress. Spouses or partners of emergency service personnel often want to share the burden of the stressful situations but may not fully understand the situations faced. At other times, family and friends may not want to hear about the emergency situations that their loved ones face. Families of emergency service workers also deal with the fears of injury or death on the job and with separation from their loved ones. Rotating shifts, late calls and on-call rotas all add to the stress of emergency work. Talk to your family about these concerns and work out the best solution for you and the family.

Critical incident stress debriefing

Although First Responders deal with stressful situations regularly, some situations cause reactions that are more severe than usual. Stress is a normal response to an abnormal situation, but sometimes the level of stress can become overwhelming. For example, the death or serious injury of a child may trigger greater stress than usual for a First Responder with a child of his or her own. For others, a casualty who dies after a long rescue attempt may cause severe stress. Even though the types of incident that cause stress vary, the result is often the same.

A critical incident is a specific situation that causes an emergency worker to experience unusually strong emotional reactions and so interferes with the worker's ability to function, either immediately or in the future. First Responders may also place undue stress on themselves if they have unrealistic expectations about their abilities to help. It is important to realise that there are limitations to how much help can be given to patients and that not every patient's situation will turn out for the best.

The well-being of the First Responder

One way of dealing with a critical incident is through a process called Critical Incident Stress Debriefing (CISD). The debriefing process is normally conducted by a team of peer (colleague) counsellors. The team may also consist of personnel from other emergency services and could include, in extreme cases, professional counsellors. The process is designed to accelerate the normal recovery process.

Debriefings are normally held within 24–48 hours of dealing with an incident that the attending personnel found to be of a critical nature. During the discussions, the participants are encouraged to discuss their fears, feelings and reactions openly and honestly. In doing so they come to realise that they are not the only ones in the group that have these fears, feelings and reactions. The newer or younger members also realise that the older, longer-serving personnel are affected by stressful situations in much the same way that they are. The debriefing is not an investigation into the incident – that comes later – nor is it an investigation into the causes of the stress, the way the event was handled or any other technical matters. It is an opportunity for the responding emergency service workers to discuss the events and their feelings with people who will listen and provide understanding and support, and who will not pass judgement or criticise.

All personnel involved in the incident, including control room personnel, should be involved in the debriefing process. Ground rules will be set stating that the debriefing session is as confidential as the group make it, that no notes or records will be made, that only those who wish to speak need do so, and that the session is not compulsory and therefore participants may feel free to leave when ever they wish. At the end of the session, the team may make suggestions for further ways of dealing with and overcoming stress; these may include one-to-one support sessions with a trained colleague, supporter or with professional counsellors.

Defusing

Another technique that is widely used in dealing with critical incident stress is defusing. A defusing session is a much shorter, less formal and less structured version of CISD. Defusing generally lasts 30–45 minutes and occurs within a few hours of the critical event. Defusing allows for an initial airing, which may eliminate the need for a formal debriefing. Defusing may also enhance the formal debriefing. Fire-fighters returning from an incident normally defuse over a cup of tea or coffee at their station without realising they are doing so. This defusing take various forms, from quiet individual thoughts to humour.

As an emergency service worker you should be aware of how you can access your service's CISD team and remember that the service is there for you to use when you need it. Emergency service workers should not feel embarrassed or uncomfortable when seeking help. We are all human and may need help in dealing with our responses to emergency situations. **Box 2.3** lists some common situations that may require CISD.

Comprehensive critical incident stress management

In addition to dealing with stress after a critical incident, systems have been developed to help emergency workers, their families and the community in general to deal with stress in a more comprehensive manner. Pre-incident stress education helps emergency service workers to understand how to deal with the stress they will face as part of their job. By knowing the signs of stress and how to find the help needed, emergency workers may be able to avoid or reduce burnout. In addition to pre-incident education, other health and welfare programmes are in place to help emergency workers stay in good physical and psychological shape. On-scene and one-to-one support provides a network of other emergency workers to rely on during times of stress. This support is focused not only on disasters and critical incidents, but also on the daily stress that emergency workers face. Families of emergency workers also learn how to deal with the stress their loved ones are facing as well as the stress they are facing themselves.

In times of disaster, support services are provided to emergency service workers, their families and the community. The community as a whole may need to have a place to turn to discuss their feelings of loss and sorrow. Mass floods, for example, not only affect those working to help the victims of the disaster, but everyone involved in the flooding.

Community outreach programmes provided by local authority emergency planning departments are designed to provide a way for the entire community to become involved in the healing process. They help members of the community to deal with their feelings. Follow-up services are provided by the outreach programmes to monitor how emergency workers are dealing with their own feelings after critical incidents and to provide additional support if necessary. Some workers may not feel the effects of their stress for weeks or even months after the incident.

Comprehensive stress management programmes are a way of dealing with the effects of stress before stressful events occur, during times of great stress, and after the events are over. Remember these situations do

Box 2.3	**Situations That May Require CISD**
	• Line-of-duty death or serious injury
	• Multiple casualty incident
	• Suicide of an emergency worker
	• Serious injury or death of children
	• Events with excessive media interest
	• Victims known to the emergency personnel
	• Event that has an unusual impact on personnel
	• Any disaster

not have to be something as big as a natural disaster to cause stress; they include any situation that involves a reaction to stress.

SAFETY

Safety should be your first priority every time you respond to a call for emergency help. As a First Responder, you are usually the source of scene safety for other emergency workers who arrive on the scene after you. In the excitement of an emergency, it is easy to rush to the aid of an injured person without taking proper steps to ensure your own safety. The following sections on scene and personal safety will highlight the important steps that should be taken to protect yourself, co-workers and the patients. Common sense and taking a moment to assess each situation play an important role in safety.

Scene safety

Every First Responder involved in an emergency call has a responsibility for safety at the scene. As a First Responder, you are responsible for your own safety, the safety of your partner or other First Responders, the safety of the patient, and the safety of bystanders, in that order. It is in the caring nature of emergency workers to begin treating an injured casualty as soon as possible. However, to be able to help anyone, you must take precautions so that you are not harmed. First Responders who are injured cannot provide care or help to anyone else and must be cared for themselves by other emergency crews arriving on the scene, thus taking away from the care that can be provided to the patient.

You must work as a team and watch out for the safety of your partners and any other First Responders or emergency personnel at the scene. You must also take responsibility for the safety of casualties and do your best to prevent further injuries. Traffic hazards, violent people and environmental factors all pose a risk to patients. With the help of the police, you must also protect bystanders by restricting them to areas out of the path of danger.

Scene safety begins when you receive a call. Scene safety includes an assessment of the surroundings that will provide valuable information to the First Responder and help ensure safety. As you arrive at every scene, ask yourself, "Is it safe to approach the patient?" In situations such as crash or rescue scenes, toxic substance scenes, unstable surfaces that slope or are covered with water or ice, all possibilities need to be anticipated and planned for. First Responders must remember to evaluate the scene before entering and beginning care. If the scene is unsafe, make it safe. If you can't make the scene safe, do not enter. Instead, call for specialised resources to assist in scene safety.

Hazardous materials

A hazardous material is a substance that poses a threat or unreasonable risk to life, health or property if not

---

---

properly controlled during manufacture, processing, packaging, handling, storage, transportation, use or disposal. Hazardous materials incidents should be controlled by specialised hazardous material teams, normally the crew of an emergency tender or other specialist vehicle mobilised by the brigade. In general, special equipment and knowledge are needed, and crews not equipped to handle the situation should leave it to the specialists. It is important that you know your brigade's procedures for requesting specialist assistance for hazardous material incidents, including radiation. Until assistance arrives, protect yourself and bystanders from harm.

For incidents involving hazardous materials, brigade procedures must be adhered to and protective clothing with breathing apparatus must be worn when recovering chemical information from buildings or vehicles. Information should be in the form of a placard displaying the Substance Identification Number and, in many cases, the Emergency Action Code. On vehicles, these placards will be displayed on both front sides and on the rear of the container (**Fig. 2.3**). Further information may be obtained by radio from the brigade control room or directly from equipment carried on certain appliances. For incidents involving hazardous materials at farms or some factories, placards may not be available or not immediately obvious. In

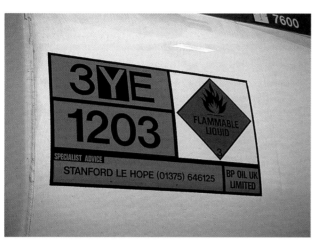

Fig. 2.3 A placard displayed on hazardous materials containers provides information about the materials inside.

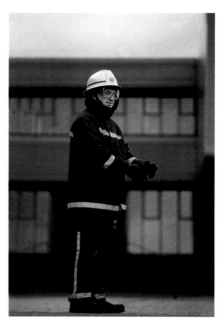

Fig. 2.4 Protective clothing is essential for all rescue situations. This equipment should include turnout gear, puncture-proof gloves, helmet with ear protection and a chin strap, eye protection (heavy goggles made specifically for working with power equipment) and boots.

these situations information should be obtained from employees on site, if available. Regardless of the material, do not attempt to enter the hazard area without sufficient protection.

First Responders provide emergency care to patients only after the scene is safe. If it is not safe to enter a scene to remove a contaminated patient, decontamination should be carried out by suitably protected personnel before treatment. Premature entry could pose a risk to the patient, bystanders and you.

Road traffic accidents

Most road traffic accidents (RTAs) involve a variety of threats to life. First Responders called to an RTA must be aware of the hazards common to these scenes. For example, along many roadways there are electricity pylons, poles and wires that may become obstacles if struck by a vehicle. High voltage electricity can be conducted through these wires and should never be touched until confirmed safe by the electricity supplier. Fires and explosions are also a possible risk. You must carry out a risk assessment of the situation before entering or committing personnel to the scene. Broken glass, sharp jagged metal and unstable surfaces are only some of the concerns at most RTAs. Traffic hazards and hazardous materials must also be dealt with.

Protective clothing must be worn when working at or near an RTA (**Fig 2.4**). The recommended protective clothing to be worn when working at RTAs is listed in **Box 2.4**.

As well as basic RTAs, there are other aspects of rescue and extrication. If you are interested in being part of these operations, you must attend the specialist courses that are organised through your brigade's training department. These courses cover safety issues, equipment and special rescue techniques. In a variety of situations, the casualty must be rescued from places that are difficult to access. Heavy rescue or speciality situations, such as water rescue or rescue from entrapment in a heavily damaged vehicle, may require

Box 2.4	**Recommended Protective Clothing for Working Near Crash Vehicles**

- Protective clothing that prevents or resists puncturing
- Puncture-proof gloves
- Helmet with ear protection and a chin strap to keep the helmet on your head (many helmets are equipped with face shields as well)
- Eye protection, such as heavy goggles made specifically for working with power equipment. Face shields and prescription glasses are not sufficient eye protection specifically when working with power equipment.
- Boots with steel toes and insoles are recommended

special rescue teams. The points covered in this section may be appropriate at any type of crash rescue scene.

Methods of extrication are dealt with in more detail in Chapter 13 ('EMS operations').

Violence

The control of violence at any incident is the responsibility of the police, and violence must be controlled before you enter to provide care to patients. Consider your own safety first. Allow the police to determine that the scene is safe for you to enter. At a suspected crime scene, disturb as little evidence as possible. Evidence that you protect at the scene of a crime may solve a criminal case. Do not disturb anything unless you have to in order to provide medical care. If you do disturb anything, make a mental note of what you have seen, where it was, how and where it was moved, by whom and why. Dealing with the scene carefully will help maintain the chain of evidence.

Once you have taken the time to ensure the scene is safe, the next step to ensure your personal safety is to follow the universal precautions.

Personal safety

Universal precautions

One of the first steps in personal protection is to prevent the spread of communicable diseases from patients to you. Some patients clearly present a disease exposure risk, but it is impossible to evaluate any casualty as safe. Patients infected with diseases such as hepatitis or human immunodeficiency virus (HIV) do not have a certain appearance or dress nor do they belong to any particular socio-economic class. Contact with the blood or other body fluid of any casualty should be considered a risk, and you should follow steps to avoid such contamination.

Universal precautions are designed to prevent you from coming into contact with a patient's body fluids. Preventative measures to avoid exposure to communicable diseases are also a part of good patient care. First Responders could transfer a disease to other patients, health-care workers, or family members if they are careless. To prevent the transmission of disease between patients, equipment should be disinfected or cleaned according to your brigade's and the suppliers' policies, and disposable items should be replaced after each patient contact.

The routine use of personal protective equipment will help reduce the risk of coming into contact with a communicable disease. Systems should include policies for the use of personal protective equipment that follow health and safety and brigade regulations regarding universal precautions. Protective equipment should be made available to you for use when there is a potential risk. To help prevent the spread of infection, take the measures described in the following sections.

Hand washing – Hand washing is the single most important procedure for preventing the spread of disease. Effective hand washing involves vigorously rubbing the hands together with lathered soap and then rinsing them under a stream of water (**Fig 2.5**). Hand washing should last for at least 10–15 seconds. You should dry your hands thoroughly with a clean cloth or a disposable towel. Be sure to wash your hands thoroughly after every patient contact, even though you are wearing gloves. There are also waterless hand-washing substitutes available for use when you do not have access to a sink and water but need to wash your hands. These solutions are usually alcohol based. The rubbing action causes friction, and the alcohol kills most surface organisms. You must thoroughly wash your hands when you have access to a sink, even if you use waterless hand-washing substitutes.

Gloves – Wear disposable vinyl or latex gloves whenever you are in contact with blood or other body fluids, when there is a high chance there will be blood or other body fluids present, or when there is a chance you will come into contact with mucous membranes or broken skin. Gloves should also be worn if you will be dealing with equipment that has been in contact with blood, other body fluids or mucous membranes. If a patient complains of nausea but has not vomited, you face a high likelihood of contact with vomit during the incident; it is too late to put on gloves once the patient has vomited. Prepare ahead and wear gloves if it seems possible that the situation could include contact with blood or other body fluids. Many First Responders find it convenient to put on gloves when they are approaching the scene, before patient contact begins (**Fig. 2.6**). Change gloves between patients to prevent cross contamination. To remove gloves, turn them inside out using the cuff to pull them off so you do not touch the outside of the glove with your hands. When cleaning

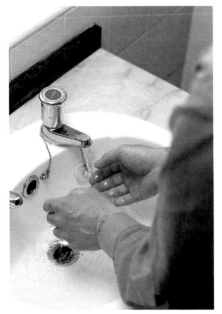

Fig. 2.5 Hand washing is the single most important procedure for preventing the spread of disease.

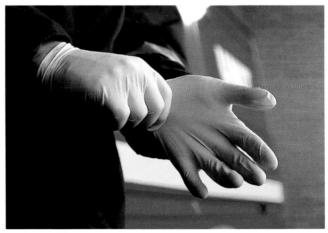

Fig. 2.6 First Responders should put on vinyl or latex gloves if it seems likely that the situation could include blood or other body fluids.

vehicles, general-duty gloves should be worn to protect your hands, and they should be washed after use.

Eye protection – Eye protection is available in a variety of forms and should be worn when there is a possibility of blood or body fluids splashing into the face or eyes. Any type of eye protection that stops fluids from reaching the eyes is sufficient. High quality, expensive goggles are not required. Remember, the splashing of body fluids can occur in many situations, not only in trauma cases. Assisting childbirth, for example, is likely to place you at risk of contact with splashing fluids. If you wear prescription glasses, you can apply removable shields to them.

Masks – Masks can be worn by emergency workers to prevent body fluids from splattering into the mouth and nose. There are masks available that also incorporate eye protection. If it is likely that body fluids will come into contact with your nose and mouth, it is likely these fluids will also contact your eyes; therefore, eye protection should also be worn (**Fig. 2.7**)

Masks can be worn by a patient who has an airborne disease. If the patient is unwilling to wear a mask, you should wear one.

Gowns – Gowns are used for calls when large amounts of blood or other body fluids are expected, such as assisting in child birth. Regular fire-fighting uniforms are also part of the protective barrier against body fluid contamination. Wearing a plastic gown keeps you from soiling your uniform. A change of uniform should always be readily available.

In addition to these universal precautions, First Responders should always use a barrier device when ventilating a patient. Barrier devices and techniques for ventilating patients are discussed in Chapter 5 ('The airway').

Advanced safety precautions

Before becoming First Responders or beginning patient contact, you should take steps to help ensure your physical well-being. Your immune status to commonly transmitted diseases such as rubella, measles, mumps and polio should be verified, and you may also choose to be vaccinated against hepatitis B. In addition you should receive a tetanus booster. Tuberculin-purified protein derivative testing should be conducted in accordance with the policy of your local health authority.

The Health and Safety at Work Act, 1974, requires employers to record exposure of their employees to substances hazardous to health. Each brigade has its own system for meeting this statutory requirement, and you should be conversant with your brigade's systems.

Scene safety is discussed in more detail in Chapter 6 ('Patient assessment').

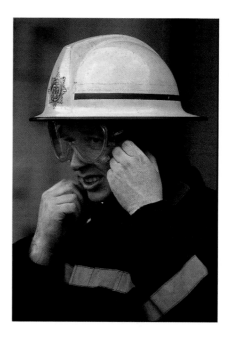

Fig. 2.7 First Responders should wear eye protection and a mask if body fluids could splash into the face.

CHAPTER SUMMARY

Emotional aspects of emergency care

First Responders face many situations, including patients and the members of their families who are dealing with dying and death. Patients respond differently to injury, illness and death. People pass through a series of stages when faced with death: denial ("Not me"); anger ("Why me?"); bargaining ("OK, but first let me...."); depression ("OK, but I haven't ..."); and acceptance ("OK, I'm not afraid").

Treat dying patients and their families with dignity and respect. Explain all your actions, and honour the patient's wishes. Patients may need to feel they have some control over the situation. The response of family members to the impending death of a loved one may be stronger than that of the patient, who may have already accepted his or her own death.

Review Questions

Safety

1. First Responders must wear gloves only in trauma situations. True of False?
2. Hand washing is one of the best defences against the spread of infectious diseases. True or False?
3. Hazardous materials signs identify the material inside the container bearing the sign. True or False?
4. First Responders should wait for the police at all scenes of crime or violence, even if the patient states the violent individual has left the scene. True or False?

1. False; 2. True; 3. True; 4. True

Almost all emergency service workers experience severe stress when responding to situations such as mass casualty incidents, paediatric patients, death, infant and child trauma, amputations, violence, abuse and death or injury of emergency service personnel. First Responders may feel the effects of stress immediately after the call, or the reaction may be delayed or cumulative.

Stress can be detected by a variety of warning signs, including irritability to co-workers, family or friends; inability to concentrate; difficulty in sleeping or nightmares; anxiety; indecisiveness; guilt, loss of appetite; loss of interest in sexual activities; loss of interest in work; and isolation.

Stress can be managed in many ways, not all of which work for all people. Some options for stress management include eating a balanced diet; not smoking; exercise; relaxation techniques; and balancing work, family and recreation. Find professional help if stress is severe and you can't manage it alone. Families of emergency service personnel also feel the effects of stress. CISD allows emergency workers to discuss their emotions and counsellors help them work through their problems.

Safety

As a First Responder, you are responsible for your own safety and the safety of your partner, colleagues, the patient and any bystanders.

First Responders should not enter any scenes that is unsafe or that requires special knowledge or equipment. Speciality crews should be called to deal with hazardous materials and hazardous rescues. You may be able to identify hazardous materials by the placards on the containers. Police personnel should be called on to control scenes of crime or violence.

Basic universal precautions include hand washing and wearing gloves, eye protection, masks and gowns. These precautions should be followed whenever there is a chance you will encounter body fluids. It is not always possible to determine at the beginning of a call if body fluids will be involved. It is often impossible to apply gloves once a patient begins to vomit or bleed, so evaluate the need for precautions early.

Emergency service personnel who come into contact with patients should be vaccinated against common communicable diseases and tested for others on a regular basis.

Chapter

Three

The human body

I. **The respiratory system**
   A. The airway
   B. The lungs
   C. The respiratory system of infants and children

II. **The circulatory system**
   A. The heart
   B. Blood vessels
   C. The blood
   D. The circulation of blood

III. **The musculoskeletal system**
   A. The skeletal system
   B. The muscular system

IV. **The nervous system**

V. **The skin**

VI. **The digestive system**

VII. **The endocrine system**

Key terms

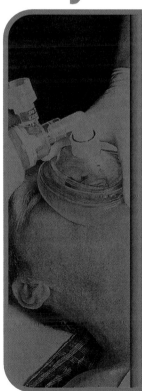

Atria The two upper chambers of the heart, which function to receive blood and pump it to the ventricles.

Diaphragm
The large, dome-shaped muscle separating the thoracic and abdominal cavities; used in breathing.

Epiglottis
A leaf-like flap that prevents food and liquid from entering the windpipe during swallowing.

Hormones
Chemicals that regulate the body's activities and functions.

Nasopharynx
The part of the pharynx that lies directly behind the nose.

Oropharynx
The part of the pharynx that is just behind the mouth and extends to the level of the epiglottis.

Perfusion
The process of circulating blood to the organs, delivering oxygen and removing waste products.

Pharynx
A muscular tube commonly referred to as the throat.

Pulse points
A location where an artery passes close to the skin and over a bone, where the pressure wave of the heart contraction can be felt.

Ventricles
The two lower chambers of the heart, which pump blood out of the heart.

Objectives

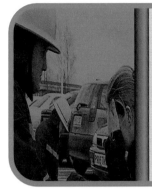

On completion of this chapter you will be able to meet the following objectives:

Cognitive objectives

1. Describe the anatomy and function of the respiratory system.
2. Describe the anatomy and function of the circulatory system.
3. Describe the anatomy and function of the musculoskeletal system.
4. Describe the anatomy and components of the nervous system.

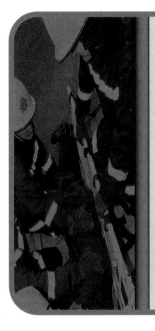

First response

IT WAS A QUIET, LANCASHIRE SUMMER EVENING. Just as the sun was going down, the paramedic unit approached the scene. A drunken driver had struck a 14-year-old boy while he was riding his bike. Police Constable Benfield saw that the boy was bleeding profusely from the wrist. With each beat of his heart, blood spurted from the wound. He feared that the boy had cut his radial artery and knew he had to stop the bleeding quickly. He put pressure on the injury and remembered that the brachial artery was the major artery supplying the arm. He put pressure on the inside of the upper arm and the bleeding slowed. The responding paramedic crew said that his quick thinking had probably saved the boy's life.

The driver of the car that had hit the boy was shaken up but uninjured. He barely remembered the accident after he sobered up and was convicted of driving under the influence of alcohol. The boy was riding his bike again 3 days later.

The human body is the envy of modern engineering. An engineer has yet to come close to creating anything as well designed and constructed. Although no body system functions independently, the complexity of the human body can be better understood by considering its separate parts. A body system is a group of organs that work together to perform a function. Although each body system is described in the following sections as an independent component, they are all interconnected.

THE RESPIRATORY SYSTEM

The respiratory system plays a crucial role in the delicate balance of life. The body is composed of trillions of cells that need oxygen to convert food into energy. This process gives off carbon dioxide as a waste product. The respiratory system takes oxygen from the air and makes it available for the blood to transport to every cell, and rids the body of excess carbon dioxide.

The airway

Air enters and exits the respiratory system through the mouth and the nose. These two structures play an important role in warming, cleaning and humidifying inhaled air. The pharynx is a muscular tube commonly referred to as the throat.

The pharynx is divided into two areas: the nasopharynx and the oropharynx. The nasopharynx lies directly behind the nose. The oropharynx is just behind the mouth and extends to the level of the epiglottis. The epiglottis is a leaf-like flap that prevents food and liquid from entering the windpipe (trachea) during swallowing. The pharynx is a common pathway for both food and air. Because air and food pass through the pharynx, it is often the location of airway obstructions by foreign bodies. **Figure 3.1** shows the upper airway.

Just below the epiglottis is the opening to the windpipe. The voice box (larynx) is just below this opening. The vocal cords are bands of cartilage that vibrate when we speak.

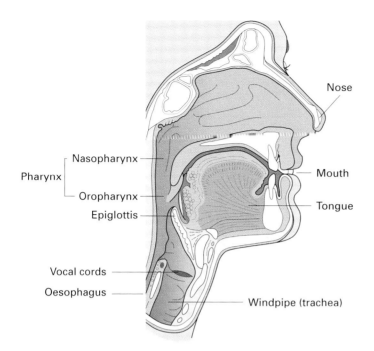

Fig. 3.1 The upper airway.

The lungs

The windpipe extends from the voice box and is the common pathway for the air that enters the lungs. The trachea splits into two branches, each leading to one lung. These branches subdivide into smaller and smaller air passages until they end at the microscopic air sacs of the lungs. These air sacs are only one cell thick and are surrounded by capillaries. This is where gas exchange actually occurs (**Fig. 3.2**).

The process of ventilating the lungs with a constant supply of fresh air uses two sets of muscles: the diaphragm and the muscles between the ribs (the intercostal muscles). The diaphragm is the large, dome-shaped muscle separating the thoracic and abdominal cavities. When the diaphragm contracts, the dome of the diaphragm flattens and lowers.

Contraction of the intercostal muscles (the muscles between the ribs) causes them to move upwards and outwards. Inhalation begins with the contraction of the diaphragm and the intercostal muscles. This increases the size of the chest, and air is pulled into the lungs through the mouth and nose, much like pulling the plunger back on a syringe. Inhalation is an active process resulting from muscle contraction, and therefore the muscles must act for inhalation to occur (**Fig. 3.3a**). The exchange of oxygen for carbon dioxide occurs, and then exhalation takes place.

Exhalation begins with relaxation of the intercostal muscles and the diaphragm. As these muscles relax and return to their resting position, the size of the chest decreases and air rushes out through the mouth and nose. Normally, exhalation is a passive process, and therefore muscle action is not needed for exhalation to occur (**Fig. 3.3b**). In some cases of disease or obstruction, exhalation becomes an active process. A cough is also an example of a forced exhalation.

Gas exchange

There are two sites for the exchange of oxygen and carbon dioxide: the lungs and the tissues. During inhalation, air is drawn into the lungs. Normally, air contains 21 per cent oxygen and almost no carbon dioxide. As this oxygen-rich air enters the lungs, blood with low levels of oxygen and high levels of carbon dioxide flows through the capillaries in the lungs.

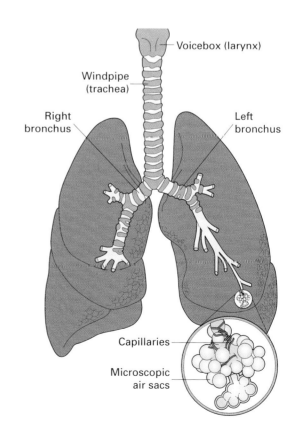

Fig. 3.2 Anatomy of the windpipe (trachea) and lungs.

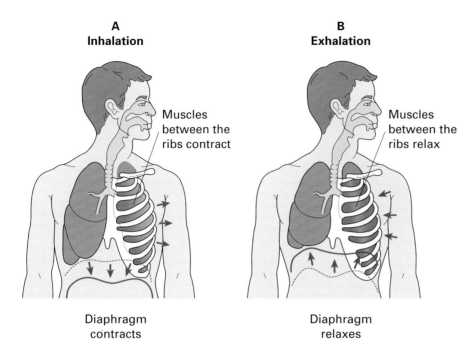

A
Inhalation

Muscles
between the
ribs contract

Diaphragm
contracts

B
Exhalation

Muscles
between the
ribs relax

Diaphragm
relaxes

Fig. 3.3 The mechanics of ventilation. **(a)** Inhalation; **(b)** Exhalation.

Oxygen enters the blood and carbon dioxide is removed (**Fig. 3.4**).

The oxygenated blood is then pumped by the heart to the rest of the body. As this oxygen-rich blood approaches its destination, the blood vessels decrease in size until they branch into thin-walled capillaries. The blood in the capillaries is highly oxygenated and low in carbon dioxide. However, the tissue is low in oxygen and high in carbon dioxide. The capillaries give up oxygen to the cells, and the cells give carbon dioxide to the blood in the capillaries (**Fig. 3.5**). The blood is then collected in the veins and returned to the lungs for re-oxygenation.

The respiratory system of infants and children

Infants and children are not just small adults. There are considerable differences between paediatric and adult patients. The most obvious difference in the respiratory system is the smaller size of the airway structures. The smaller diameter of the airway makes obstructions much more common in young patients. Airway obstruction can occur when foreign bodies are lodged in or below the trachea or with even a small amount of swelling of the airway.

Two factors combine to make infant's and children's airways more easily obstructed than those of adults. First, the tongue is much larger in proportion to the size of the mouth in infants and children. Secondly, the younger the patient, the softer and more collapsible the trachea. Because of these factors, the airway can be more easily obstructed. The most common cause of cardiac arrest in infants and children is uncorrected respiratory problems.

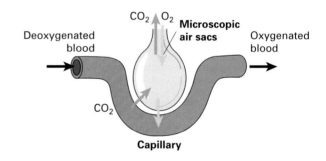

Deoxygenated
blood

CO_2 O_2 **Microscopic air sacs**

Oxygenated
blood

CO_2

Capillary

Fig. 3.4 Gas exchange in the lungs.

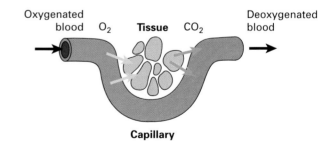

Oxygenated
blood O_2 **Tissue** CO_2

Deoxygenated
blood

Capillary

Fig. 3.5 Gas exchange in tissues.

THE CIRCULATORY SYSTEM

In the growing foetus, the heart begins to pump in the fourth week of development and, on average, will keep beating continuously for the next 75 years. Contracting over 100,000 times a day, the heart is a marvel of endurance and reliability. The heart pumps blood that contains oxygen and nutrients to the body's organs through the circulatory system. The exchange of oxygen and nutrients for waste products occurs in the smallest vessels of the circulatory system. This process is so vital to life that any interruption for more than a few minutes can mean death to the individual.

The heart

The heart is a pump consisting of four chambers. The two upper chambers are called the atria, which function to receive blood and pump it to the lower chambers of the heart. The two lower chambers are the ventricles, which pump blood out of the heart. Because of one-way valves between the chambers, heart contractions move blood in only one direction.

The left ventricle pumps blood that is rich in oxygen to the body to be used by the cells. After the oxygen is used, blood is returned from the veins of the body into the right atrium, which pumps it to the right ventricle. The right ventricle pumps this oxygen-poor blood to the lungs for oxygenation. The oxygen-rich blood from the lungs is returned into the left atrium. The left atrium pumps blood to the left ventricle, and the circuit starts all over again (**Fig. 3.6**).

The heart has specialised cells that generate electrical impulses and serve as the heart's pacemaker. Electrical signals are carried through the heart by conductive tissue. These signals give the heart the amazing ability to beat on its own. The number of times per minute that the heart beats is the heart rate. The heart rate varies with age, physical condition, situation and a number of other factors.

Blood vessels

Blood vessels are the 'pipes' of the body. These vessels carry blood to every organ. Arteries carry blood away from the heart. The major artery of the body is the aorta, which is a vessel approximately the diameter of your thumb. It originates from the left ventricle and arches in front of the spine, then descends through the chest and abdomen. The two carotid arteries are the major arteries of the neck, and pulsations can be palpated on either side of the neck. The femoral artery is the major artery of the thigh, and pulsations can be palpated in the groin. The radial artery is the artery of the lower arm, and pulsations can be palpated on the thumb side of the wrist. The brachial artery is the artery of the upper arm, and can be palpated on the inside of the arm between the elbow and the shoulder. **Figure 3.7** shows the location of the major arteries in the body.

Arteries branch as they get further away from the heart and eventually lead to capillaries, which are the smallest blood vessels in the body. Capillaries are tiny blood vessels that connect arteries to veins. The exchange of oxygen and nutrients for carbon dioxide and other wastes occurs in the thin-walled capillaries

Fig. 3.6 Normal blood flow through the heart.

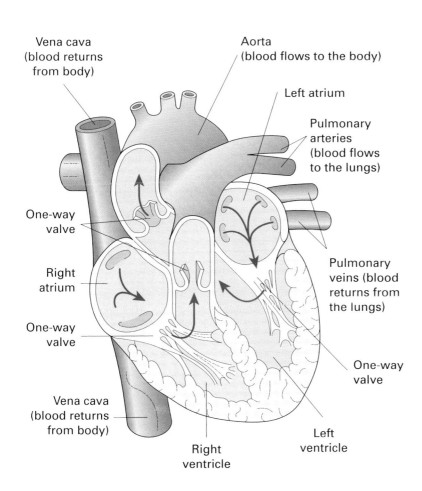

Vena cava (blood returns from body)

Aorta (blood flows to the body)

Left atrium

Pulmonary arteries (blood flows to the lungs)

One-way valve

Right atrium

Pulmonary veins (blood returns from the lungs)

One-way valve

One-way valve

Vena cava (blood returns from body)

Right ventricle

Left ventricle

The human body

(**Fig. 3.8**). The capillaries are microscopic structures, only about 1 mm in length and just one cell thick, but they are present in astronomical numbers everywhere in the body. If all of the capillaries in your body were placed end to end, they would extend for 62,000 miles!

Many capillaries join together to form veins, which return the oxygen-poor blood back to the heart. **Figure 3.9** shows the location of the major veins of the body.

The blood

An average-sized adult man has about 5–6 litres (9–11 pints) of blood circulating in his body. This complex fluid serves many functions and contains many components. One of the main functions of the blood is to deliver oxygen and remove carbon dioxide. Blood also plays an important role in clotting and in the body's defence against infection.

The circulation of blood

As the left ventricle contracts, pumping blood to the body, a wave of pressure is sent through the arteries. This pressure wave can be felt anywhere an artery passes close to the skin and over a bone. These locations are called pulse points and occur both in the extremities and near the trunk. The most common pulse points of the body are the carotid, femoral, radial and brachial pulse points (**Fig. 3.10**).

For the cells of the body to function properly, they must have a continuous supply of oxygenated blood. This supply requires adequate pressure in the heart and vessels to circulate the blood to all parts of the body. The process of circulating blood to the organs, delivering oxygen and removing wastes is called perfusion. When perfusion is inadequate, a state known as shock develops. Shock is a state of widespread decrease of perfusion (hypoperfusion).

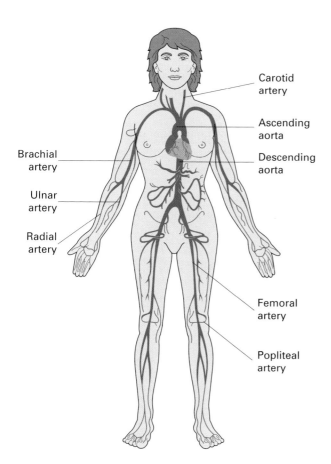

Fig. 3.7 Major arteries of the body.

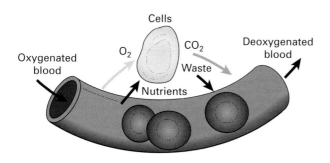

Fig. 3.8 The exchange of gases, nutrients and wastes between tissue cells and capillary blood.

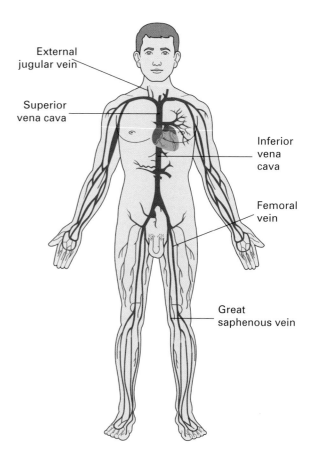

Fig. 3.9 Major veins of the body.

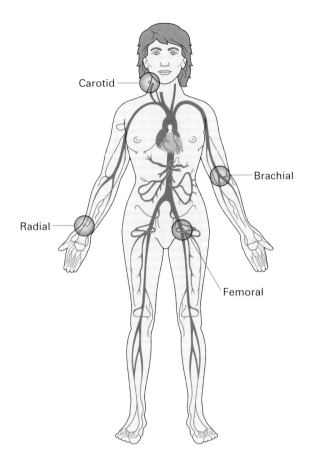

Carotid

Brachial

Radial

Femoral

Fig. 3.10 Pulse points.

Review Questions

The Respiratory and Circulatory Systems

1. What are the two main muscles of respiration?

_____

_____

2. Inhalation is an (active or passive) process, while exhalation is an (active or passive) process.

3. Where is blood reoxygenated and carbon dioxide removed?

4. Which of the following is NOT a characteristic of the respiratory system of infants and children:
   A. Proportionally larger tongue
   B. Slower respiratory rates
   C. Smaller airway structure
   D. Softer trachea

5. Place the following in order of blood flow from the right atrium:
   A. left ventricle   _____
   B. lungs   _____
   C. left atrium   _____
   D. body   _____
   E. right ventricle   _____

6. Blood carries oxygen to the _____ and carbon dioxide to the _____ for removal.

1. The diaphragm and the muscles between the ribs; 2. Active, passive; 3. The lungs; 4. B; 5. E, B, C, A, D; 6. Tissues, lungs

THE MUSCULOSKELETAL SYSTEM

The skeletal system

The skeletal system is the scaffolding of the body. Not only do bones give the body shape and rigidity, but they also protect the vital internal organs. For example, the skull completely surrounds the delicate brain and protects it from everyday bumps and bruises. The ribs, breastbone (sternum) and spinal column play important roles in protecting the heart and other important organs from damage.

Along with muscles, bones also serve as attachment points to enable the body to move. The skeleton creates levers and fulcrums throughout the body. The contracting of muscles moves these levers with incredible precision. **Figure 3.11** shows the major bones of the body.

The head, spinal column and thorax

The skull houses the brain and forms the face. The brain is the most important organ in the human body and is protected by the rigid bones of the skull. The spinal column extends from the base of the skull to the pelvis and consists of 33 small bones (**Fig. 3.12**). The bones in the neck and back each have a vertical hole in them and stack on top of each other. The holes line up to create a tube for the spinal cord. If one of these

bones becomes misaligned or damaged, it can cause permanent damage to the spinal cord.

The bones of the spinal column in the upper back serve as a point of attachment for the twelve pairs of ribs. The first ten pairs of ribs are attached in front to the breastbone (sternum). The eleventh and twelfth ribs are the floating ribs, so called because they simply extend from the spinal column. The floating ribs help protect the kidneys. The attached ribs provide protection to all of the organs in the chest and assist in breathing.

The thorax consists of the ribs and the breastbone (sternum). At the lower end of the sternum is the xiphoid process. The xiphoid process is an important landmark when performing chest compressions during cardiopulmonary resuscitation (CPR). The xiphoid process is sharp and delicate and can cause damage to internal organs (such as the liver) if your hand placement is incorrect.

The pelvis and lower extremities

The spinal column forms the back of the pelvis. Fused bones create the remainder of the pelvis, which serves as an attachment point for the legs at the socket for the hip joint.

The femur is the long bone of the thigh. One end of the femur fits into the hip joint and allows the leg to move easily. The other end meets the bones of the

The human body

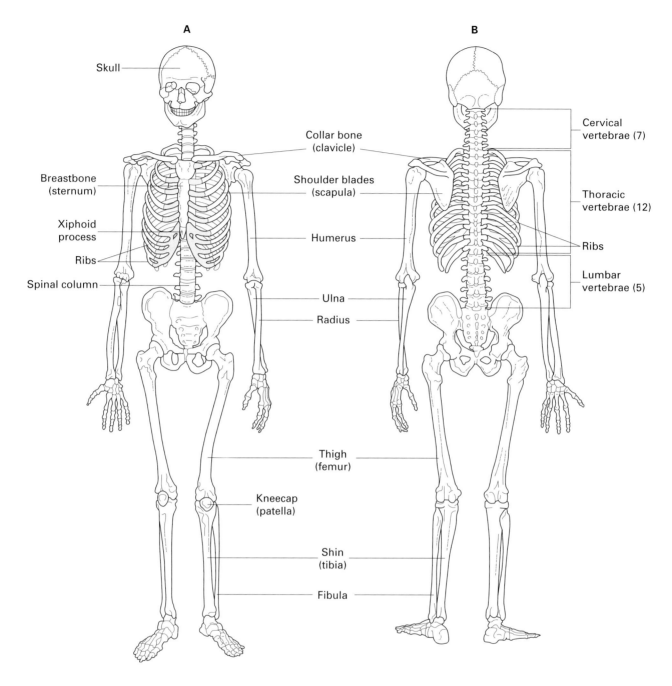

A

Skull

Collar bone
(clavicle)

Breastbone
(sternum)

Shoulder blades
(scapula)

Xiphoid
process

Humerus

Ribs

Spinal column

Ulna

Radius

B

Cervical
vertebrae (7)

Thoracic
vertebrae (12)

Ribs

Lumbar
vertebrae (5)

Thigh
(femur)

Kneecap
(patella)

Shin
(tibia)

Fibula

Fig. 3.11 (a) and **(b)** The skeletal system.

lower leg at the knee. The kneecap (patella) protects you from injury if you fall directly on to your knee.

The lower leg has two bones. The shin (tibia) is the main weight-bearing bone of the lower leg. The fibula does not bear weight but assists in the movement of the ankle. Small bones provide structure to the heel, feet and toes (**Fig. 3.13**).

The upper extremities

The arms join the trunk at the shoulder, which consists of the collar bone (clavicle) and the shoulder blade (scapula). The humerus is the bone of the upper arm. The forearm contains the radius and the ulna. Small bones make up the wrist, hand and fingers. These

small bones enable the hand and wrist to move into many intricate positions (**Fig. 3.14**).

Joints

A joint is a place where bones come together. Joints serve many functions, but most importantly they provide a system of fulcrums and levers that make movement of the body possible.

The muscular system

No movement in the body could occur without muscles. Every physical activity, from riding a bike to turning the pages of this book, occurs with the

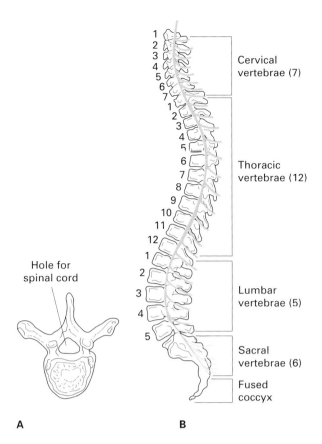

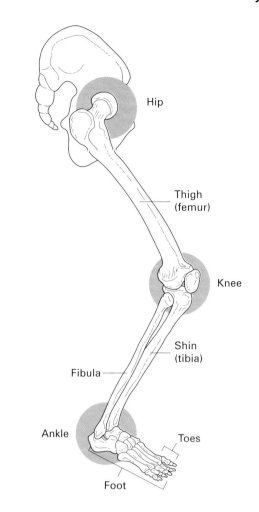

Fig. 3.12 The spinal column comprises 33 vertebrae. **(a)** Single vertebra. **(b)** The spinal column.

Fig. 3.13 The pelvis and right lower extremity.

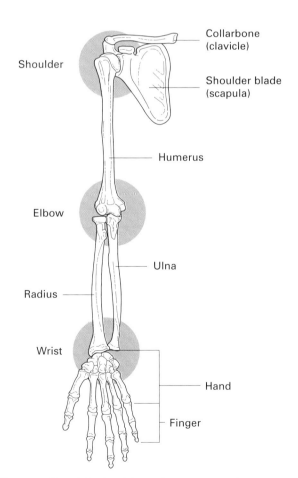

Fig. 3.14 The right shoulder and upper extremity.

contraction of muscles. Additionally, muscles protect vital organs and help give the body shape.

There are three types of muscles found in the human body: skeletal, smooth and cardiac. All three types of muscle have the unique ability to contract (shorten) (**Fig. 3.15**).

Skeletal muscles

As the name implies, these muscles are attached to bones. When these muscles shorten, they provide the force to move the levers of the skeletal system, allowing the body to move (**Fig. 3.16**). Skeletal muscles make up the major muscle mass of the body. Weight lifters and athletes exercise to strengthen and develop skeletal muscles.

Tap your right foot three times. To accomplish this task, your brain sent a signal to the muscles in your calf instructing them to shorten, so that your foot extended. Then your brain told your calf to relax and the muscles in the front of your lower leg to contract; this process was repeated twice more. Although you did not have to consciously think about each step, it was voluntary because you chose to do it. Therefore, skeletal muscles are called voluntary muscles.

31

The human body

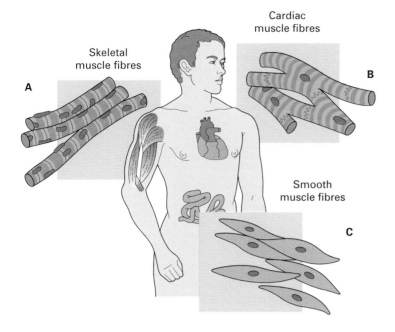

Skeletal muscle fibres

Cardiac muscle fibres

Smooth muscle fibres

A

B

C

Fig. 3.15 **(a)** Skeletal muscle attaches to the bone. **(b)** Cardiac muscle is located in the heart. **(c)** Smooth muscle is located in organs such as the stomach and intestine.

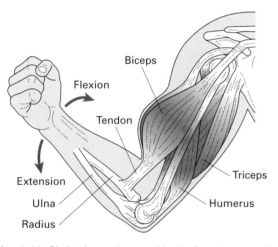

Biceps

Flexion

Tendon

Triceps

Extension

Ulna

Humerus

Radius

Fig. 3.16 Skeletal muscles provide the force to move the body.

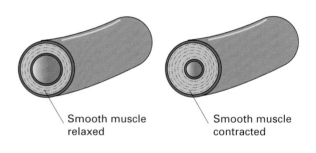

Smooth muscle relaxed

Smooth muscle contracted

Fig. 3.17 Smooth muscles are found in the walls of some tubular structures and can contract or relax to change the diameter of the tube.

Smooth muscles

These muscles are found in the walls of tubular structures in the gastrointestinal tract and the urinary system. Smooth muscles are also found in the blood vessels and the bronchi. Because they are circular, contraction changes the inside diameter of the tube (**Fig. 3.17**). This contraction is very important for controlling flow through the tubes of the body.

For instance, when you are cold, the body decreases blood flow to the arms and legs because significant body heat can be lost through the skin in these areas. The blood flow to the extremities is reduced by contracting the smooth muscles in the arteries that lead to the arms and legs.

You have no control over this process. Smooth muscles carry out many of the automatic muscular functions such as digestion, blood vessel control and modifying the diameter of your airway. Because no conscious thought is required for these activities, the smooth muscles are called involuntary muscles.

Cardiac muscle

The heart is the most important muscle in the body. The heart muscle has tremendous stamina. Imagine squeezing a tennis ball 60 times per minute. How long do you think that you could keep up with that pace? Certainly not 60 times per minute, 24 hours a day, just as the heart does. To accomplish this amazing feat of stamina, the heart must have a continuous supply of blood. The heart has its own special arteries (the coronary arteries) to deliver oxygen and nutrients to the heart muscle.

Cholesterol in the bloodstream is deposited on the inside walls of these arteries. Eventually, these deposits can decrease blood flow to the heart. If the flow of blood is interrupted for more than a few minutes, part of the heart will be damaged. The damaged muscle causes the most common sign of a heart attack – chest pain.

Cardiac muscle is the only type of muscle that has the ability to contract on its own, and it is found only in the heart. Because your heartbeat is not under conscious control, cardiac muscle is an involuntary muscle.

THE NERVOUS SYSTEM

The human nervous system is incredibly well developed and complex. It is the root of all thought, memory and emotion. It also controls the voluntary and involuntary activities of the body. Anatomically, the nervous system has two components: the central nervous system and the peripheral nervous system (**Fig. 3.18**).

The central nervous system consists of the brain, which is located within the skull and the spinal cord, which is located within the spinal column from the base of the skull to the lower back. The central nervous system is responsible for all higher mental functions, such as thought, decision making and communication, and it also has an important role in the regulation of body functions. The peripheral nervous system consists of sensory and motor nerves that lie outside the skull or spinal cord. These nerves serve as wires, carrying information between the central nervous system and every organ and muscle in the body.

Sensory nerves carry information from the body to the central nervous system. They provide information about the environment, pain, pressure and body position to the brain for decision making. Motor nerves carry information from the central nervous system to the body. Signals from the motor nerves cause contraction of skeletal muscles, which are responsible for all body movement (**Fig. 3.19**).

THE SKIN

Most people think of the skin as just a covering for the body. In reality it is a very important organ that performs many functions. The skin protects the body from the environment. Not only does it keep us from drying out, it also serves as a barrier to prevent invasion of the body by bacteria and other organisms.

The skin also plays a crucial role in temperature regulation. When you are too hot, the blood vessels dilate and the skin secretes sweat, which evaporates and cools the body. When you are cold, the blood vessels to the skin contract to decrease the heat loss to the environment.

Skin is also an important sensory organ. Special receptors in the skin can detect heat, cold, touch, pressure and pain. Information from these receptors is transmitted to the central nervous system by sensory nerves.

THE DIGESTIVE SYSTEM

Food provides our bodies with substances that cells need to produce energy and build new tissue. The digestive system breaks down food so that it can be absorbed into the blood and delivered to the cells as nutrients, vitamins and minerals (**Fig. 3.20**).

Food passes through the hollow organs of the digestive system from the mouth to the anus. The breakdown of food begins in the mouth as the food is chewed and mixed with saliva. This breakdown

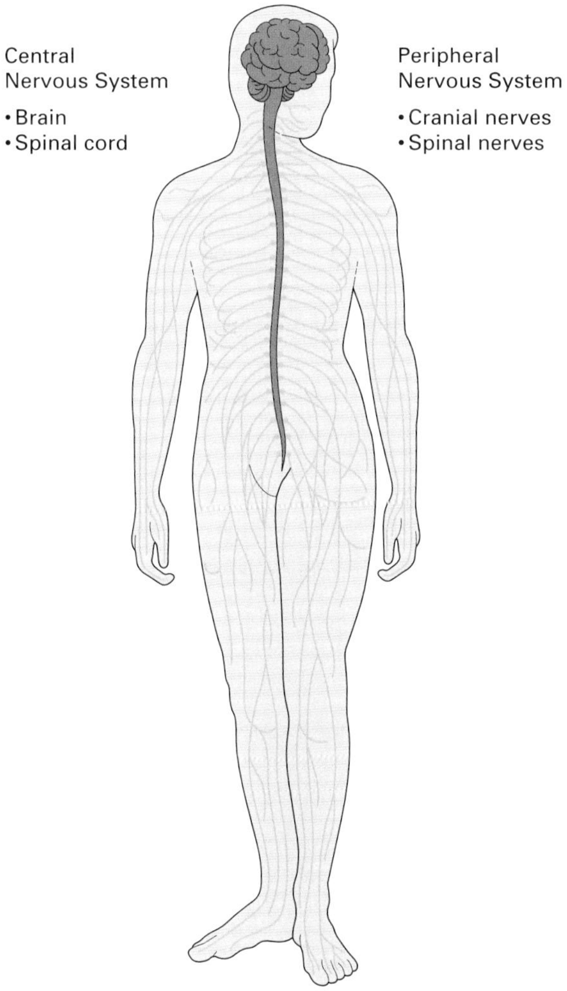

Central
Nervous System

• Brain
• Spinal cord

Peripheral
Nervous System

• Cranial nerves
• Spinal nerves

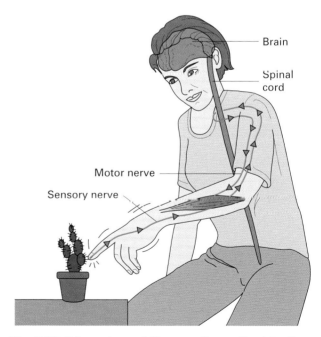

Fig. 3.18 The central nervous system consists of the brain and spinal cord. The peripheral nervous system consists of nerves that lie outside the skull and spinal cord.

Fig. 3.19 Pain, such as pricking your finger, stimulates the sensory nerves, which carry the information to the brain. The brain then signals the motor nerves to withdraw your finger.

The human body

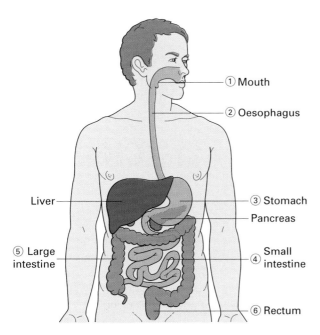

① Mouth
② Oesophagus
Liver
③ Stomach
Pancreas
⑤ Large intestine
④ Small intestine
⑥ Rectum

Fig. 3.20 The pathway food follows through the digestive system, from mouth (1) to rectum (6). The liver and pancreas secrete chemicals into the digestive system to aid the breakdown of food.

continues in the stomach, where the food is churned and combined with stomach acids. Chemicals from the liver and pancreas further break down food into its component parts. Once food has been broken down, nutrients are absorbed into the blood as the food passes through the small intestine. Liquid is removed from the food as it passes through the large intestine, which is also called the colon. Material that cannot be digested is eliminated from the body as faeces.

THE ENDOCRINE SYSTEM

The endocrine system is a very complicated system, consisting of a number of glands inside the body that produce chemicals called hormones. These chemicals, when secreted into the bloodstream, regulate the activities and functions of many body systems. Two examples of such hormones are adrenaline, which helps prepare the body for emergencies, and insulin, which is crucial for the body's use of sugars.

CHAPTER SUMMARY
The respiratory system

The respiratory system makes oxygen available to the blood and rids the body of carbon dioxide. The respiratory system can be divided into the airways, which are the passageways through which air flows, and the lungs, where gas exchange actually occurs.

The circulatory system

The circulatory system delivers oxygen and nutrients to the organs and tissues of the body and removes waste products from them. This is accomplished by pumping blood through the lungs and to the body tissues through a network of blood vessels.

The musculoskeletal system

The skeleton gives the body shape, protects vital organs and provides for body movement. The skeleton can be divided into the head, spinal column and thorax, the pelvis and lower extremities, and the upper extremities. The muscles provide movement by contracting. There are three types of muscles: skeletal muscles, which are attached to bones and move the skeleton; smooth muscles, which affect the flow of fluid or gas through the tubes of the body; and cardiac muscle, which enables the heart to beat.

The nervous system, skin, digestive system and endocrine system

The nervous system controls all voluntary and involuntary actions of the body. The skin provides a barrier for protection and interaction with the environment. The digestive system breaks down food so that it can be absorbed into the blood and delivered to the cells as nutrients, vitamins and minerals. The endocrine system regulates body function through the release of chemicals called hormones into the bloodstream.

Chapter Four

Lifting and moving patients

I.   Role of the First Responder

II. Body mechanics and lifting techniques
    A Guidelines for lifting
    B. Guidelines for carrying
    C. Guidelines for reaching
    D. Rescue board technique
    E. Helmet removal
    F. Guidelines for pushing and pulling

III. Principles of moving patients
    A. General considerations
    B. Emergency moves
    C. Non-urgent moves
    D. Patient positioning

IV. Equipment
    A. Wheeled stretcher
    B. Scoop stretcher
    C. Carrying chair
    D. Spinal boards
    E. Immobilisation extrication devices
    F. Cervical collar

Key terms

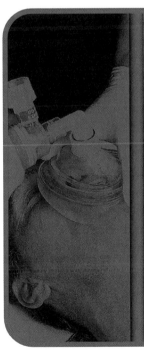

Manual handling
An activity involving the movement or support of a load by hand or other bodily force.

Emergency move
A casualty move used when there is an immediate danger to the casualty or crew members if the casualty is not moved, or when life-saving care cannot be given because of the casualty's location or position.

Non-urgent move
A casualty move used when there are no present or anticipated threats to the patient's life and care can be adequately and safely administered.

Body mechanics
The principles of effective use of the muscles and joints of your body when lifting and moving casualties.

Rescue board
A flat, rigid board of plastic, wood or aluminium, used to immobilise the entire spine; 'long-spinal board' or 'backboard' are synonymous terms.

Recovery position
Position in which the casualty is placed on his or her side, used to maintain an open airway by preventing the tongue from blocking the rear aspect of the mouth and allowing gravity to assist in draining secretions.

Objectives

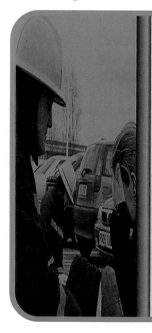

On completion of this chapter you will be able to meet the following objectives:

Cognitive objectives
1. Define body mechanics.
2. Discuss the guidelines and safety precautions that need to be followed when lifting a patient.
3. Describe an emergency move.
4. Describe a non-urgent move.

Affective objectives
5. Explain in detail the correct lifting techniques for moving patients.
6. Explain the rationale for properly lifting and moving patients.
7. Explain the rationale for an emergency move.

8. Acknowledge the importance of working with other emergency service personnel (EMS) for a patient-centred rescue.

Psychomotor objectives
9. Demonstrate an ability to immobilise the spine and carry out manual in-line stabilisation.
10. Demonstrate an emergency move.
11. Demonstrate the use of equipment to move patients in the out-of-hospital arena.

First response

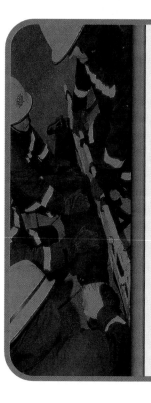

FIRE-FIGHTERS IAN AND DAVE are part of a fire crew responding to an emergency call from an 82-year-old woman who is complaining of being very ill. Control has reported that the patient believes there is carbon monoxide in her house, but that she feels too weak to get out of her bed. The patient is reported to be in the upstairs bedroom.

When Ian and Dave arrive at the scene, they use their breathing apparatus to protect themselves from carbon monoxide. They open doors and windows as they search for the patient. Ian finds her in a first-floor bedroom, and he and Dave prepare to remove her immediately from the house. The ambulance crew is on the way to the scene and will arrive within 5 minutes.

Ian and Dave take a blanket and place it on the floor next to the bed. They lift the elderly woman from the bed and gently place her on top of the blanket. They use the blanket to move her gently down the stairs and out to the front of the house to the ambulance crew that has just arrived on the scene. Ian and Dave then assist the ambulance crew to move the patient on to the stretcher and into the ambulance.

Lifting and moving a patient is a common practice for anyone involved in rescues. As a First Responder, the amount of lifting and moving that you do will be determined by the system in which you work. For the most part, the role of the First Responder is to assist other emergency service personnel with lifting and moving patients. However, for emergency situations, it may be necessary to rapidly move the patient to a safe location prior to the arrival of the ambulance service.

First Responders may be called on to move patients before the ambulance personnel arrive. Therefore, it is important that you understand the techniques involved, including how to position patients and how to best assist ambulance personnel with lifting and moving patients.

Emergency service personnel can sustain injuries while performing lifting during their duties. Most of these injuries can be prevented by using the proper lifting and moving techniques discussed in this chapter.

ROLE OF THE FIRST RESPONDER

There are three situations when First Responders commonly move patients:

1. When there is immediate danger to the patient or the crew.
2. When it is necessary to prevent further injury to the patient.
3. When assisting ambulance personnel.

In most situations, First Responders will not move patients until other ambulance personnel are on the scene. However, if there is a threat to patients' lifes, such as a fire, explosion or hazardous substance, the First Responder may move them to an area of safety. Remember, never enter a scene until it is safe. If you determine that ambulance personnel with additional training or equipment are necessary to move the patient, wait until they are available before making the move.

The patient's condition determines how he or she should be positioned. Patient positioning is discussed later in this chapter.

Once ambulance personnel arrive at the scene, you should assist them with lifting and moving. Therefore you should become familiar with the equipment used by your local ambulance services.

BODY MECHANICS AND LIFTING TECHNIQUES

One of the most common ways of injuring yourself as a First Responder is through use of poor body mechanics when lifting or moving patients. Body mechanics are the principles of effective use of the muscles and joints of your body when lifting and moving patients. Use of proper body mechanics is essential in performing your duties and greatly reduces your chances of being injured.

Guidelines for lifting

In the UK, The Manual Handling Operations Regulations 1992 came into force on 1 January 1993. These regulations were made under the Health and Safety at Work Act 1974 and implement European Directive 90/269/EEC on the manual handling of loads. They cover the following topics:

* the handler's posture;
* the individual's capability;
* the size of the load; and
* the working environment.

When lifting a patient, you should keep your back straight and your shoulders level. Bend your knees and hips, not your back – the closer you hold the patient's weight to your body, the less strain is placed on the muscles of your back. Do not twist or bend your spine and keep your chin and your elbows tucked in and

your feet one hip's width apart. Your own weight at this point can be used to counterbalance the load. Point your feet in the right direction and communicate with your partner or the patient at all times. Ensure you have divided the lift into stages and, if using equipment, ensure that it is used safely and correctly.

Incorrect lifting commonly causes back injury. The back injury may manifest itself as chronic back pain, which, although not always disabling, can limit life-style and work capabilities. A sudden traumatic back injury, such as a ruptured disc, may also occur as a result of incorrect lifting. A high percentage of this back pain and subsequent absence from work could be prevented by using the most appropriate techniques for lifting and handling (**Fig. 4.1**).

When preparing to lift a patient, always explain what you intend to do and – in appropriate circumstances – obtain their permission. Clear the working area to ensure that it is safe and that the route to be taken with the patient is clear of obstacles. If working as a team, decide who will give the instruction for the lift.

Proper lifting depends on understanding several key principles. These include, but are not limited to, the weight of the patient and number and size of crew members. Again, be sure you can handle the lift. At the very minimum, two people are required for a successful lift. Call for more help if necessary. The more help that is available, the easier and the safer the lift will be. Every First Responder has different lifting capabilities and it is your responsibility to ensure that you do not exceed your own limit. Use an even number of people to maintain the balance of both the patient and the lifting and moving device. Don't try to lift more than you can handle. Always request additional personnel if they are needed.

You must also know the weight limitation of any equipment being used. Most lifting and moving equipment has a warning label similar to that shown in **Fig. 4.2**. Check the manufacturer's guidelines for equipment weight limits. You may have to improvise if the patient's weight exceeds the capacity of the equipment. There is no set rule other than to use skilful common sense in moving the patient. If the situation appears unsafe to you, do not move the patient until you are comfortable with the method to be used.

When lifting from the ground, use the power lift position. This position keeps your back locked during the lift. The power lift is the ideal method for lifting from the ground, particularly for crew members with weak knees or thighs. If only two crew members are present, maintain balance by standing opposite each other at the sides or ends of the stretcher when lifting the patient.

Guidelines for carrying

Sometimes First Responders will be called on to assist ambulance personnel in carrying patients from the scene to the ambulance. Be sure to take your direction for this from the more advanced personnel at the scene. As a general rule, always try to wheel patients to the

Lifting and moving patients

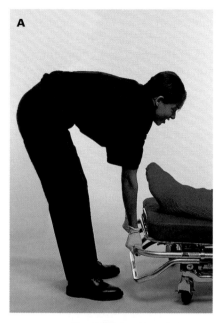

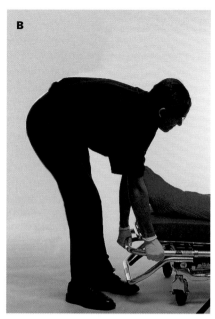

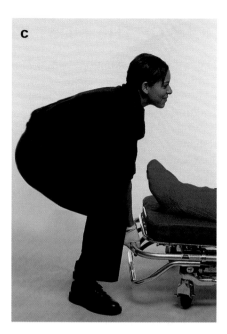

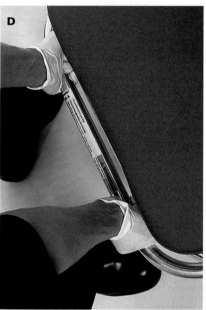

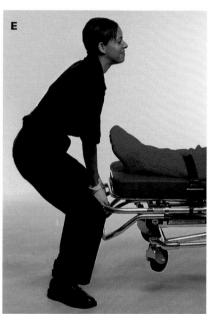

Fig. 4.1 Guidelines for proper lifting technique. **(a)** Improper lifting technique with back bent. **(b)** Improper lifting technique with the torso twisted. **(c)** Proper lifting technique with knees bent. Stand facing the stretcher with your feet shoulder width apart. This can be done at either the ends or the side of the stretcher. Squat down to the stretcher, bending at the knees. Keep your back tight, with the abdominal muscles locking your back in a normal slight inward curve. **(d)** To get the maximum force from your hands, the palm and fingers should come into complete contact with the object and all fingers should bend at the same angles. Your hands should be at least 25 cm (10 in.) apart. **(e)** Keep your feet flat and distribute your weight to the balls of your feet, or just behind them. Stand up, making sure that your back is locked and your upper body comes up before your hips.

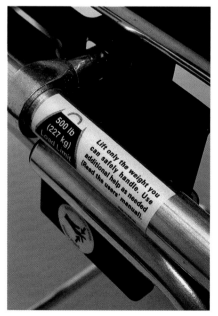

Fig. 4.2 Warning labels on lifting equipment specify weight limits.

ambulance rather than carry them. Let the stretcher wheels do the work for you. However, in some situations, such as on uneven ground or in areas with multiple obstacles, the crew needs to carry the patient and any equipment to the ambulance. In such a case, the safety precautions and guidelines are the same as for lifting a patient.

Ideally, First Responders should work with partners of similar height and strength to maintain better balance when lifting and carrying. This is often not possible, so you may have to adapt to differences in height and strength. Be careful not to hyperextend your back or to lean to either side in order to compensate for any imbalance when carrying a patient. When only two crew members are carrying a stretcher or spinal board, they should face each other in opposing positions from the sides or ends (**Fig. 4.3**).

The more people that there are available to help, the easier it is to carry the patient. If there are multiple rescuers, the stretcher or spinal board can be carried using the one-handed technique (**Fig. 4.4**). This is much safer than a two-person carry, because the stretcher or spinal board is balanced, the weight is evenly distributed and there is less weight for each person to carry.

When you assist in carrying a patient down steps or stairs, a carrying chair should be used (**Fig. 4.5**). Carrying chairs allow the crew more flexibility in handling and transporting the patient. The patient is seated in the carrying chair, and straps are applied to secure him or her to the chair. The smaller size of the carrying chair makes it easier to manoeuvre in tight, steep areas. However, it should not be used for a patient with a possible spinal injury. In this case, the patient should be transported down stairs immobilised on the spinal board.

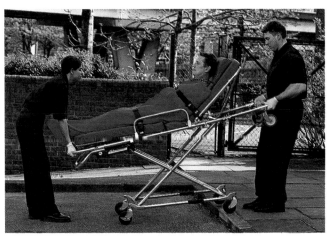

Fig. 4.3 When carrying the stretcher with only two crew members, face each other in opposing positions – from either the sides or the ends of the stretcher.

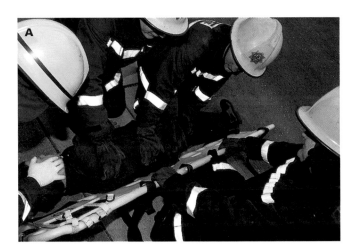

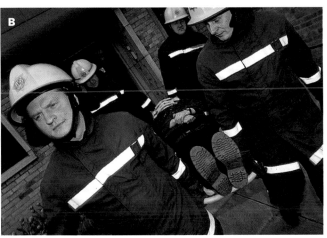

Fig. 4.4 (a) Multiple rescuers preparing to lift a backboard using the one-handed technique. **(b)** Multiple rescuers carrying a patient.

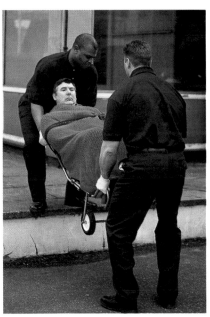

Fig. 4.5 A stair chair provides more flexibility for handling and transporting the patient in narrow or steep areas.

Review Questions

Body Mechanics and Lifting Techniques

1. Bending the back during lifting may cause serious back injury. True or False?

2. Feet should be about _____ width apart when lifting a patient.

3. It is better to _____ rather than _____ a patient.

1. True; 2. Shoulder; 3. Push; pull

Lifting and moving patients

Guidelines for reaching

Reaching for patients can also lead to injury. The actions involved in reaching range from simply reaching across the stretcher to fasten a buckle to straining in order to pull the patient on to a spinal board. Try to keep your back in a locked position, avoid leaning back over your hips and avoid twisting your back. All of these actions place strain on the spine and increase the chance of injury. Generally, try not to reach more than 0.5 m in front of you, and avoid situations where you must reach for longer than 1 minute to perform a task. Reaching for longer than 1 minute may fatigue body muscles, increasing the chance of injury. When assisting in rolling a patient on to a long spinal board, keep your back straight when leaning over the patient, lean from the hips, and use your shoulder muscles to help with the roll.

Rescue board technique

There are many ways of removing patients from a vehicle, but certain rules must always be applied. These are:

- One Responder must always hold the neck to ensure cervical spine immobilisation.
- One Responder must always support the chest of the patient, so that the thoracic spine is immobilised.
- One Responder must move the pelvis and legs, therefore supporting the lumbar aspect of the spine.
- One Responder must hold the rescue board .

When moving a patient from a vehicle, therefore, a minimum of four personnel are needed. **Figure 4.6** shows the immediate release method of removing a patient from a vehicle using a rescue board or long spinal board.

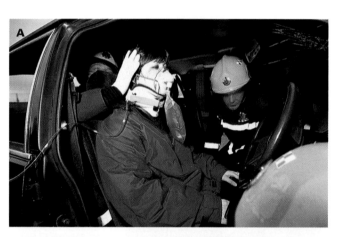

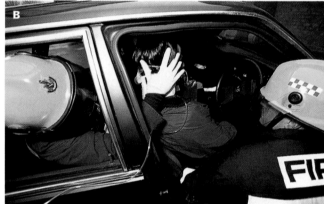

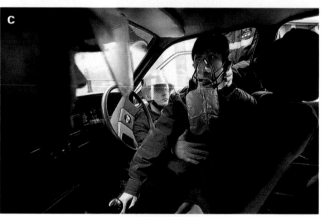

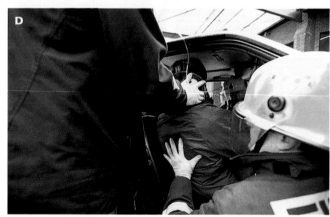

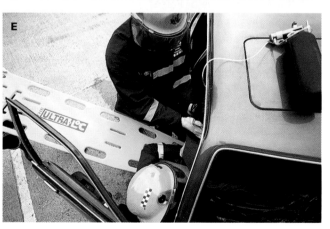

Fig. 4.6 Extrication from a vehicle using a spinal board.
(a) Three rescuers are in position, ready to evacuate the patient. The first is holding the neck of the patient, while the second has entered from the passenger side and will take control of moving the pelvis and legs. The third is in position outside the vehicle ready to support the chest of the patient. **(b)** The patient is rotated around in the seat of the vehicle so that his or her back is facing the vehicle door. One rescuer is still holding the neck, the second has rotated the pelvis and raised the legs onto the passenger seat. The third is rotating the chest in line with the neck. The first rescuer holding the neck has now reached his limitation. The second rescuer who has rotated the legs onto the passenger seat can now walk around the vehicle and take over the cervical hold, if there are insufficient rescuers available. **(c)** and **(d)** show the patient rotated around in the seat ready for extrication onto a rescue board. In **(e)**, the board has been

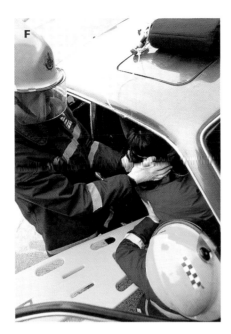

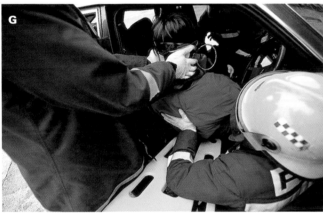

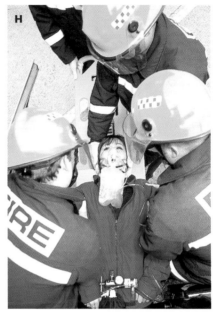

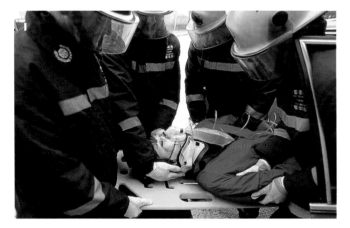

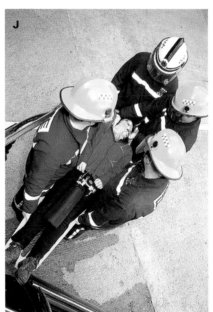

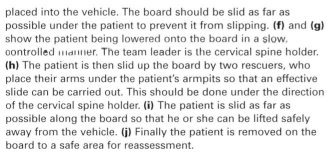

placed into the vehicle. The board should be slid as far as possible under the patient to prevent it from slipping. **(f)** and **(g)** show the patient being lowered onto the board in a slow, controlled manner. The team leader is the cervical spine holder. **(h)** The patient is then slid up the board by two rescuers, who place their arms under the patient's armpits so that an effective slide can be carried out. This should be done under the direction of the cervical spine holder. **(i)** The patient is slid as far as possible along the board so that he or she can be lifted safely away from the vehicle. **(j)** Finally the patient is removed on the board to a safe area for reassessment.

Lifting and moving patients

Helmet removal

Following an accident. it may be necessary to remove a motorcyclist's helmet if the casualty's airway is compromised. Two First Responders are needed for this technique, but as it is simple to apply and one skilled person and an unskilled person could undertake this procedure. The technique is illustrated in **Figure 4.7**.

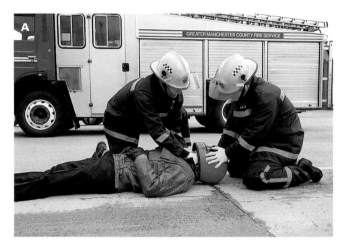

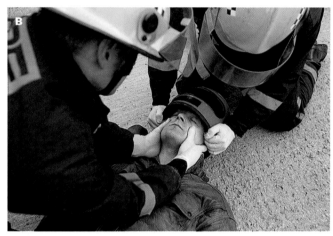

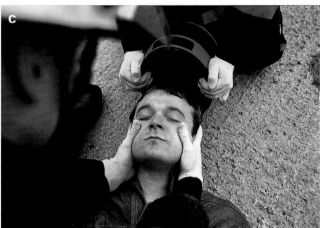

Fig. 4.7 Helmet removal. **(a)** The first rescuer approaches the patient from the head end and takes hold of the helmet. This will also immobilise the cervical spine. The second rescuer removes the chin strap and slides his hands up underneath the helmet rim, as far as possible. **(b)** The second rescuer places his hands as far as possible into the helmet, so that his thumbs are over the patient's cheek bones. The first rescuer then places his fingers inside the rim of the helmet and gently pulls the helmet apart. This creates more space so that the second rescuer can place his fingers as far as possible into the helmet. The first rescuer then pulls the helmet horizontally from the patient's head, towards himself. This is done slowly when approaching the patient's nose. **(c)** As the helmet is removed the second rescuer takes the full weight of the patient's head, and should expect a sudden heavy weight in his hands. Once the first rescuer has removed the helmet, he can take over the neck immobilisation whilst airway assessment takes place.

Guidelines for pushing and pulling

Whenever possible, it is preferable to push rather than pull a patient into position, although, in some situations, pulling may be the only option. Again, keep your back locked in position. The back is simply not strong enough to bear the weight of your body along with the added stress of the patient's weight. Keep the weight of the patient close to your body. When pulling the patient, keep the line of pull through the centre of your body by bending your knees. The line of pull is the path from the patient directly to you. Push the patient with your arms between your waist and shoulder.

Be careful whenever the weight load is below your waist level, or above the level of your shoulders. If the weight is below waist level, kneel down to prevent back injury. Keep your elbows bent with arms close to the sides when you push or pull.

Pushing and pulling should only be carried out if there is no other method of moving the patient available. This type of patient manoeuvre is not practised by ambulance personnel. Practise lifting and moving techniques with your local ambulance personnel to develop alternatives to pushing and pulling.

PRINCIPLES OF MOVING PATIENTS

General considerations

Deciding to move any patient depends on two major considerations: the seriousness of the patient's condition and the presence of any life-threatening conditions at the scene. The three basic types of patient moves are:

- emergency moves;

- non-urgent moves; and
- patient positioning.

An emergency move is required when there is immediate danger to the patient or to you if the patient is not moved, or when life-saving care cannot be given because of the patient's location or position. This includes the following situations:
- where there is a fire or a danger of fire;
- where there are explosives or the danger of an explosion;
- where the patient cannot be protected from other hazards at the scene (for example, traffic hazards or environmental factors such as extreme cold or lightning); and
- where it is impossible to gain access to other patients who need life-saving care.

It may also be necessary to move a patient to a different location or position in order to provide care. For example, if a patient is in cardiac arrest and is found sitting in a chair, he or she must be moved to the floor to begin cardiopulmonary resuscitation (CPR; see Chapter 7, 'Circulation').

A non-urgent move is appropriate when there is no threat to life, and care can be adequately and safely administered. If there is no threat to the patient's life, then the patient should not be moved until more advanced ambulance service personnel are at the scene. Remember, your role is primarily to assist with the lifting and moving of the patient.

Patients may require positioning to prevent further harm. Patients can be positioned for airway control or allowed to remain in a position of comfort. The patient should be assessed in the normal way, following the well-trodden path of AcBC (see Chapter 6, 'Patient Assessment').

If it is felt that there may be a cervical spine injury, then the patient, if conscious, should be asked if there is any neck pain or any pain or tingling in the arms or legs, and he or she should be asked to move the fingers and toes. Having noted whether the patient is conscious or unconscious and, if conscious, the patient's responses to your questions, you should proceed to stabilise the cervical spine by providing manual in-line stabilisation.

Manual in-line stabilisation – See Chapter 10, Injuries to Muscles and Bones. The head is grasped and moved to the neutral in-line position (unless contraindicated). Traction is not applied. The head should now be constantly held in this position until full immobilisation has taken place. The contraindications to in-line movement includes increased pain experienced by the patient; any tingling in the arms of the patient; and worsening airway control.

Cervical collars – Having provided in-line stabilisation the next manoeuvre is to apply a rigid cervical collar. Cervical collars do not immobilise the cervical spine but they do reduce the potential for neck movement, and manual in-line stabilisation is still required after a rigid collar has been fitted. The principal use of a rigid collar is to prevent compression of the cervical spine. Any rigid collar that is used should be correctly sized. Inappropriately sized collars are either ineffective or potentially dangerous. There are several types of collar in general use. The method of sizing and fitting varies and the manufacturer's instructions should be followed.

Following any manoeuvre of the head and cervical spine or the application of a rigid collar the patient should be assessed again to ensure that there are no changes in the patient's neurological response.

Extrication devices – There are a number of different devices available. They are used to provide support and stabilisation to the upper spine. They should be used in conjunction with the rigid cervical collar and they allow the patient to be lifted easily. Manual in-line stabilisation should be performed followed by the application of the rigid cervical collar. Manual cervical spine stabilisation should be continued throughout the rescue or until the patient is securely strapped to a spinal board or stretcher.

Emergency moves

Once you have determined that an emergency move is necessary (**Principle 4.1**), there will be no time to immobilise the spine properly, but you should attempt to protect the spine by pulling the patient in the direction of the long axis of the body while keeping the patient's body in a straight line.

A patient who is lying on the floor or ground can be moved in several ways. The general principle is to maintain as much in-line spine control as possible. The clothes drag uses the patient's clothing as the point for

Principle 4.1	**Considerations for an Emergency Patient Move**

There is an immediate danger to the patient or First Responders if the patient is not moved in the following situations:
1. Fire or danger of fire
2. Explosives or other hazardous materials
3. Inability to protect the patient from other hazards at the scene
4. Inability to gain access to other casualties in a vehicle who need life-saving care
5. Any other situation that has the potential for causing immediate injury
6. Life-saving care cannot be given because of patient location or position; for example, a cardiac arrest patient sitting in a chair

Lifting and moving patients

balance (**Fig. 4.8**). Your arms cradle the patient's head as you pull on the clothing around the shoulders. The blanket drag has the same principle, except that the patient is placed on a blanket (**Fig. 4.9**). If a patient is difficult to handle because of size or lack of co-operation, securing your arms under the patient's arms will help to maintain balance and control (**Fig. 4.10**).

Always suspect a spinal injury when moving a trauma patient, especially if the mechanism of injury involved forces that might cause spinal damage. Every precaution should be taken to protect the patient's spine from additional risk. Do not apply traction to the patient's neck and head.

Non-urgent moves

For a non-urgent move, the role of the First Responder is to assist ambulance personnel. Remember to ask for directions and listen carefully to the people who are directing the movement of the patient.

Patient positioning

The patient's condition determines how they should be positioned. An unresponsive patient without a suspected spinal injury should be placed in the recovery position to allow secretions to drain from the airway (**Fig. 4.11**). (The reader should refer to the current UK Resuscitation Council Guidelines.)

A patient without injuries but with complaints of chest pain, discomfort or difficulty in breathing should be allowed to sit in a position of comfort. Usually, the patient breathes more easily sitting than lying down. A patient who is nauseated or who has vomited should remain in a position of comfort; however, be prepared to reposition the patient to manage the airway.

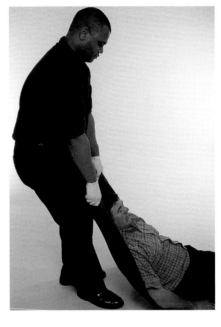

Fig. 4.9 The blanket drag technique for moving a patient.

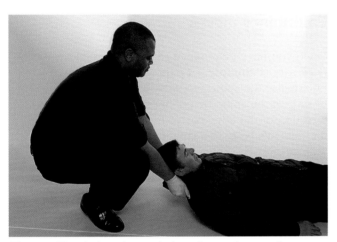

Fig. 4.8 The clothes drag technique for moving a patient.

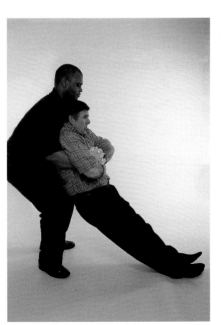

Fig. 4.10 Pulling the patient under the arms is also a technique for moving or lifting a patient.

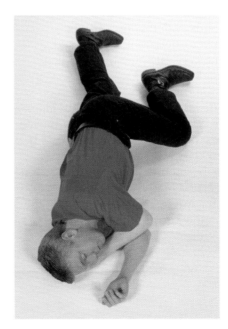

Fig. 4.11 The recovery position.

First Responder Alert

Always suspect a spinal injury when moving a trauma patient, especially if the mechanism of injury involved forces that might cause spinal damage. Every precaution should be taken to protect the patient's spine from additional risk.

EQUIPMENT

As discussed earlier, First Responders must work in conjunction with local ambulance service protocols to practise the techniques and become familiar with the equipment used to lift and move patients. Remember, your role is to assist local ambulance service personnel with lifting and moving patients, unless there is danger if the patient is not moved immediately. There are many devices used to move patients in pre-hospital care. The types of equipment that you should be familiar with include the wheeled stretcher (trolley) found in the ambulance, the scoop (orthopaedic) stretcher, the carrying chair and the spinal board.

Wheeled stretcher

The most common device used for patient movement is the wheeled 'ambulance' stretcher (**Fig. 4.12**). Whenever possible, assist in moving the patient by rolling him or her on a wheeled stretcher. This reduces the risk of injury to the crew or exhaustion caused by carrying a patient. However, a wheeled stretcher can be used only on smooth ground. Direct the stretcher by guiding the foot end, while another rescuer at the head of the patient pushes the stretcher. This prevents the patient from becoming dizzy or disorientated.

Lifting the stretcher is better than rolling it in narrow, steep spaces, but this technique requires more strength on the part of the rescuers. The stretcher must

Review Questions

Principles of Moving Patients

1. An emergency move is considered for a patient in a vehicle on fire. True or False?
2. A cardiac arrest patient should be moved immediately if you cannot provide CPR because of the patient's position. True or False?
3. An emergency move is used for a patient with a swollen, painful left ankle as long as no danger is present to the patient or crew members. True or False?
4. A non-urgent move means there is no threat to the patient's or your life. True or False?

1. True; 2. True; 3. False; 4. True

be carried over steps, because it is difficult to roll wheels over steep steps. With two rescuers, one stands at the patient's head and the other at the feet. This allows for greatest control and balance. A four-person carry is better because it provides more stability and places less strain on the rescuers. Each rescuer carries a corner. The four-person carry is considered much safer over rough terrain.

When assisting in loading the patient into an ambulance, the primary concern is safety. Follow the equipment manufacturer's directions, and ensure all stretchers and patients are secured before the ambulance moves. Be careful of traffic around the ambulance.

Scoop stretcher

A scoop stretcher (**Fig. 4.13**) is used to lift and transport a patient who is lying down to an ambulance or onto a stretcher for transport. The scoop stretcher is hinged and opens at the head and feet to 'scoop'

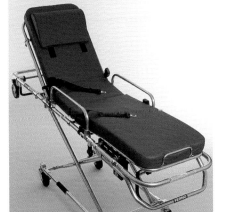

Fig. 4.12 The wheeled stretcher.

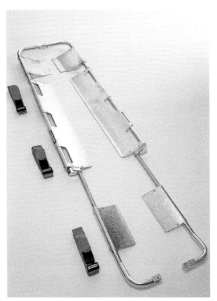

Fig. 4.13 A scoop stretcher.

Lifting and moving patients

around and under the patient. Once the scoop stretcher is fastened, the patient can be lifted on to the wheeled stretcher (**Fig. 4.14**).

A scoop stretcher should only be carried by two people, one at the head end and the other at the foot. One at either corner puts a strain on the couplings and could cause the stretcher to split.

As there is controversy regarding the use of a scoop stretcher for patients with a suspected spinal injury, follow local protocol. If you do use a scoop stretcher for patients with possible spinal injury, use it to transfer a patient to a spinal board (see **Fig. 4.14**).

Carrying chair

The carrying chair (**Fig. 4.15**) is a purpose-built piece of equipment that should be used only to transport conscious patients. It is suitable for a one-person or two-person lift. You must always reassure the patient before you tilt or move the chair. Use the proper techniques for lifting and carrying (see **Fig. 4.1**).

The carrying chair is the preferred method for transporting the patient down stairs or through narrow hallways to a stretcher. After securing the patient to this device, two emergency service personnel can safely carry the chair. Most carrying chairs have wheels at the rear, which are used to roll the patient to the stretcher.

Carrying chairs cannot be used to move unresponsive patients or patients with a suspected spinal injury.

Spinal boards

The 'spinal' or 'rescue' board (**Fig. 4.16**) is used to immobilise the entire patient. Straps must be secured across the patient's torso, waist and legs along with a head immobilisation device for the patient to be properly immobilised. There are several varieties of spinal boards available, and the manufacturer's directions for use and maintenance should be followed.

Immobilisation extrication devices

Immobilisation extrication devices are used for the immobilisation of a patient with a suspected spinal injury. Various types are available (**Fig. 4.17**). Some are collapsible for ease of use by one person. All are constructed along similar lines, with vertically aligned slats to provide the necessary rigidity to minimise the risk of further injury. Integral handgrips are provided to assist when extricating and placing a patient on a spinal board. These devices may also come with lifting slings or attachments, and some are approved for helicopter use. All immobilisation extrication devices

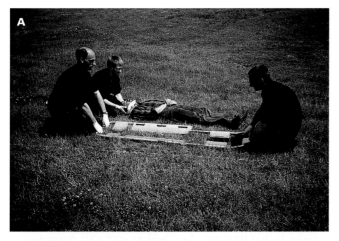
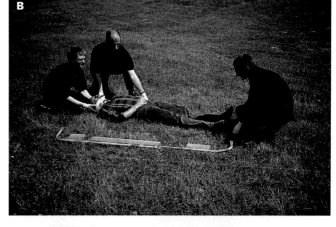
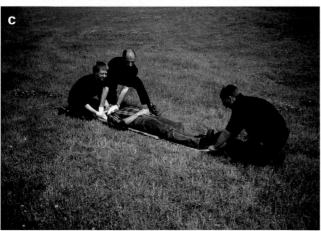
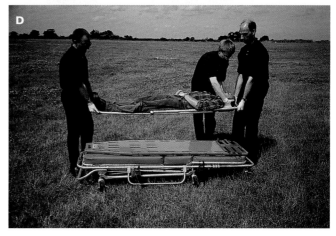

Fig. 4.14 Transfer of the supine patient from the ground to the wheeled stretcher using a scoop stretcher.

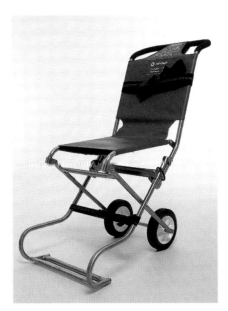

Fig. 4.15 A carrying chair.

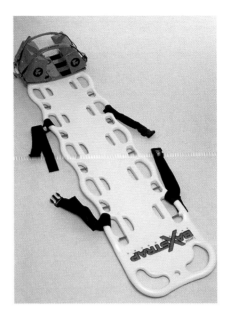

Fig. 4.16 The spinal (or rescue) board with head immobiliser and straps.

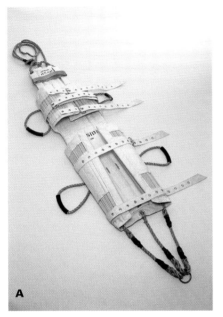

A

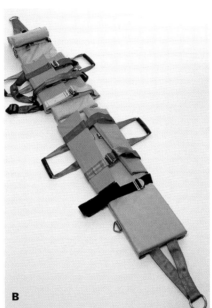

B

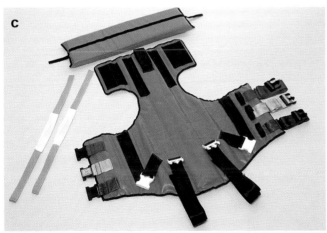

C

Fig. 4.17 (a) The Neil Robertson board; (b) The Paraguard board; (c) The Kendrick Extrication Device ('KED').

must be used in conjunction with a rigid cervical collar which together offer cervical and thoracolumbar spine immobilisation.

The main advantage of immobilisation extrication devices is that they may be fitted *in situ* with minimum movement to the patient in readiness for a controlled movement by the emergency service personnel. Care must be exercised to ensure that any torso-securing straps are not over tightened, particularly around the chest area, as this could cause further injury or discomfort to the patient and also restrict the patient's breathing.

Cervical collar

The cervical collar provides a means of supporting the neck in the neutral position in alignment with the spine. Modern collars are available in various sizes or are adjustable. Strong Velcro fasteners hold the collar in place. Full foam lining improves patient comfort and the collars fold completely flat for compact storage.

Equipment

1. The _____ is used to fully immobilise the spine of a patient.

2. When using multiple rescuers to lift or carry a stretcher, the carry will be much safer than when only two rescuers carry the stretcher. True or False?

3. An unresponsive patient without a suspected spine injury is placed in the _____ position.

1. Long backboard; 2. True; 3. Recovery

CHAPTER SUMMARY

Role of the First Responder

The role of the First Responder in lifting and moving a patient is limited. First Responders should generally move patients with ambulance personnel. First Responders should be able to move patients who are in immediate danger, position patients to prevent further injury, and assist ambulance personnel in lifting and moving patients.

Body mechanics and lifting techniques

Use your legs, not your back, to lift a patient. The power-lift method is used to minimise strain on the back when lifting. Do not attempt to lift a weight beyond your physical limitations. Carrying the patient requires excellent balance and more work by the crew than rolling the patient on a wheeled stretcher. Reaching for the patient puts stress on the back. Never try to reach overhead or hyperextend the back, as these lead to possible injury. It is preferable to push, rather than pull, a patient or stretcher into position.

Principles of moving patients

The three types of moves are emergency moves, non-urgent moves and patient positioning. An emergency move is used for patients who are in immediate danger or when life-saving care cannot be given because of the patient's location or condition. The role of the First Responder with non-urgent moves is to assist ambulance personnel. Remember to ask for directions and listen carefully to the people who are directing the movement of the patient. A patient who has no life-threatening conditions may be moved when the patient is ready for transportation. Responsive patients with no suspected spinal trauma can remain in a position of comfort. Unresponsive patients with no suspected spinal trauma should be placed in the recovery position.

Equipment

You should meet regularly with your local ambulance personnel and practise working with the following devices: wheeled stretchers, scoop stretchers, carrying chairs and spinal boards. These are all tools used to move the patient from the scene to the ambulance for transport.

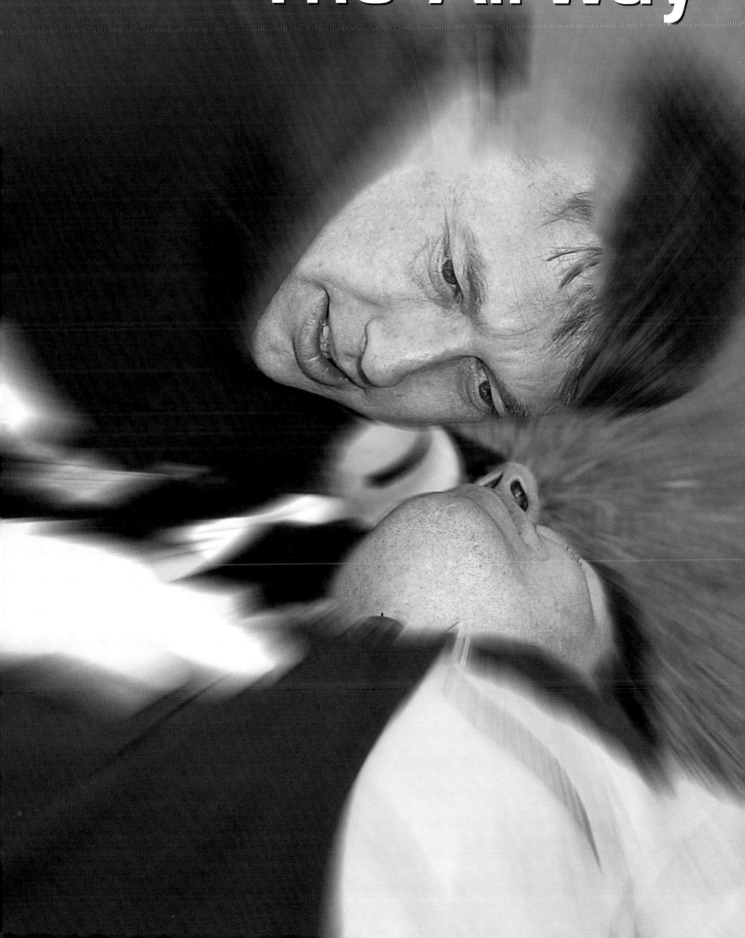

Division Two:
The Airway

Chapter
Five
The airway

I. **The respiratory system**
   A. Components and function of the respiratory system
   B. Considerations for infants and children

II. **Opening the airway**
   A. Manual positioning
   B. Inspecting the airway
   C. Airway adjuncts

III. **Clearing the compromised airway and maintaining an open airway**
   A. The recovery position
   B. Finger sweeps
   C. Suctioning

IV. **Assessing breathing**
   A. Determine the presence of breathing
   B. Determine the adequacy of breathing

V. **Artificial ventilation**
   A. Mouth-to-mask ventilation technique
   B. Mouth-to-barrier device ventilation technique
   C. Mouth-to-mouth ventilation technique
   D. Special considerations for trauma patients
   E. Assessing the effectiveness of artificial ventilation

VI. **Special situations in airway management**
   A. Patients with laryngectomies
   B. Ventilating infants and children
   C. Gastric distension
   D. Facial trauma
   E. Dental appliances

VII. **Foreign body airway obstruction (FBAO)**
   A. FBAO in the responsive patient
   B. FBAO in the adult patient
   C. FBAO in infants and children

Key terms

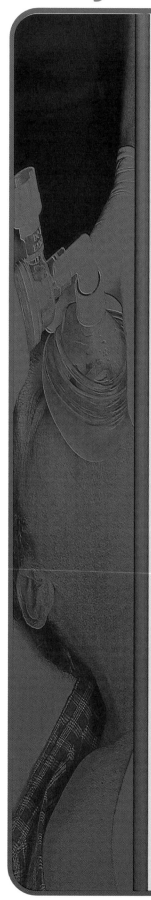

AcBC

A mnemonic for the initial protocol to be adopted by the First Responder when performing the primary assessment; it stands for 'Airway with cervical spinal control, Breathing and Circulation'.

Accessory muscles

Muscles in the neck, chest and abdomen used to assist breathing. The use of accessory muscles indicates difficulty in breathing.

Agonal respirations

Weak and ineffective chest wall movements immediately before or after cardiac arrest.

Airway

The respiratory system structures through which air passes.

Barrier devices

Typically a piece of plastic that is designed to create a barrier between the patient's and rescuer's mouth during ventilation.

Diaphragm

The large, dome-shaped muscle that separates the thoracic and abdominal cavities; the main muscle used in breathing.

Epiglottis

The flap-like structure that prevents food and liquid from entering the windpipe during swallowing.

Finger sweep

Placing a gloved finger deep into the patient's mouth to remove solids or semi-solid obstructions.

Gag reflex

A reflex that causes the patient to retch when the back of the throat is stimulated; this reflex helps the unresponsive patient protect the airway.

Heimlich manoeuvre

Abdominal thrusts used to relieve a foreign body airway obstruction (FBAO).

Laryngectomy

A surgical procedure in which the larynx is removed.

Larynx

The voice box; contains the vocal cords that vibrate during speech.

Mucus extractor

A device that is used to provide suction to the mouth and nose of infants and children.

Nasopharyngeal airway

A flexible tube of rubber or plastic that is inserted into the patient's nostril to provide an air passage.

Nasopharynx

The region of the pharynx that lies just behind the nose.

Oropharyngeal airway

A curved piece of plastic that goes into the patient's mouth and lifts the tongue away from the back of the throat.

Oropharynx

The region of the pharynx that lies just below the nasopharynx; the back of the throat.

Pharynx

Part of the airway behind the mouth and nose, divided into two regions, the nasopharynx and the oropharynx.

Resuscitation masks

Small, lightweight masks that can be used when ventilating a patient.

Stridor

A harsh sound heard during breathing, usually during inhalation, that indicates an upper airway obstruction.

Suction

Using negative pressure to remove liquids or semi-liquids from the airway.

Suction catheter

A flexible or rigid tip placed on the end of suction tubing. The suction catheter goes into the patient's mouth.

Trachea

The windpipe.

Tracheal stoma

A permanent artificial opening into the trachea.

Universal distress signal

Both hands clutching at the neck; a sign of upper airway obstruction.

Wheeze

A high-pitched whistling sound caused by narrowed air passages, which can indicate an airway obstruction.

Objectives

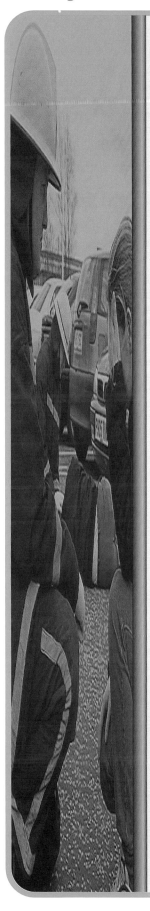

On completion of this chapter you will be able to meet the following objectives:

Cognitive objectives

1. Name and label the major structures of the respiratory system on a diagram.
2. List the signs of inadequate breathing.
3. Describe the steps in the head-tilt, chin-lift.
4. Relate the mechanisms of injury to opening the airway.
5. Describe the steps in the jaw thrust.
6. State the importance of having a suction unit ready for immediate use when providing emergency medical care.
7. Describe the techniques of suctioning.
8. Describe how to ventilate a patient with a resuscitation mask or barrier device.
9. Describe how ventilation of an infant or child is different from ventilation an adult.
10. List the steps in providing mouth-to-mouth and mouth-to-stoma ventilation.
11. Describe how to measure and insert an oropharyngeal (oral) airway.
12. Describe how to measure and insert a nasopharyngeal (nasal) airway.
13. Describe how to clear a foreign body airway obstruction in a responsive adult.
14. Describe how to clear a foreign body airway obstruction in a responsive child with complete or partial airway obstruction with poor air exchange.
15. Describe how to clear a foreign body alrway obstruction in a responsive infant with complete or partial airway obstruction with poor air exchange.
16. Describe how to clear a foreign body airway obstruction in an unresponsive adult.
17. Describe how to clear a foreign body airway obstruction in an unresponsive child.
18. Describe how to clear a foreign body airway obstruction in an unresponsive infant.

Affective objectives

19. Explain why basic life-support ventilation and airway protective skills take priority over most other bacio lifo oupport skills.
20. Demonstrate a caring attitude towards patients with airway problems who request emergency medical services.
21. Place the interest of the patient with airway problems as the foremost consideration when making any and all patient care decisions.
22. Communicate empathically with patients with airway problems, as well as with the family members and friends of the patient.

Psychomotor objectives

23. Demonstrate the steps in the head-lift, chin-tilt.
24. Demonstrate the steps in the jaw thrust.
25. Demonstrate the techniques of suctioning.
26. Demonstrate the steps in mouth-to-mouth ventilation with universal precautions (barrier shields).
27. Demonstrate how to use a resuscitation mask to ventilate a patient.
28. Demonstrate how to ventilate a patient with a stoma.
29. Demonstrate how to measure and insert an oropharyngeal (oral) airway.
30. Demonstrate how to measure and insert a nasopharyngeal (nasal) airway.
31. Demonstrate how to ventilate infants and children.
32. Demonstrate how to clear a foreign body airway ohstruction in a responsive adult.
33. Demonstrate how to clear a foreign body airway obstruction in a responsive child.
34. Demonstrate how to clear a foreign body airway obstruction in a responsive infant.
35. Demonstrate how to clear a foreign body airway obstruction in an unresponsive adult.
36. Demonstrate how to clear a foreign body airway obstruction in an unresponsive child.
37. Demonstrate how to clear a foreign body airway obstruction in an unresponsive infant.

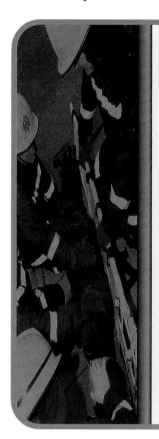

First response

MIKE ENFIELD IS A PROUD FATHER – he is constantly showing pictures of Cathy, his wife, and his two children, Julie and Jeffrey, to everybody at the station. He had just come home from a midnight shift and was eating breakfast with Cathy when Julie came running downstairs screaming for her parents to come quickly. They burst through the door to find the limp little body of their 8-month-old son, Jeffrey. He had been playing with his sister's stuffed animals when he suddenly stopped breathing.

Mike looked at his son who was blue around the lips and unresponsive, and he knew that he had to do something quickly. Cathy said, "I'll call 999; you help Jeff!'" Mike took hold of his son. He remembered what he learned from his First Responder training as he opened the little boy's airway and checked for breathing. He sealed his lips around his son's mouth and nose. When he attempted to ventilate, no breath went in. He repositioned his son's head and tried again, to no avail. He began performing back blows and chest thrusts. On the third chest thrust a button popped out of Jeffrey's mouth. He still was not breathing, so Mike performed mouth-to-mouth ventilations. Within a minute, Jeffrey started to breathe on his own. By the time the ambulance arrived, he was crying and fully responsive. Jeffrey was checked at the accident and emergency department, and they were all home before lunch.

Nothing is more immediately life threatening than something that compromises the airway or prevents a patient from breathing. One of the popular memory aids to remember the priorities in managing emergencies is AcBC – Airway with cervical spinal control, Breathing and Circulation. You will hear this many times as a First Responder and it emphasises the importance of proper airway management and ventilation. As a First Responder, the patient care skills you learn in this chapter will be the most important skills you will learn.

THE RESPIRATORY SYSTEM

The respiratory system includes the parts of the body through which air passes. These tubes and passageways make up what is known as the airway. Because the body requires a continual supply of fresh air, anything that blocks or obstructs the airway is a serious threat to life. As a First Responder, you must ensure that the patient's airway remains clear and open.

Components and function of the respiratory system

The main purpose of the respiratory system is the delivery of oxygen to the body and the removal of carbon dioxide. This process is so essential for life that any interruption of respiration can be fatal within minutes. Familiarity with the anatomy of the airway helps you understand airway management (**Fig. 5.1**).

The airway begins with the mouth and nose and continues into the pharynx. The pharynx is divided into two regions: the nasopharynx and the oropharynx. The nasopharynx is the area just behind the nose; the oropharynx lies just below the nasopharynx and is the back of the throat.

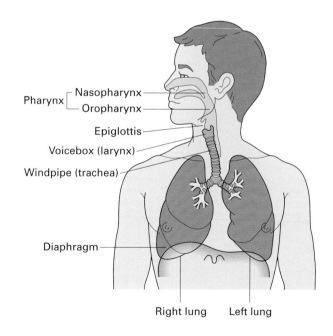

Fig. 5.1 Anatomy of the respiratory system.

Covering the passageway into the windpipe, or trachea, is the leaf-shaped epiglottis. The epiglottis is a flap-like structure that prevents food and liquid from entering the trachea during swallowing.

The voice box, or larynx, is the first part of the windpipe. The voice box forms the prominence commonly called the Adam's apple. The windpipe descends from the voice box and divides into two main branches that lead to each lung. Within the lungs, the passageway continues to divide into smaller and smaller branches, ending at tiny air sacs where the exchange of oxygen and carbon dioxide takes place (**Fig. 5.2**).

The diaphragm is the main muscle that makes breathing possible. The diaphragm is a large, dome-shaped muscle that separates the chest from the abdomen. When the diaphragm contracts, it flattens. Contraction of the diaphragm increases the size of the chest, and air is pulled into the lungs through the mouth and nose. The exchange of oxygen and carbon dioxide takes place in the lungs. During exhalation, the diaphragm relaxes and moves upward. This movement decreases the size of the chest, moving air out through the mouth and nose.

Considerations for infants and children

Because the airway structures in infants (<1 year old) and children (>1 year old) are smaller than those in adults, the airway is more easily blocked. Furthermore, the tongue is larger in relation to the size of infant's or child's mouth (**Fig. 5.3**), and the large tongue can easily fall against the back of the throat and block the airway if the patient is on his or her back.

Because the windpipe in infants and children is very narrow, it can become easily obstructed by even a small amount of fluid or swelling. The windpipe of an infant is so soft and flexible that it can be kinked by positioning the head incorrectly, especially by tilting the head back too far. Excessive head tilt can also cause damage to the spine. It is very important to maintain the airway in infants and children carefully because uncorrected respiratory problems are the primary cause of cardiac arrest in infants and children.

OPENING THE AIRWAY

Anything that interferes with the continuous flow of air into and out of the lungs is an immediate threat to life. Ensuring that the patient's airway is open and clear is your most important patient care responsibility as a First Responder.

Infant/Child

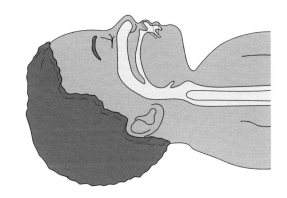

Adult

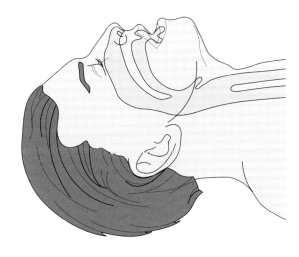

Fig. 5.3 In infants and children, the airway is more easily obstructed, and the tongue takes up proportionally more space in the mouth.

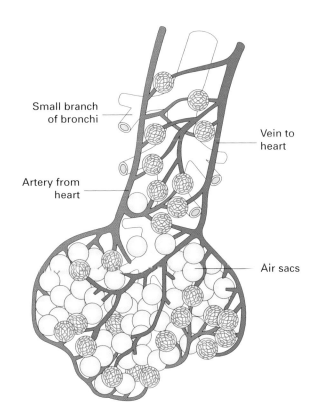

Small branch of bronchi

Artery from heart

Vein to heart

Air sacs

Fig. 5.2 In the lungs, capillaries surround the air sacs.

Manual positioning

Unresponsive patients lose muscular control of the jaw. If the patient is lying on his or her back, the jaw falls backwards and the base of the tongue touches the back of the throat (**Fig. 5.4**). This closes the airway and makes it impossible to move air from the mouth and nose into the lungs. The tongue is the most common cause of airway obstruction in the unresponsive patient.

Head-tilt, chin-lift manoeuvre

Research has indicated that the head-tilt, chin-lift manoeuvre consistently provides the optimal airway. The head-tilt, chin-lift manoeuvre is the most common method of opening the airway in the uninjured, unresponsive patient. Since the tongue is attached to the lower jaw, tilting the head back and displacing the jaw forwards will lift the base of the tongue away from the back wall of the throat. This simple technique requires no equipment and should be performed immediately whenever you are treating an unresponsive, uninjured patient.

The first step in performing the head-tilt, chin-lift manoeuvre is to place the hand closest to the head on the patient's forehead and apply firm backwards pressure to tilt the head back. Next, place the fingers of your other hand on the bony part of the patient's chin. Lift the chin forwards and support the jaw while tilting the head back (**Fig. 5.5**).

When performing the head-tilt, chin-lift manoeuvre be sure that you do not press on the soft tissues of the chin. This can push the tongue against the roof of the mouth and cause an airway obstruction, especially in children. The thumb is not used to lift the chin, but rather to keep the patient's mouth open.

When using this technique with infants and children, avoid tilting the head past the point where the nose is perpendicular to the surface upon which the patient is lying. Tilting the head too far can kink the windpipe and cause spine damage. If an elderly patient has a curvature of the upper back that places the head in a hyperextended position, you should use padding under the head to maintain the correct position.

Jaw thrust without head tilt

If the patient is injured, moving the neck can damage the patient's spinal cord. However, in many situations, you will not know if the patient has injured the spinal cord. If the mechanism of injury suggests that there may be injury, the jaw thrust without head tilt should be performed when opening the airway. Mechanism of injury is discussed in Chapter 6 ('Patient assessment').

The jaw thrust without head tilt is used to open the airway of unresponsive, injured patients. Although this technique is effective, it is technically difficult and tiring to perform. You should practice this skill often to maintain your proficiency.

To perform the jaw thrust without head tilt, place the tips of your index fingers between the jaw and the earlobe, and the meaty parts of your thumbs on the cheekbones. Lift the jaw forwards with both hands and use your thumb tips to keep the mouth open (**Fig. 5.6**).

Inspecting the airway

If there is fluid or solid material in the mouth, manual positioning techniques will effectively open the airway. Foreign material can block the passage of air from the mouth and nose and can prevent air from passing through the airway structures into the lungs. This can occur even if you have performed the head-tilt, chin-lift manoeuvre or the jaw thrust without head tilt correctly. For this reason, you should inspect the airway in any unresponsive patient and in a responsive patient who is not able to protect his or her own airway. To inspect the airway, open the patient's mouth with a gloved

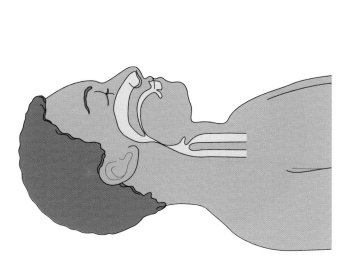

Fig. 5.4 Unresponsive patients lose muscular control of the jaw. This may cause the tongue to contact the back of the throat, so obstructing the airway.

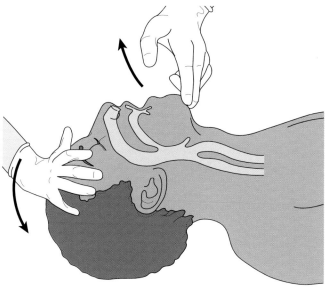

Fig. 5.5 When you tilt the head back and lift the chin, the base of the tongue and the epiglottis are lifted out of the airway.

hand and look inside it. You may find the airway to be clear (patent) or, as you inspect the airway, you may find fluids or solids (for example, sweets or food, teeth, dentures) that may block the free passage of air.

Airway adjuncts

Oropharyngeal airways and nasopharyngeal airways are airway adjuncts that help to open and maintain the airway. One of these two devices should be used when unresponsive patients are unable to control their airway.

Oropharyngeal airway
The oropharyngeal airway (**Fig. 5.7**) is a curved piece of plastic that goes into the patient's mouth and lifts the tongue away from the back of the throat (**Fig. 5.8**). It is

also called an oral airway or an OP airway. It is important to select the correct airway size.

The gag reflex causes the patient to retch when the back of the throat is stimulated. This reflex helps unresponsive patients protect their airway. Unresponsive patients who lose the gag reflex are at very high risk of airway obstruction and inhalation of material into the lungs. The oropharyngeal airway should be used only if the patient is unresponsive and has no gag reflex. If it is used in a patient who has a gag reflex, the patient may gag or vomit. This can seriously threaten the airway. **Figure 5.9** illustrates the technique for inserting an oral airway in an adult; **Figure 5.10** illustrates the technique for inserting an oral airway in an infant or child.

Nasopharyngeal airway
The nasopharyngeal airway (**Fig. 5.11**) is a flexible tube of rubber or plastic. It is inserted into the patient's nostril to provide an air passage (**Fig. 5.12**). The nasopharyngeal airway is commonly called a nasal airway or NP airway.

The nasopharyngeal airway is less likely to stimulate vomiting and is a valuable adjunct in patients who are responsive but who need assistance in keeping the tongue from obstructing the airway. This type of airway is well tolerated in patients of all ages and is the easiest airway adjunct to use if the patient is fitting. **Figure 5.13** illustrates the technique for inserting a nasopharyngeal airway in a patient of any age.

It is important to select the correct airway size. You should first consider the diameter of the nostril. If after inserting the airway 20 mm there is blanching to the skin around the nostril, a smaller size should be used. If you meet resistance, do not force the airway. Remove it from that nostril, re-lubricate it and try the other side. Even a well-lubricated nasopharyngeal airway may be uncomfortable for the patient.

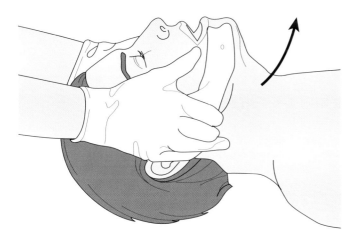
Fig. 5.6 Use the jaw thrust without head-tilt to open the airway in an injured patient.

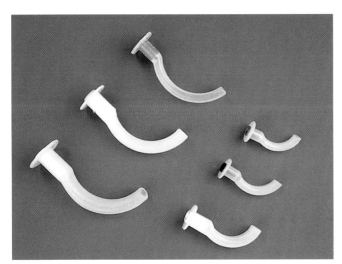
Fig. 5.7 Oropharyngeal airways are available is several sizes and types.

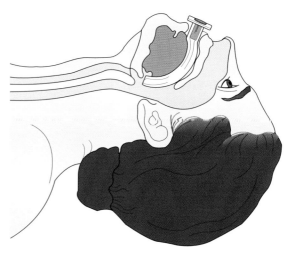
Fig. 5.8 The oropharyngeal airway displaces the tongue from the back of the patient's throat.

The airway

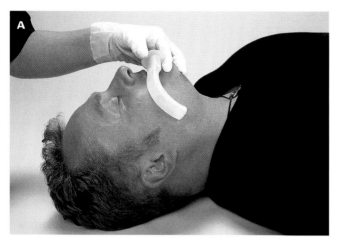

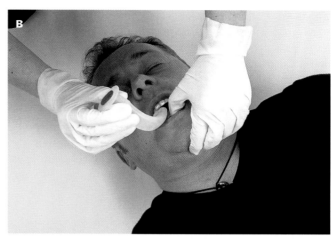

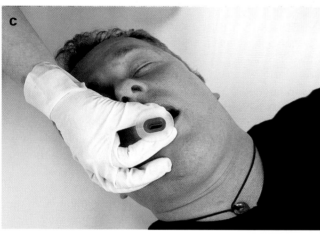

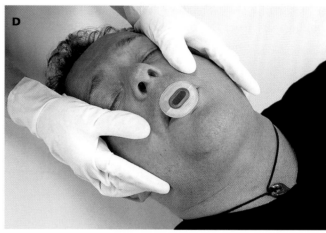

Fig. 5.9 Method for inserting the oral airway in adults. Take universal precautions. **(a)** Select the properly sized airway, which should measure from the centre of the patient's front teeth to the angle of the jaw. Position yourself at the patient's side. **(b)** Open the patient's mouth by lifting the jaw and tongue. Insert the airway upside down (with the tip facing the roof of the patient's mouth). Advance the airway gently until you feel resistance. **(c)** Turn the airway 180 degrees so that it **(d)** comes to rest with the flange on the patient's teeth. Ventilate the patient as necessary.

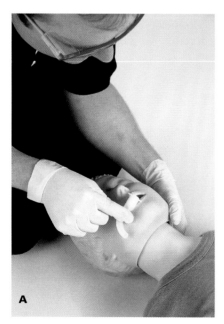

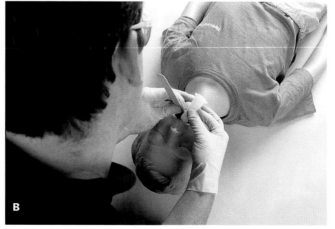

Fig. 5.10 Method for inserting the oral airway in infants and children. Take universal precautions. Select the properly sized airway, which should measure from the centre of the patient's front teeth to the angle of the jaw. Position yourself at the top of the patient's head. Open the patient's mouth and use a tongue depressor to press the tongue forwards and out of the airway. Insert the airway right side up (with the tip facing towards the floor of the patient's mouth). Advance the airway gently until the flange comes to rest on the patient's lips or teeth. Ventilate the patient as necessary.

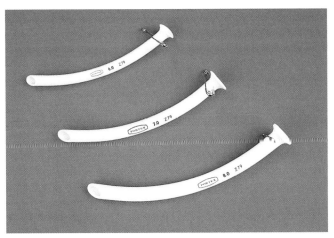

Fig. 5.11 Nasopharyngeal airways are available in several sizes and types.

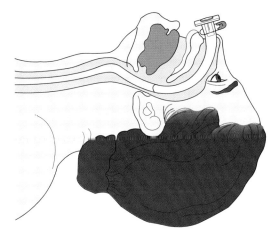

Fig. 5.12 Nasopharyngeal airways can be used in responsive and semiresponsive patients to maintain an open airway.

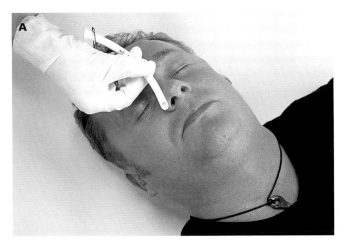

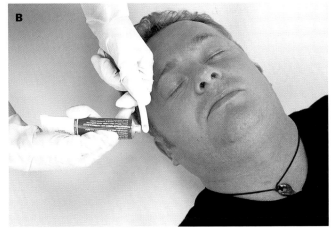

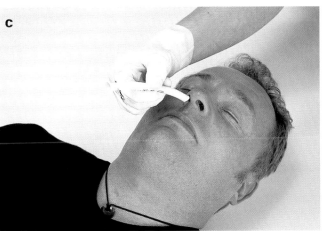

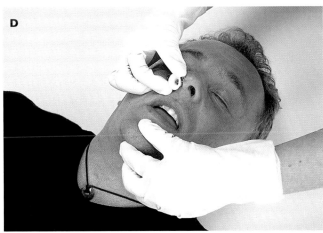

Fig. 5.13 Inserting a nasopharyngeal airway. Take universal precautions. **(a)** Select the properly sized airway by measuring from the tip of the patient's nose to the earlobe. Also consider the diameter of the patient's nostril when choosing a nasal airway. **(b)** Lubricate the airway with a water-soluble lubricant.

(c) Insert the airway into the patient's nostril with the bevel towards the base of the nostril or the nasal septum. Most nasal airways are designed to be inserted into the right nostril. **(d)** Advance the airway gently until the flange comes to rest at the patient's nostril. Ventilate the patient as needed.

Review Questions

The Respiratory System and Opening the Airway

1. What is the main muscle used in respiration?

2. Normal inhalation is a process initiated by _____ of the diaphragm, whereas exhalation is a process that occurs during _____ of the diaphragm.

3. Why is airway obstruction more common in infants and children?

   _____

4. What is the proper way to size an oral airway?

   _____

   _____

5. What is the proper way to size a nasal airway?

   _____

6. Place the following steps in order for inserting an oral airway in an adult:
   A. Advance the airway gently until you feel resistance.
   B. Select the properly sized airway.
   C. Ventilate the patient as needed.
   D. Follow universal precautions.
   E. Insert the airway upside down.
   F. Position yourself at the patient's side.
   G. Turn the airway 180 degrees so that it comes to rest with the flange on the patient's teeth.
   H. Open the patient's mouth by lifting the jaw and tongue.

1. The diaphragm; 2. Contraction; relaxation; 3. Because of the larger tongue and smaller airway structures; 4. The oropharyngeal airway is sized by measuring from the centre of the patient's mouth to the angle of the jaw; 5. The nasopharyngeal airway is sized by measuring the diameter of the patient's nostril; 6. D, B, F, H, E, A, G, C.

CLEARING THE COMPROMISED AIRWAY AND MAINTAINING AN OPEN AIRWAY

Threats to the airway are quickly fatal and therefore immediate action is required. There are three techniques that are used to clear and maintain the airway. The specifics of any situation dictate which of these techniques is most appropriate. These three techniques are not sequential; you will have to decide which is most appropriate and effective depending on the nature of the problem.

The recovery position

The recovery position is an important technique for maintaining an open airway in the unresponsive, uninjured patient who is breathing adequately. It uses patient positioning and gravity to prevent the tongue

First Responder Alert

BE AWARE that moving an injured patient into the recovery position may cause permanent spinal cord damage!

and foreign material from obstructing the airway. Placing the patient on his or her side allows fluids to drain from the mouth and prevents gravity from causing the base of the tongue to contact the back of the patient's throat. By placing the patient in the recovery position, obstructions are less likely to occur and the airway is more likely to remain open. The recovery position makes it easier to monitor the patient until additional EMS resources arrive and assume care.

A simple illustration of the effectiveness of the recovery position is the fact that most people will stop snoring if they lie on their side. Snoring is caused by the base of the tongue producing a partial obstruction to the airway. Lying on the side keeps the tongue out of the airway. **Figure 5.14** illustrates the technique for placing the patient in the recovery position.

Finger sweeps

Occasionally, solid or semi-solid objects (such as broken teeth, dentures, sweets, chewing gum or vomit) become lodged in the airway. If you see any of these objects when you inspect the airway, quickly remove them with a hooked gloved finger placed deeply into the mouth. Finger sweeps are generally more effective if the patient is on his or her side. An uninjured patient can quickly be placed on his or her side before you perform the finger sweep. If the patient is injured, you should perform the finger sweep while the patient remains in the position in which he or she was found.

Liquid or semi-liquids should be wiped out with the gloved index and middle fingers covered with a cloth. You should observe proper universal precautions since your hands will be exposed to the patient's body fluids. You should also make sure the patient is completely unresponsive so as to ensure that your fingers do not get bitten. The assessment of patient responsiveness is discussed in Chapter 6 ('Patient assessment').

Placing the fingers into the mouth of children can push the obstruction further into the airway or stimulate swelling. Never perform a finger sweep on infants or children unless you can see an obstruction. **Fig. 5.15** illustrates the technique for performing a finger sweep.

Suctioning

Fluids such as blood, vomit, mucus or saliva in the airway can obstruct the passage of air into the lungs. This fluid can also be inhaled into the lungs, causing damage to lung tissue. Suction should be used if the recovery position and finger sweeps are ineffective in draining fluid from the airway, or if the patient is injured and cannot be placed in the recovery position.

Suction devices are important emergency equipment and are often included as part of the equipment available for First Responders. If possible, have a portable suction device within reach whenever you are treating a patient. Hand- or foot-operated suction units have become very popular because of their lightweight, compact design, their reliability and their low cost (**Fig. 5.16**). Some portable suction devices are electric and have rechargeable battery systems (**Fig. 5.17**). Some suction units are capable of clearing small solid objects but are inadequate for removing larger solid objects

such as teeth, foreign bodies or food.

Portable electric suction units generate negative pressure by using a vacuum pump. The material that has been sucked out empties into a collection canister. With most devices a suction catheter is attached to the end of tubing before it is placed in the patient's mouth. A suction catheter is a flexible or rigid tip placed on the end of suction tubing that goes into the patient's mouth. Most suction catheters have a hole that must be covered with your finger during suctioning. If the material that you are suctioning is so thick that it clogs the suction catheter, use the tubing without a catheter attached. If there is a large volume of material that needs to be

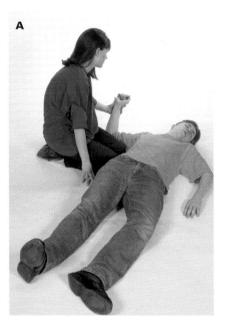
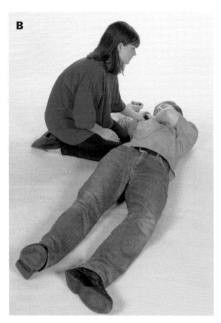
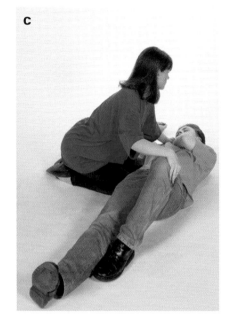

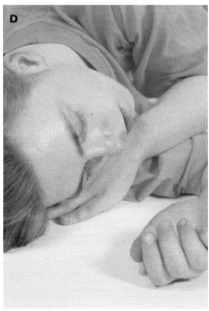
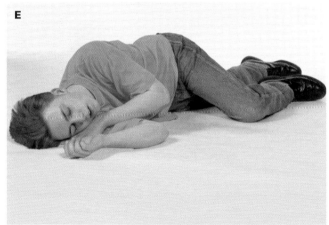

Fig. 5.14 Putting a patient into the recovery position. **(a)** Straighten the legs. Move the arm nearest to you out at right angles, with the elbow bent, and the palm facing upwards. **(b)** Bring the patient's other arm across the chest and hold the hand against their cheek with the palm facing outward. **(c)** With your other hand, get hold of the outside of the thigh furthest away from you. Pull the knee up, keeping the foot flat on the ground. Keeping the patient's hand pressed against their cheek, roll the patient towards you. Use your knees as support and to prevent the patient from turning too far forwards. **(d)** Tilt their head back to keep the airway open, adjusting the hand under the cheek if necessary. **(e)** Move the patient's upper leg so that hip and knee are at right angles. When the casualty is in the recovery position, check their breathing and pulse regularly while you wait for help to arrive.

The airway

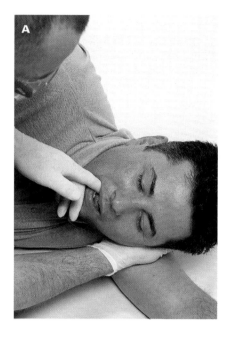 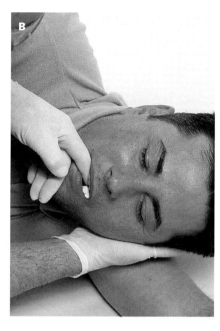

Fig. 5.15 Finger sweeps. Take universal precautions. If the patient is uninjured, turn him on his side and kneel in front of him. **(a)** Insert your index finger along the cheek, into the mouth. **(b)** Sweep your finger across the front of the tongue and attempt to hook out any foreign bodies.

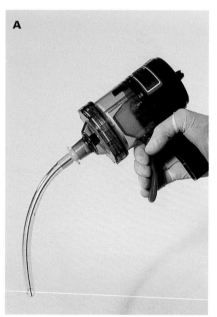 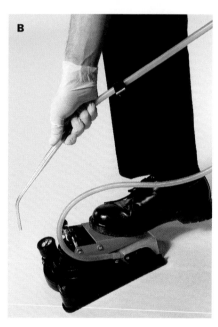

Fig. 5.16 **(a)** Hand-operated and **(b)** foot-operated portable suction units.

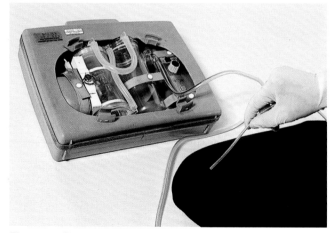

Fig. 5.17 Battery-operated portable suction unit.

First Responder Alert

Gurgling is the most common sign of liquid in the airway! If you hear gurgling:

1. Open the airway immediately.
2. If the patient is uninjured, place him or her in the recovery position.
3. If the patient is injured, suction the airway immediately.

cleared from the airway and the patient is uninjured, roll the patient on to his or side and continue suction.

There are a variety of suction catheters available, but the most appropriate ones for First Responders are rigid catheters, also called 'hard', 'tonsil-tip' and 'tonsil-sucker' catheters (**Fig. 5.18**). These hard plastic catheters are easy to control while being used. They are used to suction the mouth and oropharynx of unresponsive patients. The tip of the catheter should always remain visible when you insert it into the mouth. Never insert the catheter so far that the tip is out of sight or past the base of the tongue.

You are not able to both suction and ventilate a patient at the same time. In order to avoid depriving the patient of oxygen, be sure to limit the time of suctioning to 15 seconds for adults, 10 seconds for children, and 5 seconds for infants. Ventilate the patient between suction attempts.

The rigid catheter is used for infants and children. In younger patients, however, stimulation of the back of the throat can cause changes in the heart rate. If you use a rigid suction catheter, avoid touching the back of the airway to decrease the chances of slowing the heart rhythm. If you see a change in heart rate, stop suction and provide ventilation.

Principle 5.1 lists the key principles for using suction. **Figure 5.19** illustrates one technique for suctioning an adult with a portable electric suction unit.

A mucus extractor can be used to suction infants (**Fig. 5.20**). This simple device is effective for suctioning the nose and mouth of a newborn child and it can be used to suction an infant up to 3–4 months of age. This device is useful for clearing obstructions from the nasal passages because newborn babies and infants are not able to breathe voluntarily through their mouths. **Figure 5.21** illustrates the use of the mucus extractor.

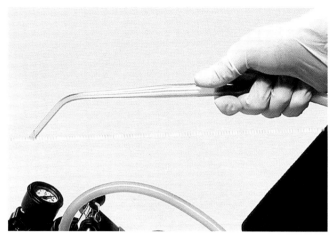

Fig. 5.18 The rigid suction catheter is the most versatile for use by First Responders.

Principle 5.1	**Principles of Suctioning**

1. Ensure the suction unit is working before use
2. Follow universal precautions
3. Use a rigid catheter
4. Do not insert the catheter further than the base of the tongue
5. Ensure that the patient does not become deprived of oxygen by limiting the time of suctioning to 15 seconds for adults, 10 seconds for children and 5 seconds for infants
6. Keep the catheter and tubing clean

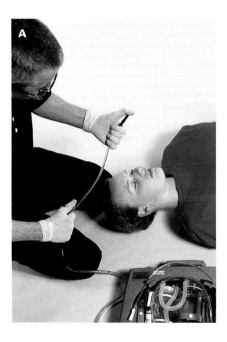

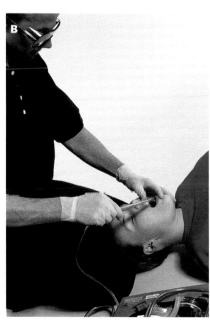

Fig. 5.19 Inspect the portable suction unit before use to ensure it is working and cleaned properly. Take universal precautions. Turn on the power. **(a)** You will hear the motor start. You should check to be sure that the suction is working by placing your thumb over the end of the suction tubing. Attach a rigid catheter to the end of the suction tubing. **(b)** Insert the catheter into the mouth without suction. To prevent the patient from becoming deprived of oxygen, never suction the adult for more than 15 seconds, a child for more than 10 seconds or an infant for more than 5 seconds. To prevent the suction catheter or tubing from becoming clogged, intermittently suction water to clear the lines.

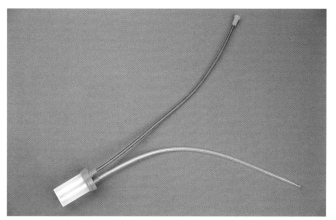

Fig. 5.20 A mucus extractor is an effective piece of equipment to clear the airway of newborns and infants.

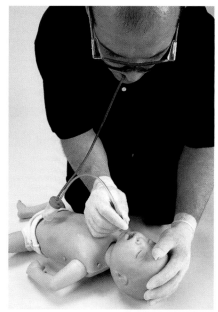

Fig. 5.21 How to use the mucus extractor.

ASSESSING BREATHING

Determine the presence of breathing

Determining if a responsive patient is breathing

Once you open the airway, the next priority is to assure that the patient is breathing. This is fairly simple in the responsive patient, because you can ask, "Can you breathe?" In order to talk, the patient must move air past the vocal cords. If the patient speaks to answer you, he or she must be able to move some air past the vocal cords. If the responsive patient is unable to speak, it is probably due to an airway obstruction. Later in this chapter you will learn how to manage the foreign body airway obstruction.

Determining if an unresponsive patient is breathing

Determining if an unresponsive patient is breathing is more of a challenge. Immediately after you open the airway, place your ear next to the patient's mouth and look at the chest (**Fig. 5.22**). Check to see if you can feel or hear any exhaled breath and watch the chest

for any rise and fall. Look, listen and feel for breathing for not more than 10 seconds

In some cases, you may see the chest rise and fall and yet feel no air moving through the mouth and nose. This is usually caused by an airway obstruction and must be managed promptly. In the first few minutes before or after a cardiac arrest, some patients have reflex gasping for air, called agonal respirations. This should not be confused with true breathing.

Determine the adequacy of breathing

Once it is determined that the patient is breathing, whether responsive or unresponsive, evaluate the effectiveness of the breathing. In order to breathe effectively, the patient must breathe at an adequate rate and depth. Normal breathing is effortless and causes the chest wall to rise and fall. In normal circumstances, the diaphragm is the major muscle of breathing. When breathing becomes laboured, the muscles of the neck and abdomen – the accessory muscles – are also used. Any use of these muscles is an indication of difficulty breathing.

The number of breaths in 1 minute is called the respiratory rate. **Box 5.1** lists the average respiratory rates for patients of different ages. Normal breathing should cause the chest to move. If the chest is not moving, or if it is moving very little, the breathing is too shallow to sustain life. **Box 5.2** lists the major signs and symptoms of inadequate breathing.

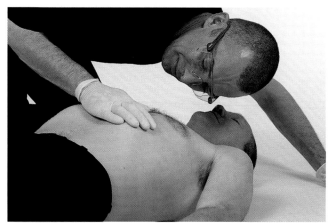

Fig. 5.22 To assess for the presence of breathing, look at the chest, listen for air movement and feel for exhalation of air against your cheek.

Box 5.1	**Normal Respiratory Rates**
Adults	12–20 breaths per minute
Children	15–30 breaths per minute
Infants	25–50 breaths per minute

Box 5.2	**Signs and Symptoms of Inadequate Breathing**

- A breathing rate that is too slow
  Less than 8/min in adults
  Less than 10/min in children
  Less than 20/min in infants
- Inadequate chest wall movements
- Increased effort of breathing
- Mental status changes
- Shallow breathing
- Bluish (cyanotic), pale, cool and clammy skin
- Gasping
- Grunting
- Slow heart rate with slow respiration

ARTIFICIAL VENTILATION

Previous sections in this chapter described how to maintain the patient's airway by positioning the head, neck and jaw, and how to keep the airway clear of obstructions. These airway management skills help keep the passageways open but do not deliver oxygen to the lungs. Once the airway has been assured and breathing is assessed, breathing for the patient may be necessary. The only oxygen that patients who are not breathing adequately have is the oxygen remaining in their lungs and bloodstream. Patients who are breathing inadequately, or who are not breathing at all, must be artificially ventilated in order to stay alive.

Techniques of artificial ventilation

There are three methods the First Responder can use to assist patients who are not breathing on their own. Each of these methods has advantages and disadvantages and they are not equally effective for all patients. The three techniques of artificial ventilation used by First Responders are:
1. Mouth-to-mask ventilation technique.
2. Mouth-to-barrier device ventilation technique.
3. Mouth-to-mouth ventilation technique.

Rate of artificial ventilation

Each of these techniques are discussed in detail, but there are some principles that apply to all methods of artificial ventilation. Whenever you artificially ventilate a patient, you are pushing air into his or her airway. This air goes both into the lungs and the stomach. The air that goes into the stomach becomes trapped and will eventually interfere with ventilation and cause the patient to vomit. In order to decrease the amount of air going to the stomach and increase the amount of air going to the lungs, deliver each ventilation slowly, during 2–4 seconds per breath for adult patients. Deliver ventilations to children or infants during 1–1.5 seconds.

Volume of air delivered in artificial ventilation

Each ventilation must deliver a proper volume of air to the patient. The average adult needs 400–500 ml of air per breath. Unfortunately, it is difficult to measure the exact volume of air you are delivering, so you should ventilate until you see the chest rise. During exhalation, you should be able to hear and feel air escape and observe the fall of the chest. Too large a volume will cause air to enter the stomach and should be avoided. Obviously, children and infants require less volume than adults.

Rate of artificial ventilation

You must also ventilate the patient at the proper rate. For adults, a good rule of thumb is that each time you feel a need to breathe, the patient needs to breathe also. This will result in a ventilation rate of approximately 10–12 breaths per minute. The younger patients are, the faster they need to breathe, so for children and infants you should ventilate 20–30 times per minute. Ventilate a newborn baby at a rate of 40 breaths per minute.

Principle 5.2 lists the key principles in ventilating a patient with any technique.

Mouth-to-mask ventilation technique

Mouth-to-mask ventilation is the preferred method for the First Responder to ventilate a non-breathing patient. It is a simple technique, and requires a minimal amount of equipment. Resuscitation masks are small,

The airway

inexpensive, and light. As a First Responder, you should always have a resuscitation mask available. They can easily fit into a first-aid kit or the glove compartment of a vehicle, and they can even be carried with you.

Mouth-to-mask ventilation is very effective because you use both hands to open the patient's airway and seal the mask to the face. Although there are a number of different makes of mask, most have similar features (**Fig. 5.23**).

Each mask has a flexible seal or gasket that creates an airtight seal with the patient's face. Resuscitation masks have an opening into which you exhale in order to breathe for the patient. You should select a mask that has a one-way valve to divert exhaled air or vomit away from the rescuer. Masks should be transparent so you can see any vomit or foreign material inside the mask and avoid blowing it into the patient's mouth. Many masks are designed to be reusable provided that they are cleaned after use.

Masks come in a variety of sizes and are designed to fit from the bridge of the nose to just below the bottom lip. If the mask is triangular, the apex of the triangle in placed towards the patient's nose. Selecting the appropriate mask size is very important, since air will leak around a mask that is too large or too small, resulting in inadequate ventilation.

Obtaining a proper seal with the patient's face is the most important part of mouth-to-mask ventilation. This can be particularly challenging in patients with facial hair or dentures or in casualties who have sustained facial trauma. Seal the mask by placing the heel and thumb of each hand along the border of the mask and compressing firmly around the margin. If there is any leakage of air when you ventilate, it will severely decrease the effectiveness of your ventilation. If you have difficulty obtaining a mask seal, lift the skin of the face up to the mask and continue ventilation. The technique of mouth-to-mask ventilation is illustrated in **Figure 5.24**.

Principle 5.2	**Principles of Artificial Ventilation**

1. Maintain an open airway
2. Use an oral or nasal airway if indicated
3. Ensure an airtight seal between the mask or barrier device and the patient's face
4. Prevent air from entering the stomach; ventilate slowly and only until the chest rises
5. Ventilate the patient with an age appropriate rate
6. Allow for complete, passive exhalation
7. Deliver the ventilation over 1.5–2 seconds for adults, 1–1.5 seconds for infants and children
8. If ventilation cannot be delivered, consider the possibility of airway obstruction
9. Turning the patient face down on the stretcher may be necessary
10. Cover the patient's mouth with a mask if he or she is biting or spitting
11. Reassess the patient frequently
12. Document all of your actions

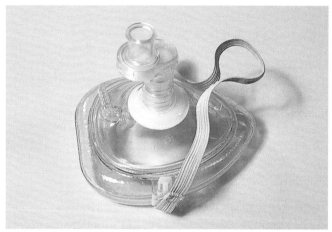

Fig. 5.23 Resuscitation mask.

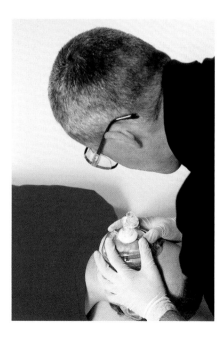
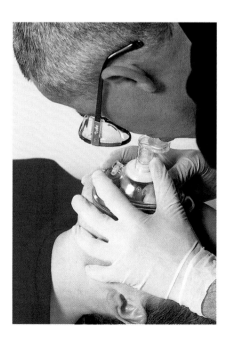

Fig. 5.24 Mouth-to-mask ventilation. Follow universal precautions. **(a)** Connect the one-way valve to the mask, if it is not already attached. Open the airway by the head-tilt, chin-lift (if no trauma is suspected) and inserting an oral or nasal airway. From a position at the top of the patient's head, place the mask on the patient. **(b)** Seal the mask to the patient's face with the heel and thumb of each hand. Place the other fingers along the bony margin of the jaw and lift the jaw while performing a head-tilt. Take a normal breath, seal your lips over the ventilation port and exhale slowly for 1.5 to 2 seconds for adult patients, and 1 to 1.5 seconds for infants or children. Stop ventilating when the patient's chest rises. Allow the patient to passively exhale between breaths. Ventilate the adult patient once every 5 seconds and infants and children once every 3 seconds.

Some manufacturers make masks that are specially designed for use on infants and children. To work effectively, the mask should fit properly. You should size the mask from the bridge of the nose to just below the bottom lip. A mask that is too large will result in inadequate ventilation, primarily because of leakage of air around the mask. If you cannot ventilate the patient, you should reposition the head, check the mask seal and consider the possibility of a foreign body airway obstruction.

Mouth-to-barrier device ventilation technique

The main advantage of barrier devices over mouth-to-mask ventilation is the size of the devices. Barrier devices are even smaller and lighter than masks. They are typically disposable and less expensive than masks. As a First Responder, you should never be in a position in which you do not have immediate access to either a mask or a barrier device. Although some rescuers prefer using a barrier device to a mask, the mask has been demonstrated to be more effective for most patients.

There are many designs of barrier devices (**Fig. 5.25**). Unfortunately, manufacturers are not required to test these products rigorously. You should fully evaluate the effectiveness of each type. Whichever device you choose, make certain it has a low resistance during ventilation. Most barrier devices do not have exhalation valves and tend to leak around the shield. With practice, you can overcome some of these limitations and use a barrier device to ventilate most patients effectively. **Figure 5.26** illustrates the technique for ventilating a patient with a barrier device.

Most barrier devices are designed for use on adult patients. Unless specifically designed and sized for paediatric patients, barrier devices should not be used when ventilating infants or children.

Mouth-to-mouth ventilation technique

Mouth-to-mouth ventilation is a quick, effective method of delivering oxygen to the non-breathing patient that does not require any equipment. Mouth-to-mouth ventilation uses the rescuer's exhaled air for ventilation. The rescuer's exhaled air contains enough oxygen to support the patient.

The decision of whether or not to perform mouth-to-mouth ventilation is a personal one, and it must be made with the understanding of the implications of your decision. Mouth-to-mouth ventilation requires direct physical contact with the patient and can place the rescuer at risk of contracting an infectious disease.

In practice, there are situations when you may want to ventilate a patient but do not have a mask or barrier device available. This should not occur in any situation in which you are functioning as a First Responder, but it may occur if you ever have to ventilate a friend or family member. For that reason, it is very important that you practice and maintain proficiency in mouth-to-

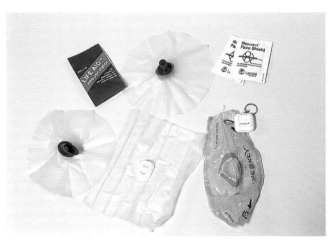

Fig. 5.25 Barrier devices.

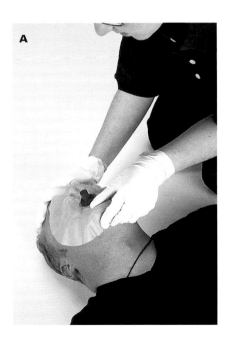
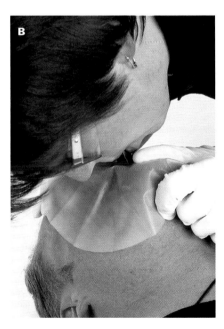

Fig. 5.26 Mouth-to-barrier device ventilation. Follow universal precautions. **(a)** Open the patient's airway with the head-tilt, chin-lift (if no trauma is suspected) and place the barrier device over the patient's face. **(b)** Pinch the patient's nose, take a normal breath, seal your lips to the barrier device and exhale slowly and constantly for 1.5 to 2 seconds. Stop ventilation when the patient's chest rises. Allow the patient to passively exhale between breaths.

mouth ventilation. **Figure 5.27** illustrates the technique for mouth-to-mouth ventilation.

Special considerations for trauma patients

Unresponsive trauma patients present a considerable challenge in airway management – there is the possibility of bleeding into the airway, and some casualties will have facial trauma. In addition, spinal injuries require special care. All techniques of ventilation have to be modified so that the head is not tilted. This is accomplished by using the jaw thrust manoeuvre without head-tilt with each ventilation technique. This can be difficult and tiring, so you should practice these skills often. These modifications are described in **Figure 5.28**.

Assessing the effectiveness of artificial ventilation

Whenever you ventilate a patient, it is very important to assess the adequacy of the artificial ventilation. Regardless of the technique, you must continually evaluate the effectiveness of the ventilation. This is accomplished mainly by watching the rise and fall of the chest, and by hearing and feeling the escape of air from the mouth and nose during exhalation. **Boxes 5.3** and **5.4** list some of the signs of adequate and inadequate ventilation.

There are a number of reasons why the chest may rise and fall inadequately. Poor ventilation most commonly results from improper opening of the airway. If you are having difficulty ventilating, the first corrective action is to reposition the airway. **Box 5.5** describes

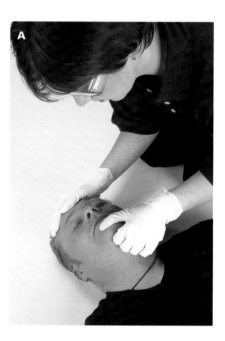
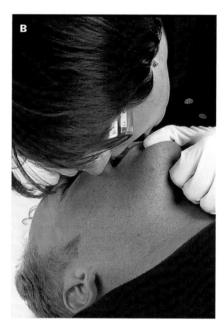

Fig. 5.27 Mouth-to-mouth ventilation. **(a)** Open the patient's airway with the the head-tilt, chin-lift (if no trauma is suspected). **(b)** Pinch the patient's nose, take a normal breath, seal your lips to the patient's lips and exhale slowly and constantly for 1.5 to 2 seconds for adult patients, or 1 to 1.5 seconds for infants and children. When ventilating an infant, seal your lips around the infant's mouth and nose. Stop ventilation when the patient's chest rises. Allow the patient to passively exhale between breaths.

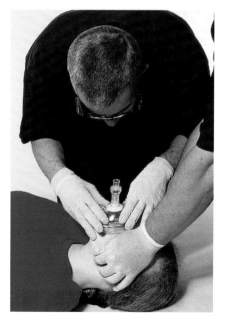

Fig. 5.28 For injured patients, all ventilation techniques are modified to open the airway with the jaw thrust without head-tilt. If at all possible, you should use two rescuers – one to open and maintain the airway and the other to ventilate.

Box 5.3	**Signs of Adequate Ventilation**

- The chest rises and falls with each artificial ventilation
- The patient is being ventilated at least 12 times per minute for adults, or 20 times per minute for infants and children
- The adult patient is ventilated over a period of 1.5 to 2 seconds; infants and children over 1 to 1.5 seconds

Box 5.4	**Signs of Inadequate Ventilation**

- The chest fails to rise and fall with each ventilation
- No air is felt or heard escaping during exhalation
- The rate is either too fast or too slow
- The abdomen is getting larger

Box 5.5	Correcting Poor Chest Rise During Ventilation	
Step	**Rationale**	
Reposition the jaw	An improperly opened airway is the most common cause of poor chest rise	
Check the mask or barrier seal	Poor seal with the face is the next most common cause of poor chest rise; you can generally hear air leaking through the sides of the mask or barrier device	
Check for an obstruction	Foreign body airway obstructions (FBAO) may cause poor ventilation. You may need to perform the age-appropriate FBAO manoeuvre or suction the patient	

other corrective actions to consider if repositioning the jaw fails to correct the situation. Always consider the possibility of a foreign body airway obstruction.

SPECIAL SITUATIONS IN AIRWAY MANAGEMENT

Patients with laryngectomies

A laryngectomy is a surgical procedure in which the voice box is removed, usually because of throat cancer. After a laryngectomy, the patient may have a tracheal stoma, which is a permanent artificial opening into the trachea (**Fig. 5.29**).

If a patient with a tracheal stoma must be ventilated, you can seal the resuscitation mask to the neck directly over the stoma. You can also ventilate by sealing your mouth around the stoma, but the use of a barrier device is preferred. Ventilate slowly, allowing time for the chest to rise and for the patient to exhale passively. Because you are more directly ventilating the lungs than when performing artificial ventilation in the usual way, the head and neck do not need to be specially positioned. If air escapes from the mouth and nose when you ventilate a patient with a stoma, close the patient's mouth and pinch the nose shut.

First Responder Alert

Evaluate the effectiveness of ventilation primarily by:

1. Observing the rise and fall of the chest.
2. Hearing and feeling the air escape during exhalation.

Review Questions

Artificial Ventilation

1. When ventilating the adult, the inspiratory time should be _____ – _____ seconds.

2. What is the primary way to assess adequate ventilation?

    _____

3. List two signs of inadequate ventilation.

    _____

    _____

4. Place the corrective actions for ventilation in order:
    A. Check the mask or barrier seal
    B. Check for an obstruction
    C. Reposition the jaw

5. What changes should you make when ventilating an injured patient?
    A. Use the head-tilt only
    B. Use only a barrier device
    C. Mouth-to-mouth ventilation cannot be used
    D. Open the airway without tilting the head

1. 1.5–2; 2. observing the rise and fall of the chest; 3. The chest fails to rise and fall with each ventilation, no air is heard or felt escaping during exhalation, the rate is either too fast or too slow, the abdomen is getting larger; 4. C, A, B; 5. D

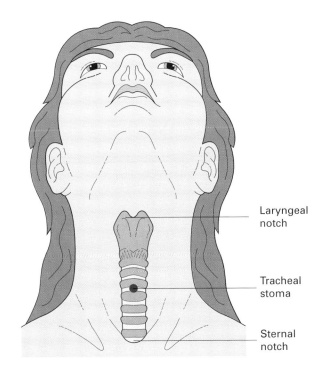

Laryngeal notch

Tracheal stoma

Sternal notch

Fig. 5.29 A tracheal stoma is a permanent artificial opening into the trachea.

Ventilating infants and children

Respiratory emergencies are quite common in children, and you need to be able to ventilate paediatric patients artificially. Because the airway is more pliable in children, you must pay particular attention to the position of the head. Infants should be ventilated without flexing or tilting the head. Since infants have a large head in comparison to the rest of their body, placing them on a flat surface causes their head to flex forwards. You may need to place your hand or a towel under their shoulders to keep the airway open. Children may need to have their head slightly tilted. Avoid tilting the head back too far in children or infants. Ventilate infants and children once every 2–3 seconds.

Gastric distension

Excessive pressure when ventilating the patient causes gastric distension by forcing air into the stomach. This severely compromises the effectiveness of ventilation and increases the possibility of the patient vomiting. Gastric distension is more common in infants and children than in adults. Gastric distension can be reduced by ensuring a patent airway and by reducing the volume of air used to ventilate the patient to that needed to be able to see the chest rise. You can use an oral or nasal airway to assist in maintaining an open airway.

Facial trauma

Facial trauma can pose considerable difficulty for managing the airway and ventilating trauma patients (**Fig. 5.30**). The head and face have a rich blood supply and injuries to the face cause significant bleeding and swelling.

Be prepared to use suction and positioning (jaw thrust without head-tilt) to keep the airway clear of blood and vomit. Use an oral or nasal airway to help maximise the airway without tilting the head. Extreme care should be exercised when using a nasal airway in patients with facial trauma because if there is significant injury to the bones of the skull it is possible to insert the airway directly into the brain.

Consider different patient positioning (for example, sitting the patient up, leaning the patient forward, or the prone position with head and face down). If you still cannot open the airway in a trauma patient and all else has failed, you must tilt the head back to ventilate the patient. Although moving the neck may cause spinal cord injury, if you do not open the airway, the patient will die.

Dental appliances

Dentures and partial dentures can create a problem for managing the airway. If at all possible, attempt to keep well-fitting dentures in place when ventilating a patient. They add form and structure to the mouth and make it easier to obtain a seal around the mask. If dentures become dislodged and make it difficult to ventilate the patient, remove them immediately.

FOREIGN BODY AIRWAY OBSTRUCTION (FBAO)

In most cases, obstruction to the airway is caused by the tongue of an unresponsive patient contacting the back of the throat. In some situations, foreign objects (such as food, gum, vomit, broken teeth, loose dentures or blood) can get into the airway and make ventilation difficult or impossible. In these cases, the foreign object must be removed from the airway if the patient is to survive. Trauma to the neck or swelling can also cause an airway obstruction. Airway obstructions can cause cardiac arrest, or they can follow a cardiac arrest if the patient has vomited or there are dentures that have slipped out of place.

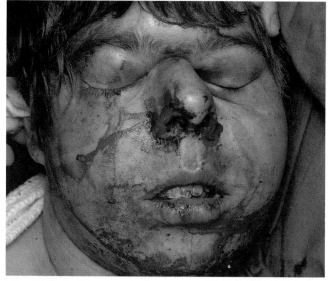

Fig. 5.30 Facial trauma can pose considerable difficulty for managing the airway and ventilating trauma patients.

The management of airway obstruction varies according to the degree of obstruction, the patient's age and whether or not the patient is responsive.

FBAO in the responsive patient

Foreign bodies that become stuck in the airway of a responsive adult are usually caused by a combination of eating too quickly, chewing incompletely, talking while eating and alcohol consumption. Typically, a piece of food that is too large to swallow becomes lodged in the back of the throat. In the responsive patient, there are three classifications of foreign body airway obstructions:
* partial FBAO with good air exchange;
* partial FBAO with poor air exchange; and
* complete FBAO.

You must be able to determine quickly the classification of airway obstruction in the responsive patient, because the management of each is different.

Partial FBAO with good air exchange

If the obstruction is small it will interfere with breathing, but the patient may still be able to get enough oxygen to remain responsive. This is called an airway obstruction with good air exchange. Such a patient will remain responsive and alert and may be able to speak and to cough forcefully. You may hear a high-pitched sound, called a wheeze, during breathing or between coughs.

Patients with airway obstruction and good air exchange will be very anxious. This creates an increase in the demand for oxygen and can cause the patient to lose responsiveness. As a First Responder, calm the patient and encourage him or her to cough forcefully. This may clear the obstruction. If you perform any additional interventions, you can worsen a partial airway obstruction. However, you should attempt to resolve an airway obstruction when the partial obstruction results in poor air exchange and in cases of complete airway obstruction.

Partial FBAO with poor air exchange

If the obstruction is large enough, it will be very difficult for the patient to breathe. These patients may have a weak, ineffective cough accompanied with a high-pitched noise on inhalation. Typically, these patients have extreme respiratory difficulty and their skin may have a blue tint.

First Responder Alert

Foreign body airway obstructions are common enough in restaurants to have been given the name 'café coronary'. Whenever you respond to an unresponsive patient or cardiac arrest in a restaurant, think of the possibility of airway obstruction.

Complete FBAO

Larger obstructions can prevent any air from being exchanged in the lungs. These patients will typically be unresponsive by the time the First Responder arrives, but you may witness a complete airway obstruction if you are with someone who chokes in front of you. The patient may clutch the neck with the thumb and fingers. This is an instinctive survival behaviour and is often referred to as the 'universal distress signal' (**Fig. 5.31**). With a complete airway obstruction, the patient will not be able to speak, breathe or cough. Death will follow quickly if prompt action is not taken.

FBAO in the adult patient

The responsive adult with FBAO

The only time you will attempt to relieve an obstruction in a responsive patient is when there is a partial obstruction with poor air exchange or a complete obstruction. Do not attempt any of these procedures on a patient with an obstruction and good air exchange, because of the possibility of making the obstruction worse. Typically, the patient with FBAO will have lost responsiveness by the time the First Responder arrives. The most common situation in which you would need to use these skills is if a friend or family member chokes in your presence.

If the patient is still responsive, you should first confirm that he or she has a complete or partial airway obstruction with poor air exchange. You should first ask the patient, "Are you choking?" If the patient can answer verbally, there is enough air exchange to stay responsive and you should encourage forceful coughing to try to dislodge the foreign body. If the patient cannot speak or can only make a high-pitched squeaking noise, you must act quickly.

The technique for relieving an obstruction in the responsive adult patient is abdominal thrusts. This technique is also known as the 'Heimlich manoeuvre', after its inventor. Abdominal thrusts are very effective because they forcefully raise the pressure in the thoracic cavity and can propel the foreign object out of the airway. To perform abdominal thrusts, approach the patient from behind. Inform the patient that you are

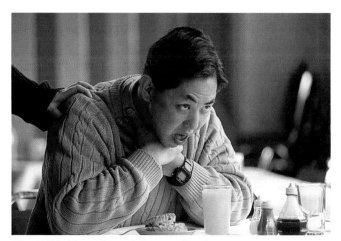

Fig. 5.31 The universal distress signal.

The airway

going to help, and have him or her relax as much as possible. Place the thumb side of the fist slightly above the navel and then grab your fist with your other hand. Quickly and sharply pull your hands towards you in an inwards and upwards fashion (**Fig. 5.32**).

Repeat the abdominal thrusts until the obstruction is relieved or the patient loses responsiveness. If the obstruction is relieved, it is usually with a dramatic exhalation and immediate relief. If the obstruction is not relieved, the patient will lose responsiveness and you should assist him to the floor and initiate the procedure for clearing an obstruction in an unresponsive patient.

The unresponsive adult with FBAO

The procedures for dealing with an FBAO in the unresponsive adult combines the use of abdominal thrusts, finger sweeps and ventilation attempts. In combination, these three techniques are very effective at relieving an obstruction. You may encounter an unresponsive patient with an obstruction as a First Responder, especially when responding to calls from restaurants and nursing homes.

In most cases, you will not realise that the patient has an obstruction until you attempt to ventilate. If the patient has an obstruction, you will meet resistance as you attempt to ventilate. Your first action should be to check to be sure you have properly opened the patient's airway. Perform the head-tilt, chin-lift manoeuvre again to be sure that the airway is open, and then attempt another ventilation. If you are still experiencing resistance, check the seal of the mask or barrier device you are using. If you are still unable to ventilate the patient, you should proceed to abdominal thrusts.

Straddle the patient and place the heel of one hand slightly above the navel, well below the xiphoid process. Place your other hand on top of the first and interlock your fingers. Be sure that your hands are clear

of the rib cage and quickly and sharply thrust inward and upwards. Just as in the responsive patient, you are attempting to push the diaphragm up and force air into the lungs to dislodge the object. **Fig. 5.33** illustrates the technique for performing abdominal thrusts in an unresponsive adult.

After the abdominal thrusts, perform a finger sweep to attempt to remove the object. To perform a finger sweep, kneel next to the patient's shoulders, and turn the head towards you. Place your gloved index finger into the patient's mouth, along the cheek. Insert your finger into the throat and attempt to dislodge any foreign objects you can feel (see **Fig. 5.15**).

After the finger sweep, attempt to ventilate the patient. It is possible that the abdominal thrusts and finger sweep will have dislodged the object from the airway and you may now be able to ventilate the patient. If ventilation is still unsuccessful, repeat the sequence of abdominal thrusts, finger sweeps and ventilations until the ambulance service arrives. If the ventilation is successful, ventilate the adult patient once every 5 seconds.

Abdominal thrusts are not performed on pregnant patients owing to the possibility of injuring the developing baby. In some cases, a patient may be so obese that you cannot get your arms around him or her. In either of these cases, you should perform chest thrusts instead of abdominal thrusts. To perform chest thrusts on responsive patients, approach them from behind, place the flat surface of your fist on the middle of the breastbone and pull sharply inward. Kneel beside unresponsive patients and place the heel of one hand in the middle of the breastbone, being sure to avoid the ribs and the xiphoid process. Place your other hand on top of the first and interlock your fingers. Lock your elbows and sharply push down 3.5–5 cm. Perform finger sweeps and ventilate as previously described.

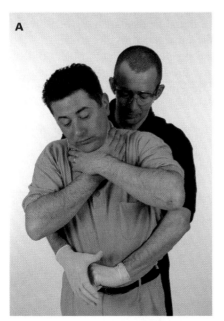 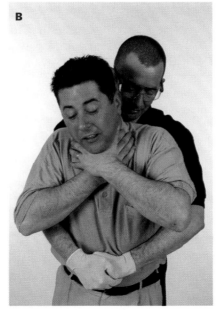 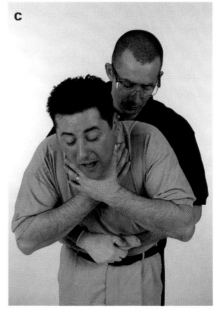

Fig. 5.32 The Heimlich manouevre. Ask the patient "Are you choking?" Inform him that you are going to help. **(a)** Approach the patient from behind and locate the belly button. Place the thumb side of the fist just above the belly button, well below the xiphoid process. **(b)** Grasp your fist with your other hand. **(c)** Pull inwards and upwards in discrete sharp blows. Repeat until the object is released or the patient loses responsiveness.

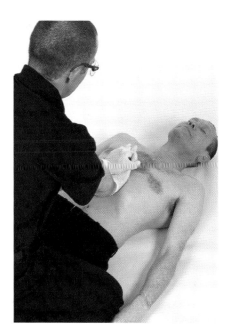

Fig 5.33 Abdominal thrusts in the unresponsive adult. Straddle the patient's thighs. Place the heel of one hand just above the belly button and well below the xiphoid process, place your other hand on top of the first and interlock your fingers. Thrust your body weight forwards in sharp, discrete blows five times.

FBAO in infants

Since infants are small enough to hold upside down, gravity can be used to help relieve an obstruction. Additionally, the abdominal organs are still developing in infants and could be damaged by abdominal thrusts. Therefore, chest thrusts are used.

The responsive infant with FBAO – If the infant has a partial FBAO with poor air exchange or a complete FBAO, a combination of chest thrusts and back blows is used. Immediately hold the infant face down with his head lower than his chest. Support the infant on your thigh and use the heel of your other hand to deliver five back blows between the shoulder blades (**Fig. 5.34**).

If the obstruction is not relieved, place two fingers on the breastbone, one finger's breadth below the nipple line. Sharply depress the breastbone five times by approximately 2 cm each time (**Fig. 5.35**). Repeat this sequence of five back blows and five chest thrusts until the obstruction is removed, or the infant loses responsiveness.

FBAO in infants and children

Anybody who has ever spent time around children knows that they have a tendency to place objects in their mouths. More than 90% of childhood deaths from foreign body airway obstruction are in children below the age of 5 years, and 65% of these deaths are in infants. Airway obstructions in children are often caused by objects that are not supposed to be eaten, such as toys, balloons, coins and other small objects that may be lying around.

When children are progressing from baby food to solid food, they are prone to airway obstruction from incomplete chewing. Foods such as hot dogs, sweets, nuts and grapes are common causes of FBAO. Airway obstruction should be suspected in any infant or child who suddenly demonstrates respiratory difficulty with a cough, gagging, stridor or wheezing.

Just as in adults, in children you should attempt to clear only a partial FBAO with poor air exchange or a complete FBAO. The procedure for clearing an obstruction is slightly different for infants and children from the procedure for adults. Also remember that airway obstructions in paediatric patients can be due to swelling of the airway caused by infection. Since stimulation of the throat with your finger could make this situation worse, blind finger sweeps are never performed on infants or children. You should only perform fingers sweeps in infants and children if you can see the foreign object that is causing the obstruction.

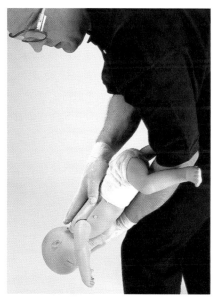

Fig. 5.34 Back blows for FBAO management in the infant. Hold the patient face down with the head lower than the chest, supported on your thigh. Perform firm back blows with the heel of your hand to the area just below the shoulder blades five times.

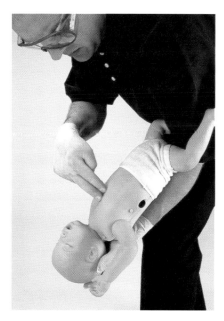

Fig. 5.35 Chest thrusts for FBAO management in the infant. Hold the patient face up with the head lower than the chest, supported on your thigh. Place two fingers on the breastbone, one finger-breadth below the nipples. Depress the breastbone 1 to 2 cm five times.

First Responder Alert

Never perform blind finger sweeps on infants or children. Remove objects from the mouth using finger sweeps only if the object can be seen.

The airway

The unresponsive infant with FBAO – Once again, you will generally not realise that your patient has an airway obstruction until you attempt ventilation after confirming that there is no breathing. If you meet resistance during your initial ventilation, reposition the airway to ensure it is open. If you are not able to ventilate, perform five back blows and five chest thrusts. After the five chest thrusts, look into the airway for any obstructions. If you see the object that is occluding the airway, perform a finger sweep to remove it. If not, attempt to ventilate. Give five rescue breaths lasting 1–1.5 seconds each. Repeat the sequence of back blows, chest thrusts and inspection of the airway. Continue to ventilate until the ambulance service arrives.

FBAO in children

Children are too large to be held upside down, so back blows and chest thrusts cannot be easily performed. Children with airway obstructions are managed in almost the same manner as adults, with cycles of chest thrusts and abdominal thrusts (**Fig. 5.36**).

The responsive child with FBAO – Children with complete or partial obstructions with poor air exchange are managed like adults. Use the upright position in the conscious child. Administer five back blows to the middle of the back between the shoulder blades. You must ensure that the head is lower than the chest. If these back blows are unsuccessful in relieving the airway obstruction, then proceed to five chest thrusts. These are carried out sharply and vigorously to a depth of approximately 3 cm with the heel of one hand placed two fingers' breadth above the xiphisternum. Then check the mouth and remove any visible foreign bodies. Open the airway and reassess air entry. If there is no breathing, provide five rescue breaths.

After the second round of back blows, proceed to five abdominal thrusts. Approach the patient from behind and place the thumb side of the fist slightly above the navel and well below the xiphoid process. Grab your wrist with your other hand and sharply pull inwards until the obstruction is relieved or the patient loses responsiveness.

The unresponsive child with FBAO – Lie the unconscious patient supine, preferably with the head lower than the chest. Once you have determined that the patient has an obstruction, reposition the airway and attempt to ventilate. Follow the same sequence of actions as for the responsive child with FBAO. If you are still unsuccessful after five chest thrusts, straddle the patient's thighs and place the heel of one hand slightly above the navel and well below the xiphoid process. Push quickly inwards and upwards towards the diaphragm five times. Look into the mouth for any foreign objects. If you see the object causing the obstruction, perform a finger sweep to remove it. Ventilate and repeat the sequence of back blows, chest or abdominal thrusts in alternate cycles, inspecting the airway and providing ventilation until the ambulance service arrives.

Responsive to unresponsive FBAO management

If you are attempting to relieve an obstruction in a responsive patient who loses responsiveness during treatment, lower the patient gently to the floor. Whether the patient is an adult, a child or an infant, the first step is to open the airway manually with the head-tilt, chin-lift manoeuvre. Since you know that the patient is not breathing, you should immediately attempt to ventilate. If you are unable to ventilate, go directly to the appropriate technique: abdominal thrusts, chest thrust, or back blows. From this point, the sequence is exactly the same.

CHAPTER SUMMARY
The respiratory system

The respiratory system maintains the delicate balance of oxygen and carbon dioxide in the body. The airway consists of the passageways from the mouth and nose to the lungs. Airway structures include the nose, nasopharynx, mouth, oropharynx, epiglottis, windpipe

---

First Responder Alert

If you know that the patient has an airway obstruction, do not waste time checking for breathing or repositioning the airway. Go directly to the appropriate technique after attempting to ventilate.

Review Questions

Foreign Body Airway Obstruction (FBAO)

1. The most common cause of airway obstruction in the unresponsive adult is the _____.

2. First Responders should not use abdominal thrusts to attempt to relieve an FBAO for an adult patient with good air exchange. True or false?

3. To relieve an obstruction in the unresponsive adult patient, the First Responder should perform _____ abdominal thrusts, then perform a _____ _____, and then attempt to ventilate.

4. When attempting to clear the airway of a responsive infant with a complete obstruction, perform 5 _____ _____ followed by 5 _____ _____.

1. Tongue; 2. True; 3. 5, finger sweep; 4. Back blows, chest thrusts

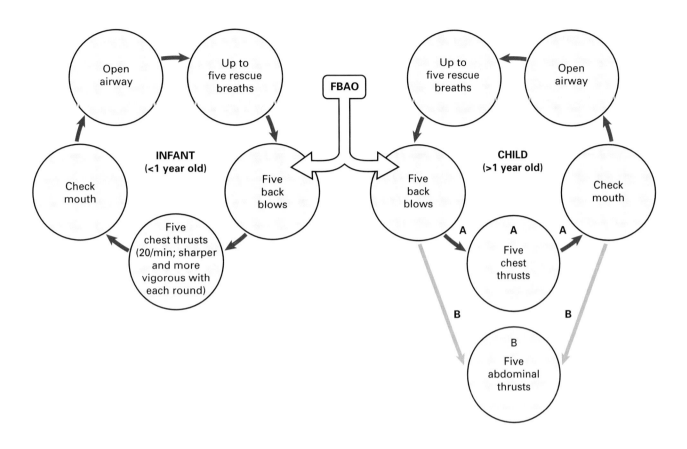

Fig. 5.36 Flow chart illustrating the technique for FBAO (foreign body airway obstruction) management in the child and infant. (Derived from Zideman D, *et al.* Guidelines for Paediatric Life Support. *Resuscitation* 1994; **27**:91–105.)

(trachea), voice box (larynx), lungs and diaphragm. Air is moved in and out of the lungs by the contraction and relaxation of the diaphragm.

Opening the airway

Ensuring an open airway is the most important patient care role of the First Responder. Many circumstances can prevent the free passage of air from the mouth to the lungs. In an unresponsive patient, the base of the tongue resting against the back of the throat can cause an airway obstruction. The head-tilt, chin-lift manoeuvre is a simple airway technique that should be performed immediately on any unresponsive, uninjured patient. The jaw thrust without head tilt should be used on casualties who have suffered trauma. Nasal and oral airway devices are very useful in helping to maintain the airway.

Clearing the compromised airway and maintaining an open airway

The primary method of keeping the uninjured patient's airway open is placing the patient in the recovery position. This position keeps the tongue away from the back of the throat and allows fluids to drain from the airway. Foreign bodies (such as teeth, gum and dentures) can create airway problems. They can usually be cleared with finger sweeps. Fluid (such as blood, saliva and vomit) should be suctioned from the airway immediately.

Assessing breathing

Once you have opened the airway, you should determine if the patient is breathing. If the patient is breathing, you must then assess the adequacy of breathing. Normal breathing causes the chest to rise and fall, and the patient must be breathing at an adequate rate and depth for breathing to be adequate.

Artificial ventilation

Once the airway has been opened, the next priority in patient management is artificial ventilation. First Responders use one of three methods for providing artificial ventilation. Mouth-to-mask ventilations are the preferred method of ventilating a patient. In this technique, the First Responder seals the mask to the patient's face with both hands and exhales into the mask until the chest rises. The next option is to use the

The airway

mouth-to-barrier technique, in which the First Responder exhales through a barrier device into the patient's mouth. The third method of ventilating a non-breathing patient is the mouth-to-mouth technique. Although this technique does not require additional equipment, it subjects the First Responder to the risk of infectious diseases.

Special situations in airway management

Special situations present challenges when managing the airway and ventilating certain patients. Patients with stomas can generally be ventilated directly through the stoma. The airways of infants and children are easily compromised by head position, swelling or fluid. Facial injuries can cause considerable bleeding and swelling.

If they are a good fit, dental appliances should be kept in place during artificial ventilation.

Foreign body airway obstruction

Foreign body airway obstruction (FBAO) is particularly common in infants and children, but they are an immediate threat to life in patients of any age. Responsive patients with airway obstruction and good air exchange should be encouraged to cough forcefully to dislodge the object. Responsive patients with an obstruction and poor or no air exchange should be managed immediately. Depending on the age of the patient, a combination of back blows, chest thrusts and abdominal thrusts may be used to relieve an airway obstruction.

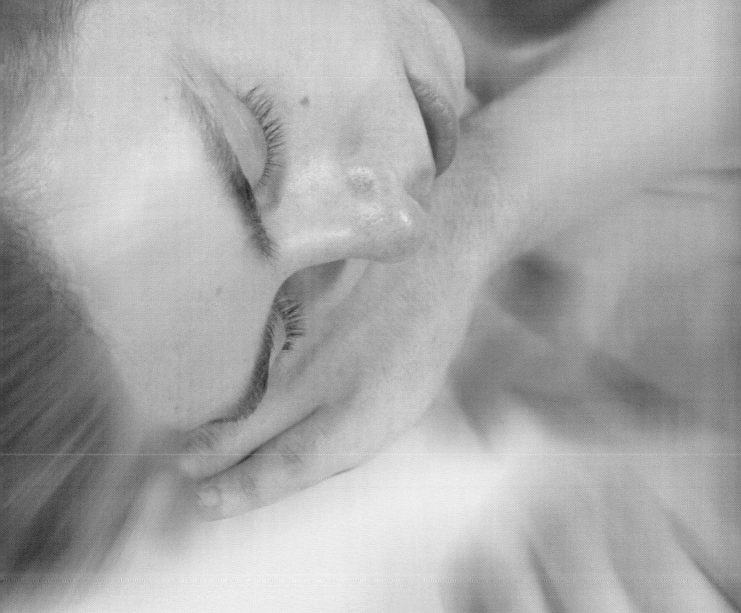

Division Three:
Patient Assessment

Chapter Six

Patient Assessment

I. **Scene assessment**
   A. Universal precautions
   B. Scene safety
   C. Nature of illness and mechanism of injury
   D. High-speed deceleration injuries
   E. Number of patients and need for additional help

II. **Triage**
   A. Triage sieve

III. **Primary assessment**
   A. General impression of the patient
   B. Assess responsiveness
   C. Assess the airway

D. Assess breathing
E. Assess circulation
F. Report to responding ambulance crews

IV. **First Responder physical examination**
   A. Performing a physical examination
   B. Medical patients and patients with no significant injury or mechanism of injury

V. **Patient history**
   A. The AMPLE history

VI. **Secondary assessment**

Key terms

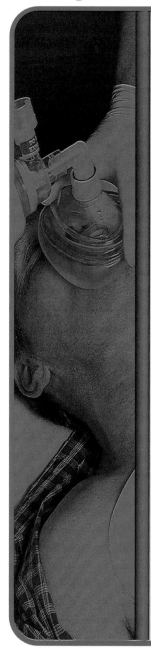

AcBC A mnemonic for the initial protocol to be adopted by the First Responder when performing the primary assessment; it stands for 'Airway with cervical spinal control, Breathing and Circulation'.

AMPLE history
A mnemonic used in the secondary assessment; it stands for the history of allergies, medications, pertinent history, last oral intake and events leading to illness or injury.

Casualty
A term used to describe a person requiring treatment, specifically as a result of trauma.

Chief complaint
The patient's description of the medical problem.

DOTS An acronym for the information that is identified when the First Responder performs the secondary assessment; it stands for deformities, open injuries, tenderness and swelling.

First Responder physical examination
A hands-on evaluation performed by the First Responder to obtain information about the illness or injury.

General impression
The First Responder's immediate assessment of the environment and the patient's chief complaint, accomplished in the first few seconds of contact with the patient.

Mechanism of injury
The event or force that caused the casualty's wounds.

Nature of illness
The event or condition leading to the patient's medical complaint.

Patient
A general term used to describe a person requiring treatment.

Primary assessment
The first step in the evaluation of every medical patient and trauma casualty used to identify immediate threats to life.

Scene assessment
The evaluation of the entire environment for safety, the mechanism of injury or the nature of illness, the number of casualties and the need for additional help.

Secondary assessment
The final step in the process of assessing the patient; it involves repeating the primary assessment and then continues until patient care is transferred to the arriving EMS personnel.

Objectives

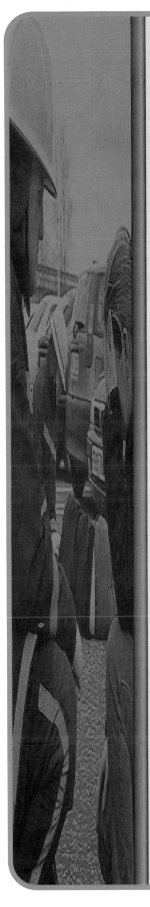

On completion of this chapter you will be able to meet the following objectives:

Cognitive objectives

1. Discuss the components of scene assessment.
2. Describe common hazards found at the scene of a trauma incident.
3. Determine if it is safe to enter the scene.
4. Discuss common mechanisms of injury and nature of illness.
5. Discuss the reason for identifying the total number of patients at the scene.
6. Explain the reason for identifying the need for additional help or assistance.
7. Summarise the reasons for forming a general impression of the patient.
8. Differentiate between a patient with adequate and inadequate breathing.
9. Describe the methods used to assess circulation.
10. Differentiate between obtaining a pulse in an adult, a child and an infant.
11. Discuss the need for assessing the patient for external bleeding.
12. Discuss methods of assessing mental status.
13. Differentiate between assessing mental status in an adult, a child and an infant.
14. Describe methods used for assessing if a patient or casualty is breathing.
15. Explain the reason for prioritising a patient for care and transport.
16. Discuss the components of the physical examination.
17. State the areas of the body that are evaluated during the physical examination.
18. Explain what additional questioning may be asked during the physical examination.
19. Explain the components of the AMPLE history.
20. Discuss the components of the secondary assessment.
21. Describe the information included in the First Responder 'hand-over' report.

Affective objectives

22. Explain the rationale for crew members evaluating scene safety prior to entering.

23. Serve as a model for others by explaining how patient situations affect your evaluation of the mechanism of injury or illness.
24. Explain the importance of forming a general impression of the patient.
25. Explain the value of an initial assessment.
26. Explain the value of questioning the patient and family.
27. Explain the value of the physical examination.
28. Explain the value of a secondary assessment.
29. Explain the rationale for the feeling that patients might be experiencing.
30. Demonstrate a caring attitude when performing patient assessments.
31. Place the interests of the patient as the foremost consideration when making all decisions relating to patient care decisions during assessement of the patient.
32. Communicate empathically with patients as well as with the patient's family and friends of the patient during patient assessment.

Psychomotor objectives

33. Demonstrate the ability to differentiate various scenarios and identify potential hazards.
34. Demonstrate the techniques for assessing the airway.
35. Demonstrate the techniques for assessing if the patient is breathing.
36. Demonstrate the techniques for assessing if the patient has a pulse.
37. Demonstrate the techniques for assessing the patient for external bleeding.
38. Demonstrate the techniques for assessing the patient's mental status.
39. Demonstrate the techniques for assessing the patient's skin colour, temperature and condition, and capillary refill.
40. Demonstrate questioning a patient to obtain an AMPLE history.
41. Demonstrate the skills involved in performing the physical examination.
42. Demonstrate the secondary assessment.

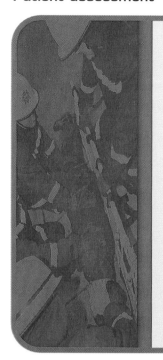

First response

POLICE OFFICERS DAVE AND TONY, both First Responders, were dispatched to a one-car crash on Salford Road, Manchester. They arrived before the ambulance and immediately began to assess the scene. The scene assessment revealed that one car had crashed head-on into a telegraph pole. Two casualties were in the car and power lines had fallen across the bonnet. Dave called his Control Room to notify the electricity company of the situation and to have them respond to the scene immediately. He then asked his Control to contact the ambulance service and gave them preliminary information about the scene as well as requesting that the fire service attend the scene because of the fire risk.

Recognising an unsafe scene, Dave and Tony did not approach the car. While waiting for the electricity company and other emergency services, Tony directed traffic and kept bystanders away from the scene. Although they were unable to assess or begin to care for the casualties, Dave and Tony's scene assessment kept them from entering a dangerous situation.

Patient assessment is the process by which First Responders gain information about the patient's condition. There are several steps in the patient assessment process:

- the scene assessment;
- the primary assessment;
- the First Responder physical examination; and
- the secondary assessment.

Each stage of this assessment reveals information that will help the First Responder decide how best to care for the patient. Let's begin by discussing the scene assessment.

SCENE ASSESSMENT

The scene assessment is the First Responder's first look at the patient and the surrounding situation. Scene assessment incorporates the knowledge, attitude and skills necessary to stay alive and well. It includes checking scene safety, determining the mechanism of injury or the nature of illness, finding out how many patients are involved, and determining whether you need additional help.

Universal precautions

Before beginning the scene assessment, always consider the need for universal precautions. Universal precautions protect health-care professionals from contact with blood and other body fluids. It is your responsibility to take the necessary precautions to protect yourself from contagious diseases. Chapter 2 ('The well-being of the First Responder') discusses universal precautions and how and when to use gloves, masks, aprons and eye protection. Many health-care professionals choose to take universal precautions before they enter the scene so they are never in a

situation in which they are exposed to blood or other fluids and are unprotected.

Scene safety

The goal of evaluating scene safety is to ensure that you, other First Responders, the patient and bystanders are not harmed while you are providing care. During the beginning of the scene assessment, you should evaluate the entire incident for any risks (**Fig. 6.1**). This assessment provides valuable information to help you stay alive and well. To protect yourself and your crew, use your senses of smell, vision and hearing to evaluate every situation.

As a First Responder, your primary responsibility is your own safety. Rushing into a scene before evaluating it for personal safety may result in your injury or death. First Responders who do not carefully evaluate situations before entering the scene not only create a danger for themselves but also put their fellow

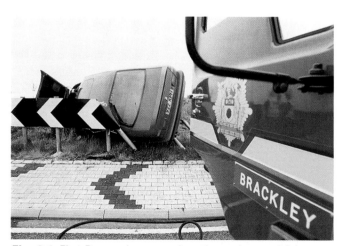

Fig. 6.1 First Responders may place themselves at risk by not checking for hazards, such as approaching this unsecured car.

health-care professionals at risk. The goal of the First Responder is to provide early care for the patient. Additional responding personnel should not have to confront a situation in which they have to provide care for both the patient who initially needed emergency medical treatment and also for a First Responder who has become injured.

Your responsibility is to ensure your own safety before addressing the safety of the patient or bystanders. Use your good judgement and experience to decide whether a scene is safe. If you decide that a scene is unsafe, do not enter until you can implement safety measures.

Everything you see and hear at the scene indicates whether the scene is safe. Trauma scenes with broken glass, torn metal and spilled hazardous fluids are not the only scenes that can result in injury. Other factors such as dangerous animals or people, fumes or toxic substances or even over-zealous bystanders can place the First Responder in danger. Any First Responder may encounter special situations such as rescue situations, toxic substances and crime scenes. A simple situation such as an icy street can place the First Responder in danger of being injured. If a dangerous situation is found, take the necessary measures to make the scene safe before proceeding. Part of making the scene safe prior to providing first aid is to wear the appropriate clothing when working around crash scenes (**Fig. 6.2**).

After checking that the scene is safe for you and other First Responders to provide care, you are responsible for ensuring the safety of the patient. Your role as a First Responder includes protecting the patient from additional injury that may occur from traffic or other hazards. Bystanders who park their cars inappropriately close to the scene create hazards for themselves, the patient and you. Exhaust fumes from vehicles (including emergency response vehicles) with engines left running may present a hazard to the patient or other personnel. An approaching vehicle that swerves to avoid hitting a bystander might end up in

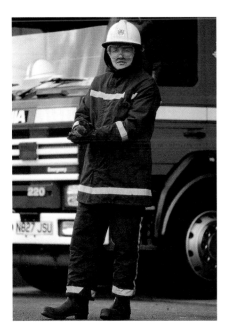

Fig. 6.2 First Responders should wear appropriate clothing when working around incident scenes.

First Responder Alert

If the scene is not safe and you cannot make it safe, do not enter.

the patient care area. In rescue and extrication operations, you must protect the patient from metal, flying glass, or sparks created by extrication tools. Patients also need protection from the environment, such as extreme heat or cold.

In some situations you need to ensure the safety of bystanders at the scene after protecting yourself and the patient. Usually police officers have this role but, if you are first on the scene, you may have to assume this responsibility. Bystanders become so engrossed in the emergency that they sometimes fail to watch out for themselves. You should move bystanders away from the immediate area for their own safety.

Remember that scene safety is not performed only during your initial approach to the incident; rather, it should be continually monitored throughout the incident to ensure continued safety as the situation changes or develops.

Nature of illness and mechanism of injury

After ensuring safety at the scene, the First Responder should evaluate the nature of illness (in the case of the medical patient) or the mechanism of injury (in the case of the trauma patient). The nature of illness is the event or condition that has lead to the patient's medical condition. The mechanism of injury is the event or force that has caused the casualty's injury.

Nature of illness

To determine the nature of illness, speak with the patient to learn more about the situation (**Fig. 6.3**). The patient, if responsive, is usually the best source of information. In some cases, the patient may be unresponsive or unable to provide information. A

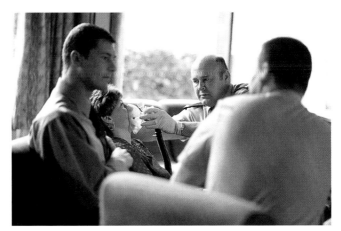

Fig. 6.3 Talk to the patient and the patient's family to gain more information about the nature of the patient's illness.

family member or a bystander who witnessed the situation or knows the patient's medical history may provide information about the patient.

The appearance of the patient or the clinical signs may make the nature of illness obvious, or you may determine it shortly after your arrival as the patient describes the symptoms to you.

The patient's chief complaint is their description of the medical problem. The nature of illness is the general cause of the problem. For example, if the patient describes the chief complaint as, "I have chest pain", the nature of illness is likely to be a cardiac problem. If the patient describes the problem as, "I can't catch my breath", the nature of illness is likely to be a respiratory problem.

Ask patients about their chief complaint and provide care based on this information and your assessment findings. Ask questions such as, "Why did you call for medical assistance?" and "How do you feel?".

Mechanism of injury

For trauma patients, after ensuring scene safety and taking universal precautions, determine the mechanism of injury. The mechanism of injury is determined by looking at the scene to see what forces caused the casualty's injury. Sometimes you can tell by looking at the casualty and the surroundings. On other occasions, you will need to get information from the casualty. If the casualty is unresponsive or cannot provide information regarding the mechanism of injury, obtain this information from family, friends or bystanders who witnessed the incident. The situation may not be what it seems at first. Ask specific questions about the situation and do not jump to conclusions. The following are examples of questions to consider or to ask others when determining the mechanism of injury after motor vehicle crashes, falls and shooting incidents.

Motor vehicle crashes – How fast was the vehicle travelling? What did the vehicle hit? How much damage was done to the vehicle? Were the occupants wearing seat belts? Were motorcyclists wearing helmets? Is the steering wheel bent? Is the windscreen cracked? An example of the mechanism of injury to report to arriving medical personnel might be: "A 7-year-old female, unrestrained front-seat passenger in a two-car head-on collision; minor damage to the car; no damage to the windscreen."

Falls – How far did the casualty fall? What did the casualty land on? What part of the casualty's body hit the ground first? An example of the mechanism of injury for a casualty who has fallen might be: "A 28-year-old male patient who fell three floors, landing feet first on a grassy surface."

Shooting incidents – What kind of gun was used? At what distance was the gun fired? An example of the mechanism of injury for a casualty who has been shot might be: "A 17-year-old male shot in the abdomen with a pistol from 2 m away."

The casualty may have sustained injuries besides the ones you first see. Often internal injuries are far more serious than the obvious external injuries to the casualty. Evaluating the mechanism of injury helps you to know when to suspect hidden injuries and guides you towards providing the most appropriate patient care. First Responders should maintain a high index of suspicion for a casualty who seems uninjured but who has undergone a serious mechanisms of injury (**Fig. 6.4**). Some examples of serious mechanism of injury are listed in **Box 6.1**. You should treat any casualty who is unresponsive following a traumatic incident as though they have severe injuries, even if you find no injuries during the physical examination.

In recent years, much work has been carried out into the mechanics of injury. This work has led to improvements in the ability to predict the type of injuries that are likely to occur to casualties. Two main types of trauma occur to a casualty – they are:
* penetrating trauma; and
* blunt trauma.

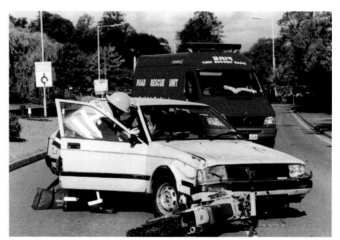

Fig. 6.4 You should expect both the motorcyclist and the driver of this car to have significant internal injuries, based on the serious mechanism of injury.

Box 6.1	**Mechanisms of Injury Considered High-Risk for Hidden Injury**

* Ejection of driver or passenger from a vehicle
* Driver or passenger in the same passenger compartment where another patient has died
* A fall of more than 6 m (20 ft)
* Vehicle rollover
* High-speed vehicle collision
* Vehicle pedestrian collision
* Motorcycle crash
* Penetrating trauma to the head, chest or abdomen

Penetrating trauma – This usually occurs from missiles such as shrapnel or bullets (these cause high-velocity penetrating trauma), or by knives (these cause low–velocity trauma). These mechanicisms of trauma cause tearing of the internal organs, and the injuries generally bleed at a faster rate than those caused by blunt trauma.

In the case of high-velocity trauma, the First Responder must suspect a high incidence of injury owing to the velocity of the projectile. Many organs can be damaged by fragmentation of the projectile or by the heat caused by the missile. Because of the speed of the missile, an exit wound is likely and should also be looked for. (The exit wound is sometimes larger than the entry wound.)

Blunt trauma – This form of energy transfer causes compression and shearing of the internal organs. This compression injury generally causes a slower internal bleeding rate, and a slower deterioration of the casualty may therefore be seen.

High-speed deceleration injuries

These are caused by:
- cars that are travelling faster than 30 miles per hour coming to an instant stop (for example, a car hitting a tree or another vehicle);
- motorcycles that are travelling faster than 20 miles per hour coming to an instant stop (for example, a motorcycle hitting a tree or another vehicle);
- pedestrians being hit by a car;
- falls from a significant height (in the case of children, 2.5 times their height).

There are in effect three decelerations in any vehicle crash:
1. The external framework of the vehicle hits an object.
2. The casualty hits the interior of the vehicle.
3. The internal organs of the casualty continue to travel forwards either until they hit the skeleton or until the ligaments that the organs are attached to are stretched to the point where they break and internal bleeding of the organ occurs.

In road traffic accidents (RTAs) in the UK, head injuries are the biggest cause of fatalities. The brain is generally damaged when it hits the skull, which is like a hard shell, and then slides back and hits the opposite side of the skull causing further damage to another part of the brain.

Road Traffic Accidents can be broken down into five types of collisions. (However, the First Responder must be aware that multiple forces occur if the vehicle is hit by numerous vehicles or if it rolls over or spins). The five basic types of impact are:
- frontal impact
- side impact
- rear impact
- rollover
- ejection

Frontal impact – This can cause major injury because the casualty continues to travel forwards until coming into contact with the restraint belt or the interior of the vehicle. This type of impact causes serious internal brain injury because the brain hits the front of the skull and then slides back into the rear portion of the skull. The organs of the chest are compressed and sheared, causing damage to the heart and the great vessels such as the aorta. The pelvis transfers forwards until it is stopped and the bowels are compressed and sheared. The lower limbs strike the lower dashboard and cause lower femoral and pelvic injuries.

Side impact – This generally causes a hyperflexion–rotation injury to the neck. This gives a 50–80% chance of a cervical spine injury. It is also the most common form of injury to the thoracic and lumbar areas of the spine. Serious chest injuries can also occur if the vehicle is deformed into the passenger area.

Rear impact – These incidents often occur at a lower speed or, in the case of two-car accidents, when both vehicles are moving in the same direction. This means that there is a longer period for the deceleration of both cars and of occupants. This type of crash causes hyperextension and hyperflexion of the neck. This common form of injury is known as 'whiplash'.

Rollover – This can cause severe injuries, but the mechanism of injury is not so clearly recognisable. Both shearing and compression of the organs can occur especially if the occupants are unrestrained. In the UK, this occurs mostly commonly to rear passengers. This is because the routine restraint of rear passengers has not yet become part of society's culture, despite it being illegal not to wear a restraint belt in the rear of a car.

Ejection – Since the introduction of seat belt legislation in the UK, ejection from a vehicle is becoming less common. Ejected casualties have a high death rate and a 1 in 13 chance of sustaining spinal injuries. Motorcyclists have a high incidence of thoracic spine injury. Again many forces are at work causing catastrophic damage to the body. Anyone found ejected from a vehicle must be considered seriously ill by the First Responder and should be moved quickly to an appropriate hospital.

Since the introduction of frontal and side airbags, the incidence of serious and life-threatening head and chest injuries has started to decrease in the UK. However, it is noticeable that, although the casualties are now more likely to survive, severe trauma to the extremities and the abdomen is likely to occur. This is because casualties now often survive many of the head and chest injuries that used to prove fatal, and they then require treatment for injuries to the lower limbs and the abdomen.

The introduction of 'crumple zones' in most cars is also causing more severe damage to the vehicle but

Patient assessment

less damage to the casualty. Therefore, casualties now sometimes 'walk out' of what appears to be an extensively damaged car or are entrapped by the crumpling effect of the vehicle. This informs the First Responder that the vehicle itself has absorbed much of the damage and therefore protected the occupant.

First Responders should always be aware of the unseen injuries.

In summary, many types of accident have a direct correlation with the injuries that the casualty will sustain. However, with changing technology, the science of predicting injury from the observation of the vehicle is becoming more difficult. It is important to establish the type of impact and at what speed it occurred. It is also important to understand whether or not the casualties were restrained and if airbags were deployed. This information should be passed onto other EMS providers on their arrival.

Number of patients and need for additional help

Calls to incidents involving a medical problem usually involve only one patient. However, trauma calls such as RTAs often involve more than one casualty. When evaluating the scene, you should also determine whether additional casualties are present. If you see a child car safety seat in or outside the vehicle, an infant or child casualty may be present somewhere on the scene. Gender-specific articles (such as a woman's purse or a man's wallet) may suggest the presence of an unseen casualty. Look all around the scene to determine the total number of casualties. Do not forget to ask casualties or bystanders at the scene how many people were in the vehicle when the accident occurred.

If there are multiple casualties, you must inform the responding ambulance service and request additional help if necessary (**Fig. 6.5**). Do not delay the call for assistance. Having extra help arrive and return unneeded is better than needing extra help and not having it available. If more casualties are present than your ambulance service can care for, you must begin triage and activate a major incident plan, as described below and in Chapter 13 ('EMS operations').

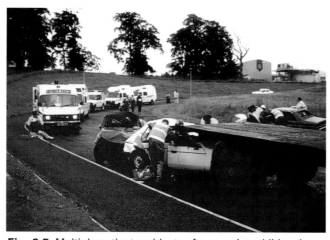

Fig. 6.5 Multiple-patient accidents often require additional EMS assistance.

TRIAGE

The word 'triage' is derived from a French word meaning 'to sort' and was first documented during the Napoleonic wars, when triage allowed the most salvageable soldiers to be treated and then sent back to the front lines. Many types of triage have now been documented and many differing coding systems, using colours, letters or numbers, have been developed in recent years.

The fundamental aim of any triage system is to ensure that the maximum number of casualties are treated with the least interventions. For example, it would be detrimental to the management of a mass casualty incident for a First Responder to spend 10 minutes dealing with one casualty when another 15 could have been treated, only to find that the casualty you have decided to stay with may die.

In the 1990s two systems of triage based on a military model were introduced. They are broken down into triage 'sieve' and triage 'sort'.

Triage 'sieve' allows a First Responder to sieve casualties by carrying out minimal interventions and taking minimal observations. This system is described in greater detail below.

Triage 'sort' is described as a medical assessment and is generally beyond the abilities of the average First Responder. It allows an in-depth assessment based on physical parameters and allows the casualty to be sent to the appropriate hospital (for example, to a burns unit).

Triage 'sieve'

Triage sieve has four priority systems, known as Red (P1), Yellow (P2), Green (P3) and Black (P4), where P stands for priority. Each casualty is placed into one of these four categories. The categories can be defined as follows:

- red – any casualty requiring immediate life-saving interventions; these could be as simple as an airway manoeuvre or a medical procedure such as chest decompression;
- yellow – any casualty who requires surgery within 6 hours;
- green – any walking casualty (if a casualty is walking and then collapses to the floor they are then reassessed);
- black – any casualty who has an obstructed airway and cannot be maintained.

Black is the most contentious priority for the First Responder. However, if the incident is one where the manpower availability is high, no casualties need to be placed into this category. However, it can be utilised if you are first on a scene where there are numerous casualties.

The next stage for the First Responder (now knowing the colour coding of the casualties) is to measure the breathing rate and the capillary refill. If the weather is cold then the First Responder needs to measure his own breathing rate first and use this as the normal variant. **Figure 6.6** illustrates the protocol to follow when initiating triage sieve.

By using this flow diagram the First Responder can see that anyone who is walking is automatically a 'green' priority. These casualties can be sent to a further clearing station.

The next stage for the First Responder is to check the casualty's airway. If it cannot be opened and then maintained by the casualty himself then he should be placed into the 'black' category (and therefore not treated). In a mass casualty situation these casualties will die if they are not already dead.

If the airway is opened and then maintained by the casualty, the respiration rate is counted. A respiration rate below 10 breaths per minute or over 29 is an indication that a serious injury should be suspected, and the casualty is given a 'red' priority. If, however, the breathing rate is between 10 and 29 breaths per minute, then the capillary refill is measured. If capillary refill is delayed (over 2 seconds), then the casualty is placed into the 'red' category. If it is normal (less than 2 seconds), then the casualty is placed into the 'yellow' category.

Remember that triage is a dynamic process and casualties must be constantly reassessed to determine any change in their condition and, consequently, in their triage categorisation

Sometimes you may require additional help for actions other than casualty care. For example, you may need help to lift a large casualty; you may need police officers to deal with traffic problems, unco-operative bystanders, or potentially violent scenes; you may need special assistance from the fire service, other voluntary rescue organisations or utility companies. When possible, call for additional help before beginning casualty care or as soon as you realise you need assistance. Avoid getting into a situation in which you become so involved in casualty care that you do not remember or have time to call for additional help.

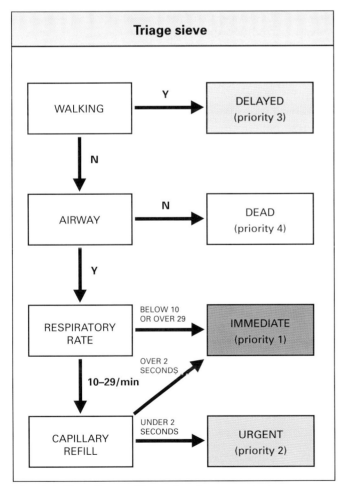

Fig. 6.6 Flow diagram illustrating the protocol when initiating triage sieve. (Reproduced, with permission, from Advanced Life Support Group: *Major Incident Medical Management and Support. The Practical Approach.* London: BMJ Publications, 1995.)

Review Questions

Triage

Place each of the following casualties into the correct priority using the triage sieve template.

1. Male in his 30s trapped in a car involved in an RTA. Airway is maintained, breathing rate is 9 breaths per minute, capillary refill is 2 seconds.

2. Female in her 20s trapped in a car involved in an RTA. Airway is maintained, breathing rate is 20 breaths per minute, capillary refill is less than 2 seconds.

3. Teenager of 15 years of age who was sitting in the back of car involved in an RTA but was not entrapped, and is now walking around at the scene.

1. Red; 2. Yellow; 3. Green.

PRIMARY ASSESSMENT

The first decisions about patient assessment and care are typically made within the first few seconds of seeing the patient. The primary assessment is completed to help the First Responder identify immediate threats to the patient's life.

During the primary assessment, you quickly evaluate the patient to:
- form a general impression;
- assess mental status;
- assess the airway;
- assess breathing rate and quality;
- assess circulation;
- identify any life-threatening injuries; and
- provide care based on those findings.

After completing the primary assessment, you should report to the responding ambulance crew with a brief report summarising the patient information.

Life-threatening injuries include airway obstruction, inadequate breathing, major bleeding, inadequate circulation and a variety of other conditions, which are discussed in later chapters. If you identify a life-threatening injury, you must correct it immediately. For example, if blood, vomit, or teeth are present in the airway of a trauma patient, you must clear the airway before performing any other assessment or care. If a patient has no pulse, cardiopulmonary resuscitation (CPR) must begin immediately. By looking at, listening to and touching the patient, you can identify threats to life.

General impression of the patient

After completing the scene assessment and taking the appropriate universal precautions, the first thing to do as you approach the patient is to form a general impression. The general impression is your immediate assessment of the environment and the patient's problem. This process takes place in seconds. The general impression usually allows you to determine the priority of care for the patient. Once you have completed the general assessment, you can form a plan of action for continuing to assess the patient and providing care. As you form your general impression, you will determine the nature of illness or mechanism of injury, the sex of the patient and his or her approximate age.

The nature of illness or the mechanism of injury guides your general impression of the patient's general appearance. For example, if a casualty was in a rollover car crash that caused severe damage to the car, the casualty has potential for serious injury. Even if the casualty seems stable or has only minor injuries, you should be suspicious that the casualty may have severe internal injuries.

If you are unsure if the patient has a medical problem or an injury, treat the patient as though he or she has sustained trauma.

Assess responsiveness

After forming a general impression and before continuing the assessment, you must stabilise or immobilise the spine if the mechanism of injury suggests that there may be a spinal injury. Specific techniques for stabilising and immobilising the spine are discussed in Chapter 10 ('Injuries to muscles and bones'). At this stage, just remember that you should not move casualties with potential spinal injuries before appropriate immobilisation has taken place, unless an airway obstruction dictates that you will have to move the casualty into a neutral alignment to clear the obstruction.

To assess the patient's responsiveness, begin by speaking to the patient. Introduce yourself, tell the patient that you are a First Responder and explain that you are there to help and to provide care until additional help arrives. Note the patient's response. Patients may be alert, they may not be fully alert but still respond to verbal stimuli, they may respond only to painful stimuli, or may be completely unresponsive. The acronym AVPU (alert, verbal, painful, unresponsive) is a reminder of these four categories, which are described in more detail below, and in Chapter 10, ('Injuries to muscles and bones'). The normal mental status is alert. If the patient is only responsive to verbal or painful stimuli or is unresponsive, then they have an altered mental status.

An **alert** patient is one who interacts with you without prompting. Alert patients know their name, where they are, what time it is and the reason they called for assistance. Some patients may know their name but be unsure of where they are or what time it is. These patients are still alert but are considered disorientated. In a child, alert responses depend on the child's developmental stage. An alert child of almost any age clearly prefers being with their usual caretakers than strangers such as you. Remember that sick and injured children often regress in behaviour. For example, children of 3 years of age who can usually say their name may not be able to do so when they are hurt or scared. Assess how well they interact with the environment and with their parents.

Some patients may appear to be sleeping but respond when you talk to them. These patients are responsive to **verbal** stimuli. Some patients may respond only to loud verbal stimuli. Responses in children of any age may range from following a command, to actively trying to find a parent's voice, to crying after a loud noise.

Patients who do not respond to a verbal stimulus may respond to a **painful** stimulus (**Fig. 6.7**). Squeezing the patient's thumbnail using the barrel of a pen, or pinching the patient's skin between the neck and shoulders, are both adequate painful stimuli. Patients may respond to a painful stimulus by making a noise, trying to remove the painful stimulus or trying to pull away from the stimulus.

If a patient does not respond to verbal or painful stimuli, the patient is **unresponsive**. Few patients are completely unresponsive. Most patients with decreased responsiveness have some response to pain.

To assess the patient's level of responsiveness, first determine if the patient interacts with you without prompting. If so, the patient is alert. If not alert, will the patient respond to verbal stimuli? If not, will the patient respond to painful stimuli? A patient who does not respond to any stimulus is unresponsive.

Note the responsiveness of the patient in your first interaction and note any later changes. If there is a change in the patient's responsiveness, discuss the trends with the arriving ambulance personnel in your verbal report. Be prepared to provide airway support or to treat the patient for signs and symptoms of shock if you note that the patient's responsiveness is deteriorating.

Assess the airway

You will assess the airway in one of two ways, depending on whether the patient is alert or has an altered mental status. Alert patients may be talking or crying. If they are, the airway is open and you should move immediately to evaluate their breathing. If the patient is responsive to verbal or painful stimuli only and is not talking or crying, you may need to open the airway.

The airway is opened in one of two ways, depending on whether the patient has a medical condition or an injury. For medical patients, perform the head-tilt, chin-lift. For trauma casualties or patients with an unknown nature of illness or mechanism of injury, manually stabilise the spine with your hands and perform the jaw thrust without head-tilt (**Fig. 6.8**). Refer to Chapter 5 ('The airway') for a review of these procedures.

Once the airway is open, check to be sure it is clear. You may need to use suction or finger sweeps or to re-position the patient in order to maintain an open, clear airway. After the airway is open and clear, the next step is to assess breathing.

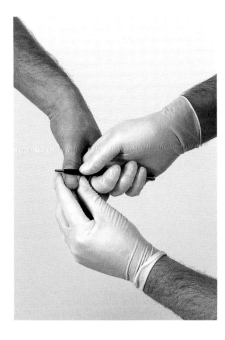

Fig. 6.7 If the patient does not respond to verbal stimuli, check the patient's response to painful stimuli by squeezing the patient's thumbnail using the barrel of a pen

Assess breathing

Assess the patient's breathing efforts to determine how much effort they are exerting to breathe. Responsive patients should be asked if they can speak as a way of assessing the effort of breathing. In unresponsive patients, remember to look, listen and feel for breathing (**Fig. 6.9**). Assess the rate and quality of the breathing. Most adults breathe between 12 and 20 times a minute and take in a volume of air based on size and weight. You should become concerned if the respiratory rate drops below 10 per minute or is greater than 29. A respiratory rate of less than 10 per minute or greater than 29 may not provide enough oxygen to support the patient's oxygen demands.

Responsive patients with respiratory rates below 10 per minute or greater than 29 should be coached to increase or decrease the respiratory rate, as appropriate. Patients who are breathing too quickly may require

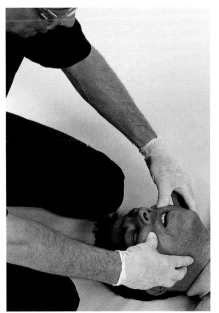

Fig. 6.8 Use the head-tilt, chin-lift for medical patients, the jaw thrust without head-tilt for trauma patients.

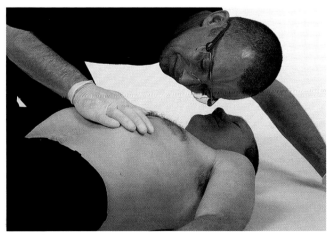

Fig. 6.9 Assess breathing by looking for chest rise, listening for air movement, and feeling the movement of exhaled air against your cheek.

oxygen administration. Patients who are breathing too slowly require artificial ventilation. Chapter 5 ('The airway') and Appendix B ('Advanced First Responder ventilation techniques') describe the techniques of ventilation and oxygen administration. The First Responder assessing the patient should not stop the assessment to administer oxygen, but should let another person perform this task. Not all First Responders have the equipment needed for oxygen administration, but when oxygen is available it should be administered at the earliest opportunity. You should follow your local protocols regarding the use of oxygen and ventilation.

Priorities for assessing breathing and providing necessary treatment are the same for infants and children as for adults. Normal breathing rates depend on the patient's age (see Appendix C, 'Vital signs'). Younger children breathe more quickly than adults. A child who is breathing too slowly is much sicker than one who is breathing too fast. As a child begins to fatigue, his or her breathing rate begins to slow. This usually represents a child in severe distress. Closely monitor children breathing at a rapid rate. Their rates may begin to drop as fatigue sets in. Provide oxygen and ventilate the patient following your local protocol.

Assess circulation

After evaluating the patient's level of responsiveness, airway and breathing and providing interventions as necessary, assess the circulation. This assessment involves:

• checking the pulse;
• looking for major bleeding; and
• assessing perfusion (skin colour and temperature).

Pulse

For responsive adult patients, assess the circulation for rate and quality by palpating (feeling) the radial artery. If you cannot feel a radial pulse, palpate the carotid pulse. If the patient is unresponsive when you arrive at the scene, you should assess for airway obstruction and breathing and then the carotid pulse.

When assessing a responsive child, palpate the brachial or radial pulse first. For an unresponsive child, palpate the carotid or femoral pulse. For infants, whether responsive or unresponsive, assess the brachial pulse (**Fig. 6.10**).

When evaluating the pulse, note the rate and quality of the pulse. The pulse rate may be rapid, normal or slow. The quality can be normal or weak. For patients who have a pulse, palpate the distal (farthest from the trunk of the body – such as the radial or brachial) and central pulses (pulses on the trunk of the body – such as the carotid or femoral) simultaneously (**Fig. 6.11**). If the distal pulse is absent or weaker than the central pulse, the patient is showing a sign of shock.

If no pulse is present, begin CPR. For certain medical patients an automated external defibrillator (AED) can also be used. AEDs are most appropriately used for adult medical cardiac emergencies. However they can

be utilised in trauma casualties, but their use is usually ineffective owing to the heart rhythm found in this type of casualty. AEDs and their use are discussed in Appendix D ('Automated external defibrillation').

Major bleeding

Next, evaluate the patient for major bleeding. You may have detected major bleeding earlier in the assessment,

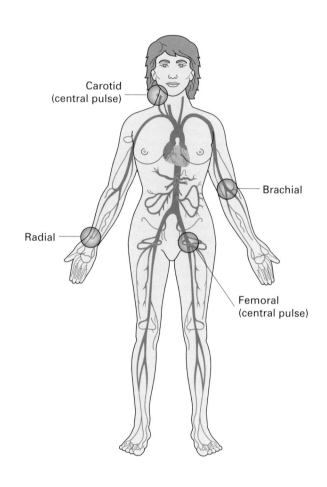

Fig. 6.10 Location of radial, carotid, brachial and femoral pulses.

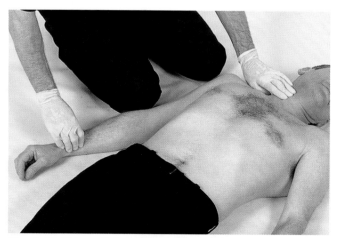

Fig. 6.11 Take radial and carotid pulses simultaneously for comparison.

while you were assessing for life-threatening conditions. As part of the assessment of the patient's circulation, check again for major bleeding. You may need to expose injured areas by removing clothing to assess for bleeding. For casualties with major trauma, you should remove all clothing to assess properly for injury and bleeding. If you see significant bleeding as you assess the patient, treat it as a life-threatening condition as described in Chapter 9 ('Bleeding and soft tissue injuries').

Assess perfusion

By assessing the patient's skin colour and temperature, the First Responder can assess the patient's perfusion. Perfusion is the process by which blood is circulated to the organs of the body, delivering oxygen and removing waste products. Assess the patient's colour by looking at the nail beds or inside the lips or at the skin inside the eyelids. Normally, the colour of these areas is pink in people of any race. Abnormal colours include pale, blue–grey, flushed or red, and jaundice or yellow.

Assess skin temperature by putting the back of your hand against the patient's skin. Normal skin is warm to the touch. Abnormal skin temperatures are hot, cool or cold. Also note if the skin is dry or moist. Taking the patient's temperature with a thermometer in pre-hospital settings is not necessary; the basic assessment with your hand is sufficient. If the patient's skin is cool and moist, the patient may be in a state of hypoperfusion (shock). If the skin is hot and dry, the patient may be suffering from a medical condition or having a heat-related emergency.

Reporting to responding ambulance crews

After completing the primary assessment, when possible you should contact the ambulance service that will be transporting the patient and provide a brief report about the patient's condition. Be sure to speak clearly and provide as much detail as possible concerning your findings (**Box 6.2**).

Ask the responding Ambulance Control to estimate how long it will take the ambulance to arrive at the scene.

Box 6.2	**Patient Information for Radio Report to Ambulance Crew**

- Age and sex
- Chief complaint
- Responsiveness
- Airway and breathing status
- Circulation status

FIRST RESPONDER PHYSICAL EXAMINATION

So far we have discussed the scene assessment that takes place before beginning patient care and the primary assessment. Following the primary assessment, your next step is to perform the First Responder physical examination. The goal of the First Responder physical examination is to find the casualty's injuries or to find out more about the signs and symptoms of the patient's illness, and to begin to manage the condition. All patients receive a First Responder physical examination, but the examination differs depending on whether the patient has a medical condition or has suffered trauma. Most patients fit into one of these categories. If you are not immediately sure which category the patient fits into, treat the situation as trauma.

The First Responder physical examination is a methodical head-to-toe evaluation of the patient. To evaluate the patient you will inspect (look) and palpate (feel) for the following signs of injury:
- deformities;
- open injuries;
- tenderness; and
- swelling.

The mnemonic DOTS is helpful in remembering the signs of injury. Deformities occur when bones are broken, causing an abnormal position or shape. Open injuries break the continuity of the skin. Tenderness is sensitivity to touch. Swelling is a response of the body to injury that makes the area look larger than usual. Be sure to evaluate the following areas: head, neck, chest, abdomen, pelvis and all four extremities.

Alert and responsive adult patients can usually tell you a great deal about the nature of their illness or how they were injured. Infants and children may not describe their symptoms accurately, although their parents or carers may be helpful in explaining their behaviour. Some older patients also may not clearly describe their illness or how they became injured. Listen

Patient assessment

carefully to what all patients tell you and ask questions to clarify if you are unsure what their responses mean.

All patients should receive a physical examination. However, if you are spending all of your time keeping the airway clear or assisting ventilation, do not interrupt care of the airway, breathing or circulation to perform the First Responder physical examination.

Performing a physical examination

Beginning at the head, inspect and palpate for DOTS. Remember, for a trauma patient, you must stabilise the spine. Palpate the head beginning on the top surface, running your hands towards the back of the head (**Fig. 6.12**). Bring your hands around to the patient's forehead and feel the face. Note any unstable areas.

Next, evaluate the patient's neck (**Fig. 6.13**). Feel around the back, the front and the sides of the neck for DOTS and look for signs of injury.

Next evaluate the chest inspecting and palpating for DOTS (**Fig. 6.14**). An easy way to perform this evaluation is to start at the clavicles (collar bone) and move to the sternum (breastbone). While inspecting and palpating the ribs, move your fingers as far around the sides towards the back as possible. Check for signs of blood on your gloves to detect an open posterior chest wound. Ask a responsive patient to take a deep breath. The chest should rise and fall equally on both sides.

Evaluate the abdomen (**Fig. 6.15**). Because some patients are particularly sensitive about having their abdominal area touched, inform all patients of what you are about to do before you begin. After placing your hand on the abdomen, allow the patient to relax the abdominal muscles so that you can better determine whether the abdomen feels soft or rigid. The abdomen is normally soft. If the abdomen is hard or distended, there may be bleeding into the abdomen caused by an internal injury. While you are evaluating

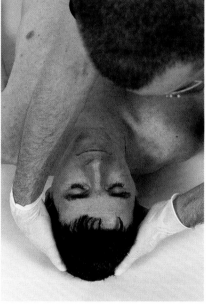

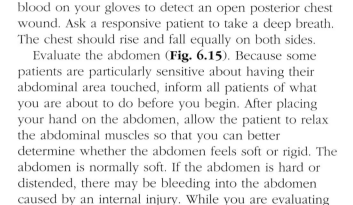

Fig. 6.12 Palpate the patient's head.

Fig. 6.13 Palpate the neck.

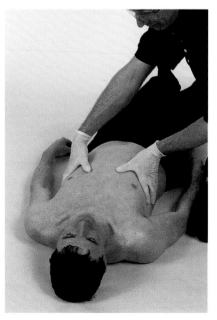

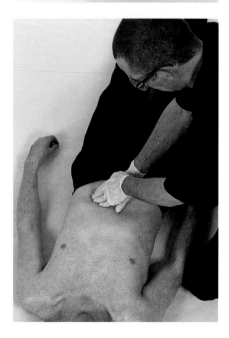

Fig. 6.14 Expose and palpate the chest.

Fig. 6.15 Palpate all four quadrants of the abdomen.

the abdomen, watch the patient's facial expression for grimaces.

If you do not suspect that the patient has a pelvic injury based on the mechanism of injury and the patient does not complain of pain, you can also gently palpate the pelvis (**Fig. 6.16**). If the pelvis appears unstable, do not reassess this area. Further movement of the pelvis could aggravate injuries to the spine, nerves or blood vessels. If the patient complains of pain in the pelvis, or if the mechanism of injury suggests a pelvic injury (for example, a casualty who has been hit by a vehicle), assume an injury is present and do not assess the pelvis.

Finally, check the four extremities. As you have just evaluated the pelvis, move on to check the lower extremities first. Do not exert pressure with your thumbs only, but use your entire hand to assess the patient's extremities. As you move down the extremity from the pelvis, start high on the thigh of the patient's leg closest to you and run your hands down the entire

extremity (**Fig. 6.17**), then assess the opposite leg. Continue the assessment by moving to the patient's upper extremities. Evaluate the arm closest to you, starting at the shoulder and moving to the finger tips. Then check the arm on the opposite side (**Fig. 6.18**).

After checking each extremity you should check for distal pulse, motor function and sensation. Pulses can be felt in the feet either on top of the foot or behind the ankle. Motor function is the ability to move and sensation is the ability to feel a touch against the skin. Ask responsive patients if they can wiggle their toes and if they can feel you touching them. You probably cannot assess sensation and motor function in unresponsive patients, because these patients may not react to a touch on the extremities. Make note of the patient's ability or inability to feel or move any of the extremities and reassess for changes in their condition.

The steps of the First Responder physical examination are the same for infants and children as

A

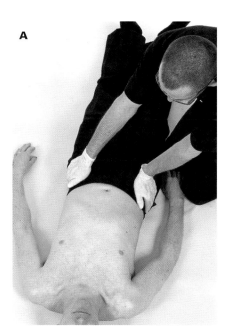

B

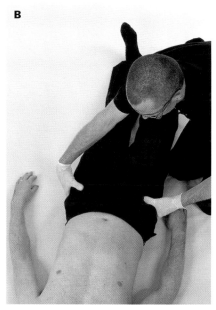

Fig. 6.16 Palpate the pelvis by gently pressing **(a)** towards the floor, and **(b)** towards the midline.

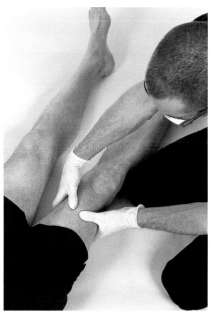

Fig. 6.17 Palpate the lower extremities.

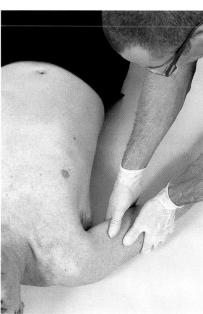

Fig. 6.18 Palpate the upper extremities.

they are for adults, though you may wish to use a 'trunk-to-head' approach, as discussed later in Chapter 12 ('Infants and children').

Medical patients and patients with no significant injury or mechanism of injury

If the patient has a medical complaint, such as chest pain, you may not have to assess the patient from head-to-toe. Ask the patient if any recent trauma may be causing the pain. If there has been no trauma, you should inspect and palpate the area involved in the patient's chief complaint.

For patients with a minor injury and no significant mechanism of injury (for example, a patient who has cut his finger, or a patient who twisted her ankle while stepping off a kerb) begin the physical examination at the site of the injury, using the same components (DOTS). Remember, however, that if the casualty has sustained a serious mechanism of injury, there may be underlying injuries of which the casualty is not aware. Patients are often aware only of their most painful injury, which is not necessarily the most serious. If you suspect other injuries, or there is a serious mechanism of injury, perform the entire physical examination.

A comparison of two cases will help clarify this principle. In the first case, a casualty is in a motor vehicle collision that results in severe damage to the car and the tree that it hit. The casualty complains only of pain in the right ankle. This casualty has sustained a serious mechanism of injury and should receive a head-to-toe physical examination. In the second case, a patient who was jogging suffered a twisted ankle when stepping off a curb. The patient did not fall and complains only of ankle pain. The First Responder physical examination for this patient can be directed towards the ankle only, because the mechanism of injury is not serious.

Remember that the patient evaluation always begins with the scene assessment followed by a primary assessment. You do not need to complete the First Responder physical examination before you begin to treat the patient. Manage any life-threatening conditions when they are found.

Patients experiencing medical emergencies are often scared, anxious or nervous. Remember that this situation is stressful for the patient and the patient's family. Your role is to care for the patient as a whole person and not just to treat the medical condition. Listen carefully to what patients tell you about their illness or injury and always treat them with respect. Do not be judgemental about the severity of their illness – if they did not feel there was an emergency, they would not have called for assistance.

PATIENT HISTORY

Another role of the First Responder is to obtain the patient's pertinent medical history. The history you should obtain is a concise set of information relating to

the current medical problem or injury. You should obtain the history from the patient, but you may have to ask family members or friends if the patient can't tell you.

Medical condition identification insignia

When assessing a patient or giving care, you may come across a medical condition identification insignia on a necklace, bracelet or even ankle bracelet (**Fig. 6.19**). Its purpose is to inform health-care providers of the wearer's medical condition in case the person is unresponsive or cannot communicate directly. Patients wear such devices because they have a potentially serious medical condition, such as diabetes, severe allergies, epilepsy or asthma, that requires rapid intervention. A symbol is sometimes engraved on one side and the patient's medical problem on the other. There may also be an identification number or telephone number for obtaining more information about the patient's medical condition.

The AMPLE history

When questioning the patient about the medical history, First Responders should take an AMPLE history. AMPLE is a mnemonic that stands for five elements of the patient history:

- allergies;
- medications;
- pertinent past medical history;
- last oral intake (solid or liquid); and
- events leading to the injury or illness.

Signs and symptoms are indications of a possible medical problem. A 'sign' is any medical or trauma condition that First Responders can observe in the patient and can identify. Examples include information the First Responder can see (such as skin colour), information the First Responder can feel (such as pulse rate or skin temperature) and information the First

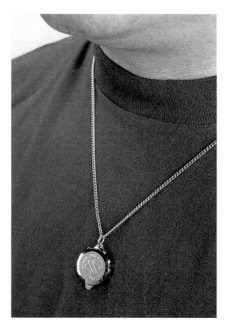

Fig. 6.19 The 'SOS' insignia informs health-care providers of the wearer's medical condition if the person is unresponsive or cannot communicate directly.

Responder can hear (such as respiratory effort). A 'symptom' is any non-observable condition described by the patient. For example, patients may state that they feel nauseated, have a headache or just feel sick. You cannot see these symptoms and can only ask the patient about them. To determine what symptoms the patient has, ask him or her, "How are you feeling?" and "Why did you call for an ambulance today?" Signs and symptoms are important because they form the basis for patient care.

Allergies

Ask the patient about any allergies to medications, foods or environmental factors (for example, dust, moulds, grass) and always look for a medical alert tag. Some people are allergic to certain medications, such as penicillin. Other people may be allergic to shellfish or other foods. This information may lead you to suspect that an allergic reaction has occurred and will act as a guide to the appropriate treatment. In addition, if the patient's mental status changes on the way to the hospital and the patient becomes unresponsive, you can provide the receiving facility staff with this valuable information.

Medications

Identify any medications the patient is taking. Ask the patient if the medications are current or recent and if they have been prescribed by their doctor or if they are over-the-counter (OTC). Ask if the patient has taken their medications as prescribed by their doctor.

Pertinent past medical history

Ask for pertinent past medical history including recent or past medical problems, surgery and injuries. Keep the patient focused on recent or pertinent medical history. Surgery on a patient's ankle 20 years ago, for example, is usually not related to the patient's chief complaint. However, heart surgery 5 years ago might be important to the patient's current problem. This information may guide you to look for subtle signs and symptoms that might not be obvious at first. In addition, give this information to the arriving ambulance crew. Ask if the patient is currently seeing a doctor for any medical condition. Also ask if the patient has been in hospital recently.

Last oral intake

Last oral intake includes the time and quantity of both solid and liquid food. Get specific information about any recent change in eating habits or lack of eating. Some patients may intentionally either not eat or overeat. Also, consider alcohol intake or ingestion of other non-food substances. The time and quantity of last oral intake is relevant in case the patient needs emergency surgery. Any solids or liquids in the patient's stomach have the potential to compromise the airway if the patient is unable to protect his or her own airway. Ask the patient, "Have you had anything to eat or drink recently?" If the answer is yes, find out what was eaten or drunk and when.

Events leading to the injury or illness

Identify events leading to the injury or illness. Ask the patient what he or she was doing when the event happened and any associated symptoms concerning the situation. For example, if the patient complains of chest pain, note if the pain began while the patient was at rest or during exertion. Other symptoms such as dizziness or confusion may also give the receiving facility important information. Sometimes the order in which the symptoms occurred is important. For example, dizziness may be the chief complaint, but the patient may state that it occurred after chest pain began.

For medical patients, the AMPLE history may be completed before the First Responder physical examination. The information you gather in the AMPLE history can help you provide care to the patient. Should a patient become unresponsive after the initial contact with the ambulance service, you will have gained valuable information to help the receiving facility.

SECONDARY ASSESSMENT

The purpose of the secondary assessment is to re-evaluate the patient's condition and to check the adequacy of each intervention. Frequent evaluations allow you to notice subtle changes in the patient's condition. The secondary assessment occurs while you are waiting for additional ambulance or medical personnel to arrive at the scene. This allows you to continue to interact with the patient and note changes or trends in the patient's mental status or vital signs. Trends in a patient's mental status can provide valuable information to the health-care professionals who will assume care of the patient.

Patient assessment

Once you have responded to a call and have performed the scene assessment, the primary assessment and the First Responder physical examination, continuous evaluation of the patient must take place. The secondary assessment repeats the primary assessment (reassess airway, breathing, circulation and mental status) and the First Responder physical examination. During the secondary assessment you will also assess the effectiveness of any interventions performed as part of the patient care process (**Fig. 6.20**). If you are artificially ventilating the patient, make sure the ventilation is adequate by watching the chest rise and by monitoring the patient. You must also assess any measures that have been taken to control bleeding. Any intervention that no longer meets the needs of the patient must be corrected immediately. **Box 6.3** summarises the elements of the secondary assessment.

For stable patients, repeat the secondary assessment and record the results every 15 minutes. For unstable patients, repeat the assessment and record the results every 5 minutes or even more frequently.

Stable patients are those medical patients or trauma casualties who have simple, specific injuries (for example, a patient who has injured an ankle while playing football). Unstable patients are those medical patients in severe distress and trauma casualties who have significant injuries or who have sustained a significant mechanism of injury, even if they seem stable.

Some patients may have life-threatening conditions that require all of your attention. If you are so busy maintaining an open airway by suctioning, you may not have time to assess the patient's skin temperature or colour. The secondary assessment for a patient with life-threatening injuries is almost constant.

Elderly patients also require special attention. Additional considerations when dealing with elderly patients are summarised in **Box 6.4**.

An important role that cannot be ignored in caring for the patient is calming and reassuring them that you are doing everything you can while additional help is

Box 6.3	**Components of the Secondary Assessment**

Repeat the initial assessment
• Check mental status
• Check airway patency
• Assess breathing rate and quality
• Assess circulation
   Pulse rate and quality
   Skin colour, temperature and condition
Repeat the First Responder physical examination
Evaluate all interventions

on the way. Remember that the patient is not the only individual who may need reassurance – the patient's family may also require comfort. However, do not provide any sense of false hope to the patient or the family if the situation is serious; you are not able to determine outcomes.

Finally, when the ambulance crew arrive on the scene, you should provide a 'hand-over' report (**Fig. 6.21**). The report to arriving ambulance crew is an essential component of your role in the care of the patient. You will need to give these people all the pertinent information that you have obtained about the patient as you transfer care to them. Speak clearly and slowly, and provide all information in a logical order. Provide the following information:

• the patient's name, age and sex;
• the chief complaint;
• the level of responsiveness;
• airway and breathing status;
• circulation status;
• findings from the physical examination;
• information from the AMPLE history;
• details of care that you have provided and the results; and
• any other information that you believe may be beneficial to assure appropriate continued care.

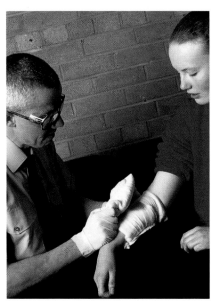

Fig. 6.20 Assess interventions to make sure they are still effective.

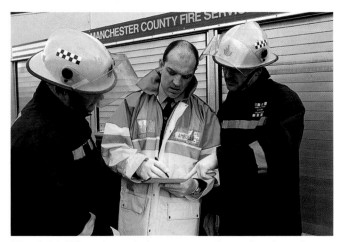

Fig. 6.21 When the ambulance crew arrive, a 'hand-over' report will update them about the patient's condition and care already provided.

	Additional Considerations When Dealing With Elderly Patients
Box 6.4	

- When maintaining an airway ensure that any false teeth are securely in place in the correct position in the mouth, or that they are removed. When false teeth are removed, flaccid muscle control to the face may cause further difficulties in maintaining an airway manoeuvre
- Because of osteoarthritis, the neck of an elderly patient is more prone to injury when exposed to extreme extension and flexion
- Injuries to the hips are common in falls in the elderly. When any external rotation and shortening of an elderly patient's leg following a fall is noted, the First Responder must suspect a hip fracture
- When using spinal boards, the First Responder must be aware that the elderly patient's skin is more prone to break down owing to the poor blood circulation to the extremities. Prolonged immobilisation on a spinal board will increase the chance of pressure sores. This in turn can lead to generalised infection and sometimes death. The elderly patient should, where possible, be placed on a spinal board for no longer than 20 minutes. If the time on a spinal board exceeds this, the receiving hospital should be informed as soon as possible.

Review Questions

Ongoing Assessment

1. How often are ongoing assessments performed on stable patients?
2. List the components of the ongoing assessment.

_____

_____

1. Every five minutes; 2. Repeat the primary assessment, repeat the First Responder physical examination, check interventions

CHAPTER SUMMARY

Scene assessment

First Responders must take precautions to prevent or reduce contact with a patient's blood or other body fluids. Gloves, eye protection, aprons and masks should be worn as necessary. After taking care of themselves and other First Responders on the scene, First Responders should next protect the patient and then bystanders. Protect patients from further injury from traffic hazards, rescue operations, heat, cold or any other danger.

If the patient has a medical condition, determine the nature of illness. If the patient has sustained a traumatic injury, determine the mechanism of injury. Determine the number of patients and whether additional help is necessary.

Primary assessment

Form a general impression of the patient during the first few seconds of contact. Determine the mechanism of injury or the nature of illness while forming the general impression. Identify and correct life-threatening conditions. Determine the approximate age of the patient. Assess the airway, breathing, circulation and mental status.

First Responder physical examination

The First Responder physical examination is designed to locate the signs and symptoms of illness and injury and begin the initial management. All patients will receive a First Responder physical examination; however, you may alter the examination to meet the needs of the patient's situation and condition. During the First Responder physical examination, evaluate the head, neck, chest, abdomen, pelvis and extremities for DOTS (deformities, open injuries, tenderness and swelling).

Patients with a minor mechanism of injury and an isolated injury do not always require a complete First Responder physical examination, and in these cases First Responders may evaluate the injury only.

Patient history

When assessing a patient or giving care, you may come across a medical condition identification insignia. Its purpose is to inform health-care providers of the wearer's medical condition in case the person is unresponsive or cannot communicate directly. The information you gather in the AMPLE history can help you to provide care for the patient. The mnemonic AMPLE stands for five elements of the history: allergies, medications, pertinent past medical history, last oral intake (solid or liquid) and events leading to the injury or illness.

Secondary assessment

All patients receive a secondary assessment, which repeats the components of the initial assessment and physical examination. Evaluate stable patients at least every 15 minutes; evaluate unstable patients every 5 minutes or more frequently. The secondary assessment is also an opportunity to check interventions.

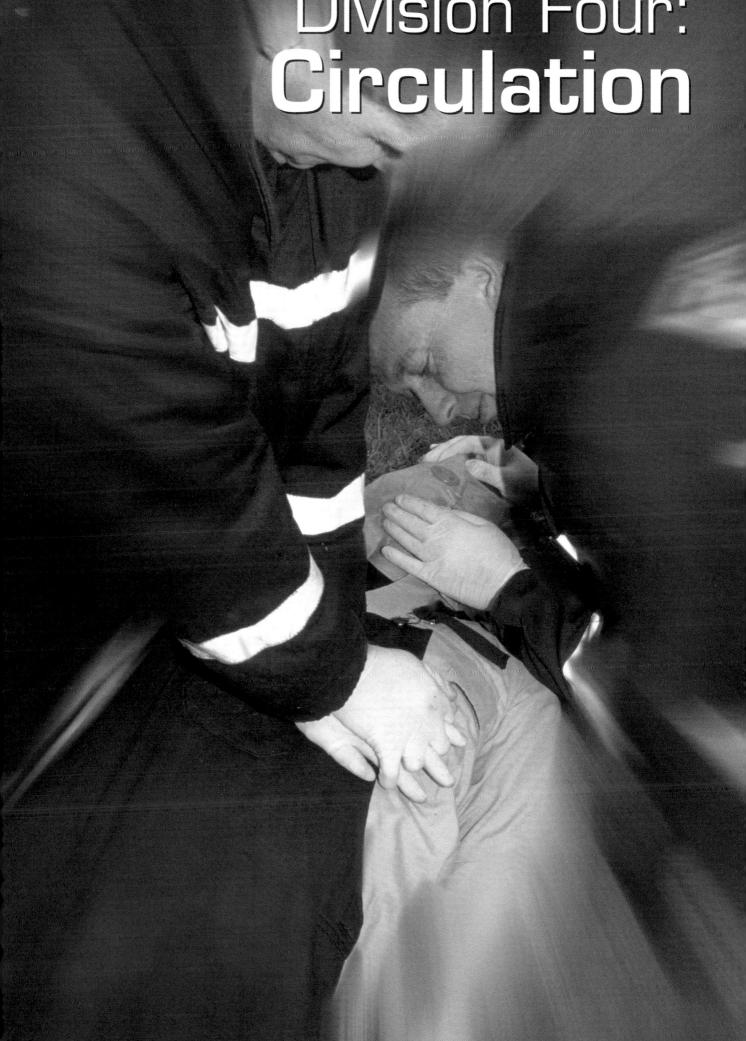

Division Four:
Circulation

Chapter
Seven
Circulation

I. Review of the circulatory system
    A. Function
    B. Anatomy
    C. Physiology

II. Cardiopulmonary resuscitation
    A. Definition
    B. Chain of survival

III. Techniques of adult CPR
    A. Steps of adult CPR

B. Hand position for chest
    compression in the adult
C. Two-rescuer CPR

IV. Techniques of infant and child CPR
    A. Steps of infant and child CPR
    B. Hand position for chest
        compression in the infant
    C. Hand position for chest
        compression in the child

V. Interacting with the patient's family
    and friends

Key terms

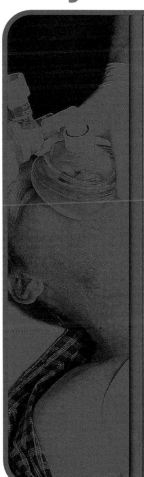

AcBC A mnemonic for the initial protocol to be adopted by the First Responder when performing the primary assessment; it stands for 'Airway with cervical spine control, Breathing and Circulation'.

Advanced life support (ALS)
Cardiopulmonary resuscitation using various medical and paramedical procedures, including intravenous drug administration and using specialised artificial ventilation equipment.

Automated external defibrillator (AED)
Machine used by basic level rescuers to provide an electrical shock to a patient who is not breathing and is pulseless; they are either automatic or semi-automatic.

Basic life support (BLS)
Maintaining an airway and supporting breathing and the circulation without the use of equipment other than a simple airway device or protective shield.

Cardiopulmonary resuscitation (CPR)
The process of one or two rescuers providing artificial ventilations and external chest compressions to a patient that is pulseless and not breathing.

Chain of survival
The term for the optimum process that should be followed for saving a life. The chain consists of: early access, early BLS, early defibrillation and early ALS.

Defibrillation
Delivering an electric shock to the patient's heart to stop a chaotic heart rhythm.

Rescue breathing
The artificial ventilations provided to a non-breathing patient by a rescuer during CPR.

Xiphoid process
The bony protrusion that extends from the lower portion of the sternum.

Objectives

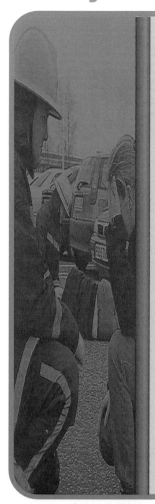

On completion of this chapter you will be able to meet the following objectives:

Cognitive objectives
1. List the reasons for the heart to stop beating.
2. Define the components of cardiopulmonary resuscitation (CPR).
3. Describe each link in the chain of survival.
4. List the steps of one-rescuer adult CPR.
5. Describe the technique of external chest compressions on an adult patient.
6. Describe the technique of external chest compressions on an infant.
7. Describe the technique of external chest compressions on a child.
8. Explain when the First Responder is able to stop CPR.
9. List the steps of two-rescuer adult CPR.
10. List the steps of infant CPR.
11. List the steps of child CPR.

Affective objectives
12. Respond to the feelings that the family of a patient may have during a cardiac event.

13. Demonstrate a caring attitude towards patients with cardiac events who request emergency ambulance services.
14. Place the interests of the patient with a cardiac event as the foremost consideration when making any patient care decision.
15. Communicate empathically with family members and friends of the patient with a cardiac event.

Psychomotor objectives
16. Demonstrate the proper technique of chest compressions on an adult.
17. Demonstrate the proper technique of chest compressions on a child.
18. Demonstrate the proper technique of chest compressions on an infant.
19. Demonstrate the steps of adult one-rescuer CPR.
20. Demonstrate the steps of adult two-rescuer CPR.
21. Demonstrate child CPR.
22. Demonstrate infant CPR.

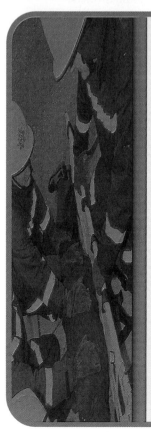

First response

A YOUNG BOY ran into the fire station, shouting, "I can't wake my grand-dad." The crew rushed the short distance to the house.

Upon their arrival, a woman met them at the door and said that her father, Sam, had just collapsed. The man was quickly assessed for responsiveness by gently shaking him and shouting his name. There was no response. A radio message was sent requesting an ambulance and informing the ambulance service that the patient was unresponsive. A fire-fighter opened Sam's airway and assessed that he was not breathing. She used her pocket mask to administer two rescue breaths. She checked his carotid pulse. There was no pulse.

For the next 4 minutes, they performed two-rescuer cardiopulmonary resuscitation (CPR) until the paramedic unit arrived. The crew helped the EMS personnel as they defibrillated the patient and administered medication. Two minutes after the paramedic personnel had arrived, Sam's pulse returned. The rescuers all knew that if Sam had not received effective CPR when he did, his chance of survival would have been drastically reduced.

Almost 170,000 people die in the UK each year from cardiovascular diseases; half these deaths occur outside hospital, with sudden death (collapse) being the first sign of cardiac disease in 20% of the cases. Early CPR, covered in this module, is a major determinant of survival in cardiac arrest.

REVIEW OF THE CIRCULATORY SYSTEM

Function

The circulatory system functions to deliver oxygen and nutrients to the tissues of the body and to remove the waste products from these tissues. Without the continuous beating of the heart, the tissues cannot receive the oxygen and nutrients from the blood that are vital to survival. Later in this chapter, you will learn how chest compressions act to pump the heart and distribute blood to the body when the heart is not beating on its own.

Anatomy

The heart has four chambers. The two upper chambers are the atria, and the two lower chambers are the ventricles. The right atrium receives oxygen-poor blood from the veins of the body and pumps it to the right ventricle. The right ventricle pumps the blood to the lungs, where it is oxygenated. The oxygen-rich blood flows from the lungs into the left atrium and is pumped to the left ventricle. The left ventricle pumps the oxygen-rich blood to the body. Valves in the heart between the chambers and major blood vessels prevent backflow of blood (**Fig. 7.1**)

Arteries are vessels that carry blood away from the heart to the rest of the body. The aorta is the main artery of the body; it originates from the heart and passes in front of the spine in the chest and abdominal cavities. The carotid arteries are the major arteries in the neck; they supply the head and brain with blood. The pulsations of these arteries can be felt on either side of the neck. The artery of the upper arm is the brachial artery. You can palpate its pulsations on the inside of the arm between the elbow and the shoulder. The major artery of the lower arm is the radial artery, and its pulsations can

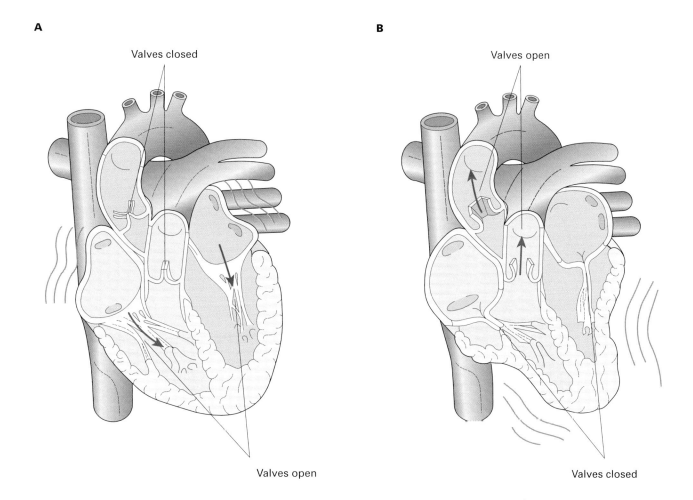

A

Valves closed

Valves open

B

Valves open

Valves closed

Fig. 7.1 Blood flow through the heart. **(a)** The atria pump blood into the ventricles.
(b) The ventricles pump blood into the lungs and the rest of the body.

Circulation

be felt on the thumb side of the wrist. The femoral artery is the major artery of the thigh; it supplies the groin and the lower extremity with blood. You can palpate pulsations from the femoral arteries in the groin (the crease between the abdomen and thigh) on either side of the body (**Fig. 7.2**).

Capillaries are the tiny blood vessels that connect arteries to veins. They are found in all parts of the body and allow the exchange of oxygen and carbon dioxide.

Veins begin at the capillary beds and carry blood back to the heart from the body. Veins carry deoxygenated blood containing waste products (such as carbon dioxide) to the heart, and the heart pumps it to the lungs where the carbon dioxide is eliminated.

Blood is the fluid portion of the circulatory system and it carries oxygen and nutrients to the tissues and carbon dioxide from the tissues. Blood also contains cells that fight disease and infection, and cells that help the blood to clot.

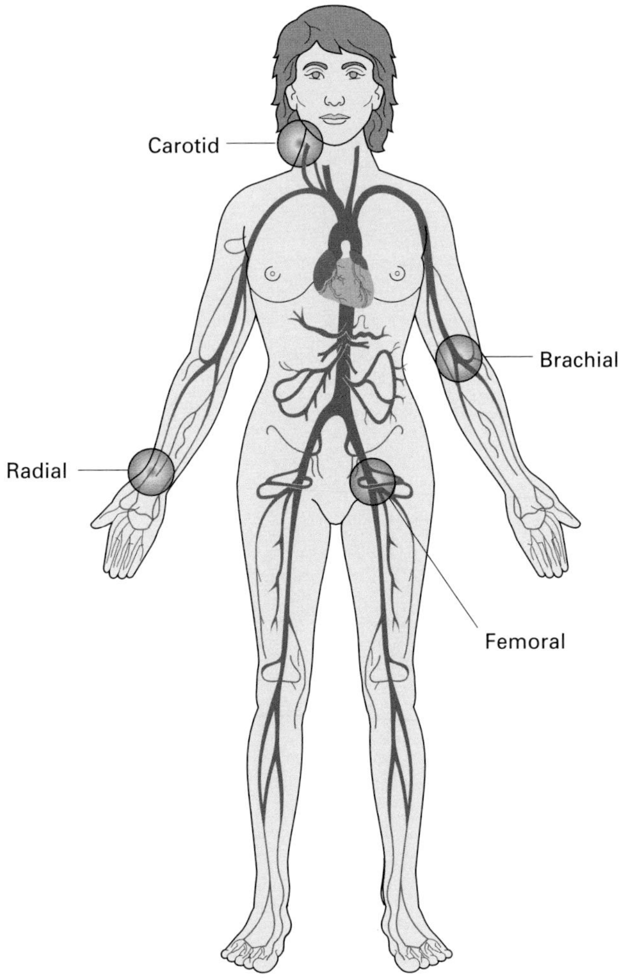

Physiology

When the left ventricle contracts, sending a wave of blood through the arteries, a pulse can be felt. You can palpate the pulse anywhere that an artery passes near the skin surface and over a bone. The most common sites for palpating pulses are the carotid artery in the neck, the radial artery in the wrist, the femoral artery in the groin and the brachial artery in the upper arm.

If the heart stops beating, no blood will flow and the body will not survive. When a patient has no pulse, he or she is in cardiac arrest. Organ damage begins very quickly without blood flow. Brain damage begins within 3-4 minutes of cardiac arrest. Within 8–10 minutes, brain damage becomes irreversible. First Responders use a combination of external chest compressions and artificial ventilations to circulate and oxygenate the blood whenever the heart is not beating. This combination of compressions and ventilations is called 'cardiopulmonary resuscitation' (CPR).

Reasons for the heart to stop beating include heart disease, respiratory arrest (especially in infants and children), drowning, suffocation, congenital heart abnormalities, trauma and bleeding. Some medical emergencies, such as stroke, epilepsy, diabetes, allergic reactions, electrical shock and poisoning, can also result in cardiac arrest. Whatever the reason, First Responders should perform CPR on any patient in cardiac arrest.

Fig. 7.2 Key pulse sites in the body.

Review Questions

Review of the Circulatory System

1. Which of the following arteries can be palpated in the neck?
   A. Carotid
   B. Radial
   C. Brachial
   D. Femoral

2. The ventricles of the heart pump blood to the lungs and the body. True or False?

3. The First Responder's emergency medical care for all patients in cardiac arrest is _____.

4. CPR is a combination of _____, to circulate blood, and _____, to oxygenate the blood.

5. Of the following, which statement is TRUE?
   A. First Responders can do nothing if the patient is in cardiac arrest.
   B. Organ damage is rare in cardiac arrest patients.
   C. Brain damage begins 4–6 minutes after cardiac arrest.
   D. You should only start CPR if you know the cause of cardiac arrest.

1. A; 2. True; 3. CPR; 4. compression, ventilations; 5. C

CARDIOPULMONARY RESUSCITATION

Definition

Cardiopulmonary resuscitation (CPR) combines artificial ventilation and external chest compressions in order to oxygenate and circulate blood when a patient is in cardiac arrest. By performing external chest compressions, the rescuer depresses the sternum (breast bone) to change the pressure in the chest. This causes enough blood flow to sustain life for a short time.

CPR cannot sustain life indefinitely and is only effective for a short period. The effectiveness of oxygen delivery to the body decreases the longer CPR is performed. Often, the patient needs an electrical shock to the heart, called defibrillation, in order to survive. CPR increases the amount of time after cardiac arrest that defibrillation will be effective. Therefore, you must start CPR as early as possible. This keeps the heart pumping and the blood circulating until a defibrillator is available.

Chain of survival

The successful resuscitation outside the hospital of a patient in cardiac arrest depends on the links in the chain of survival. The chain of survival consists of:
* early access;
* early basic life support (BLS);
* early defibrillation; and
* early advanced life support (ALS).

Weak links in the chain lower survival rates.

Early access

Early access is dependent upon public education and awareness of cardiac emergencies and the EMS system. The public must be informed of the signs and symptoms of a cardiac emergency and know when and how to contact emergency medical services. Rapid recognition of the emergency and rapid notification of EMS is key to this link in the chain of survival. **Box 7.1** lists signs and symptoms of a cardiac emergency.

For adult patients, members of the public are taught to 'phone first', even before they start CPR, provided that the adult casualty has not sustained a cardiac arrest from trauma or near-drowning. Having EMS personnel able to provide advanced life support on the way to hospital is important. By gaining early access into the system, callers can also receive pre-arrival instructions and advice on CPR. Callers may be given instructions on how to handle the situation and what they can do to help.

Early basic life support (BLS)

The lay public and First Responders provide early BLS. Public education provides family members, workmates and bystanders with the knowledge to begin CPR on a patient in cardiac arrest. First Responders trained in CPR are responsible for ensuring that CPR is done promptly and effectively.

Box 7.1	Signs and Symptoms of a Cardiac Emergency

* Squeezing, dull pressure or pain in the chest that commonly relates to the arms, neck, jaw or upper back
* Sudden onset of sweating
* Difficulty breathing
* Anxiety or irritability
* Feeling of impending doom
* Abnormal and sometimes irregular pulse rate (high or low)
* Abnormal blood pressure (different from the patient's normal blood pressure)
* Pain or discomfort in the abdomen (severe indigestion)
* Nausea or vomiting

Early defibrillation

An automated external defibrillator (AED) is a machine used by basic-level rescuers to provide an electrical shock to a patient who is pulseless and not breathing. Early defibrillation can make the difference between life and death for patients in cardiac arrest, even more so than early BLS. Check your local protocols to find out if this skill is part of your First Responder curriculum. Refer to Appendix D ('Automated external defibrillation') for details on the use of the automated external defibrillator.

Early advanced life support (ALS)

Early advanced life support (ALS) by paramedics is the final element in the chain of survival. If you are a single rescuer of an adult patient with a cardiac arrest that is not due to trauma or near drowning, the European Resuscitation Council advises that you telephone 999 *before* starting CPR. This provides the shortest time between the cardiac arrest and the arrival of personnel trained in ALS, who can use defibrillation and medications to help the patient. If the adult patient has suffered cardiac arrest that is due to trauma or near drowning, activate EMS *after* administering one minute of CPR. If each link in the chain of survival is completed, the better the chance of survival for the patient. The resuscitative effort is a continuum of care beginning at a basic level and progressing towards an advanced level as soon as possible.

Some First Responders will also learn the skills of early defibrillation using an AED. As a First Responder, you must learn what responsibilities you have in the chain of survival according to your local protocols.

TECHNIQUES OF ADULT CPR

CPR is indicated when a patient is not breathing and does not have a pulse. CPR is performed in several steps of assessment and intervention – the 'AcBCs of

Circulation

CPR'. Many techniques of CPR are similar in the adult, child and infant. When no differences are described, the technique is the same for all patients.

The reasons for beginning CPR are very specific: the patient must be pulseless and not breathing. There are also specific situations when you can stop CPR once you have started. Refer to **Box 7.2** for the reasons to discontinue CPR after you have started.

Steps of adult CPR

Step 1: Assess responsiveness and activate EMS

The First Responder arriving on the scene may be the first person to encounter and care for the patient. Advanced level rescuers should also be on their way to the scene. If they are not, the First Responder should request the attendance of an ambulance. As always, assure a safe scene before approaching the patient. Be sure to follow universal precautions while performing CPR.

First, the rescuer must determine unresponsiveness in the patient. This can be done by gently shaking the patient and asking, "Are you OK?" If there is no response in an adult patient, the First Responder should activate EMS immediately. If there is only one rescuer, the patient is adult and the cause of unconsciousness is not drowning or trauma, call the ambulance service after it has been established that the patient is not breathing. If you are alone with a casualty whose injuries are related to trauma or who has suffered near-drowning, perform CPR for 1 minute before calling an ambulance. If there are two rescuers, one can contact the ambulance service while the other continues the assessment. If paramedic personnel are already on their way, you can skip this step.

If the patient is responsive, monitor the airway and interact with the patient to find out why he or she needs help. Always have an understanding and caring attitude towards patients needing your care. Keep the patient calm and reassure him or her that an ambulance is on the way. Complete the First Responder physical examination.

Step 2: 'Ac' is for airway with cervical spine control

The next step in the assessment of the unresponsive patient is opening the airway (**Fig. 7.3**). The patient must first be lying on the back on a firm surface. If the patient is lying face down, roll the patient on to the back. If you suspect the patient has been injured, take precautions to stabilise the cervical spine as you roll the patient. Move the patient so that the spinal column remains in a straight line. Techniques for moving patients with possible spinal injuries are discussed in Chapter 10, 'Injuries to muscles and bones'.

In a medical situation the rescuer kneels by the patient's side and uses the head-tilt, chin-lift manoeuvre to open the airway, as described in Chapter 5 (The airway).

Box 7.2	**When to Discontinue CPR**

CPR started by a First Responder should be continued until:
- Effective circulation and breathing have been restored
- Care is transferred to another provider who is trained to First Responder level or higher
- Care is transferred to a physician
- The rescuer is unable to continue CPR because of hazards, exhaustion or the endangerment of others

---

In situations where trauma is suspected, use the jaw thrust without head tilt to open the airway, which is also described in Chapter 5.

Step 3: 'B' is for breathing

Determine if the patient is breathing adequately on his or her own or if assistance is required. Once the airway is opened, the rescuer places his or her cheek and ear close to the patient's mouth, while looking towards the patient's chest. Look to see if the chest is rising, listen for breathing and feel any air that may be coming from the patient's mouth (**Fig. 7.4**). This should be done for not more than 10 seconds.

If the patient is breathing adequately and there is no trauma, place the patient in the recovery position (**Fig. 7.5**). Carefully move the patient on to the side without compromising the integrity of the spine. The patient's airway remains open much more easily in this position, and fluids drain from the mouth.

If the patient is not breathing at all or is not breathing adequately, rescue breathing should be provided (**Fig. 7.6**). Providing artificial ventilations to a patient who is not breathing is called rescue breathing. Rescue breathing can be accomplished by mouth-to-mouth ventilations, mouth-to-barrier device ventilations or mouth-to-mask ventilations. Refer to Chapter 5 ('The airway') for a review of these techniques. If you are trained and have the

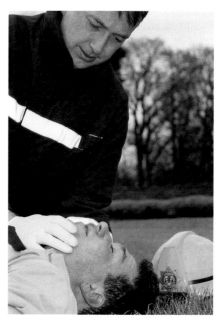

Fig. 7.3 If the patient is unresponsive, the next step is to open the airway.

equipment, you can also ventilate the patient with a bag–valve–mask or flow-restricted, oxygen-powered ventilation device, as described in Appendix B ('Advanced First Responder ventilation techniques').

Ventilate the adult patient with about 400–500 ml of air for each breath, at a rate of 10–12 breaths per minute. Each ventilation should take 1.5–2 seconds. If the air does not go in on the first attempt at ventilation, reposition the airway to assure that it is open. If the air still will not go in, then refer to the foreign body airway obstruction manoeuvre (see Chapter 5, 'The airway'). Make up to a total of five attempts to achieve two effective breaths.

Step 4: 'C' is for circulation

After the airway is open and breathing has been assessed, determine the circulatory status. The rescuer checks the carotid pulse in the neck of the adult patient for not more than 10 seconds. Maintain the head-tilt,

chin-lift manoeuvre throughout this process. Find the prominence (Adam's apple) on the patient's neck and place your index and middle fingers on it. Slide the fingers to the side of the neck that is closest to you until they are in the groove between the trachea and the muscles. This is where you can gently palpate the carotid pulse (**Fig. 7.7**).

If a pulse is found, but the patient is not breathing, the rescuer should perform rescue breathing at a rate of 10–12 breaths per minute (one breath every 5 seconds) for the adult patient. Stop about every minute to reassess the status of the patient's breathing and circulation. Take no more than 10 seconds each time.

If no pulse is found, the patient is in cardiac arrest and you must begin external chest compressions. Again, the patient should be supine on a firm, flat surface for the compressions to be effective. The rescuer's hand position for chest compressions varies with the age of the patient.

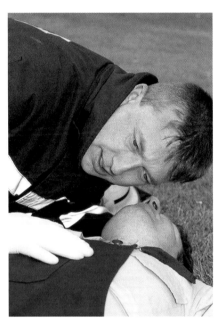

Fig. 7.4 Look, listen and feel for breathing.

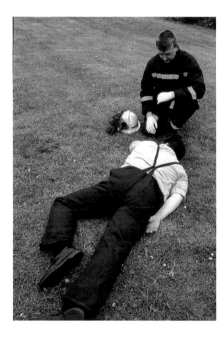

Fig. 7.5 If no trauma is suspected and the patient is breathing, place the patient in the recovery position.

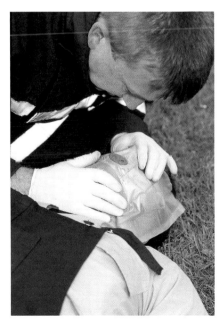

Fig. 7.6 If the patient is not breathing, provide artificial ventilations.

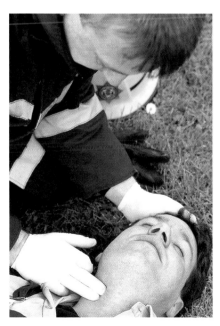

Fig. 7.7 Assess the carotid pulse in the adult patient.

Circulation

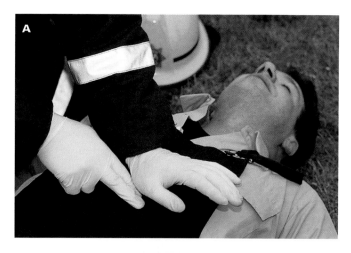

Hand position for chest compressions in the adult

To find the correct hand position for chest compressions on the adult patient, locate the edge of the ribs on the side of the patient closest to you. Trace the ribs to the centre of the patient until the ribs meet the sternum and the xiphoid process. (The xiphoid process is the end of the sternum closest to the patient's abdomen.) Place two fingers on the xiphoid process with one hand and the heel of the other hand over the lower half of the sternum (beside the two fingers, not on top of them). Then lace the heel of the other hand on top of the one placed on the sternum. The fingers may be interlaced or simply rested on one other, but they should be off the chest (**Fig. 7.8**).

To perform compressions, the rescuer leans directly over the patient, so that his or her shoulders are over the patient's sternum so as to be able to provide compressions that are straight down. The rescuer's knees should be one shoulder's width apart to provide a stable base. The arms are kept straight and locked (**Fig. 7.9**). Leaning forward and bending at the hip joint, the rescuer should exert enough pressure to compress the sternum 4–5 cm for the adult patient. Release pressure between each compression to let blood flow to the heart. The compression and relaxation phases should be equal. The hands should remain on the chest at all times so that the correct position is not lost. Movement should be rhythmic, rather than jerky or bouncing. The rate of compressions should be 100 per minute for the adult patient. **Box 7.4** lists the steps for adult one-rescuer CPR.

The chances of the heart returning to effective cardiac output without ALS skills are remote, and therefore time should not be wasted by further checks of pulse unless there are definite signs of circulation, such as movement (including swallowing or breathing if more than an occasional gasp). A pulse check should then be made, taking no more than 10 seconds.

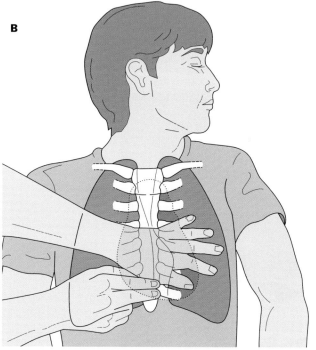

Fig. 7.8 (a) and **(b)** Correct hand positioning for chest compressions in the adult patient.

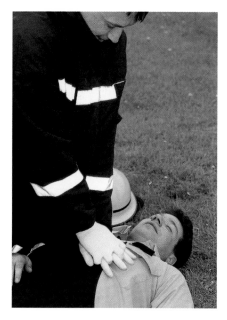

Fig. 7.9 Correct position to perform chest compressions on an adult patient.

Even when CPR is performed properly, chest compressions can cause broken ribs, bruising or other injuries. Do not stop CPR even if you suspect that there may be an injury to the ribs or chest wall. If the patient is in cardiac arrest, always perform CPR.

Two-rescuer CPR

Adult CPR can be performed with one or two rescuers. Two-rescuer CPR is much more efficient and less tiring than one-rescuer CPR. In two-rescuer CPR (**Fig. 7.10**), one rescuer performs rescue breathing while the other performs chest compressions. **Box 7.5** lists the steps for adult two-rescuer CPR. If the rescuer who is performing compressions becomes fatigued, the rescuers may switch positions at the direction of the rescuer at the chest. During two-rescuer CPR, the rescuer at the airway can palpate for a pulse at the carotid artery while the other rescuer is doing compressions. If the compressions are effective, a pulse should be felt. Refer to **Table 7.1** for a summary of adult CPR.

The chances of the heart returning to effective cardiac output without ALS skills are remote, and therefore time should not be wasted by further checks of pulse, unless there are definite signs of circulation such as movement (including swallowing or breathing if more than an occasional gasp). A pulse check should then be made, taking no more than 10 seconds.

Fig. 7.10 Two-rescuer CPR is more efficient and less tiring than one-rescuer CPR.

Box 7.4	**Steps of Adult One-Rescuer CPR**

One-rescuer adult CPR should follow these guidelines:
1. Determine unresponsiveness
2. Activate the ambulance service.
3. Position the patient and open the airway
4. Assess breathing for up to 10 seconds
5. If the patient is breathing and there is no trauma, place him or her in the recovery position. If the patient is not breathing, give two rescue breaths
6. Assess circulation for up to 10 seconds. If the patient has a pulse, but is not breathing, perform rescue breathing at 10–12 breaths per minute
7. If the patient does not have a pulse, find hand position and begin chest compressions
   - Perform 15 chest compressions at a rate of 100 per minute
   - Open the airway and deliver two rescue breaths
   - Begin 15 more chest compressions
8. Perform four cycles of 15 compressions to two ventilations
9. Reassess the pulse for up to 10 seconds. If the patient has a pulse, reassess breathing:
   - If breathing is present, keep reassessing the patient and place him or her in the recovery position
   - If breathing is absent, continue rescue breathing at 10–12 breaths per minute
   - If the patient does not have a pulse, begin a cycle of 15 chest compressions
10. If CPR is continued, stop to reassess the patient every few minutes

Box 7.5	**Steps of Adult Two-Rescuer CPR**

1. Rescuer 1 assesses responsiveness. If the patient is unresponsive, Rescuer 2 activates additional EMS personnel
2. Rescuer 1 opens the airway and assesses breathing:
   - If breathing is present, rescuers place the patient in the recovery position
   - If breathing is absent, Rescuer 1 performs two rescue breaths over 1.5–2 seconds each
3. Rescuer 1 assesses circulation:
   - If a pulse is present, but breathing is absent, Rescuer 1 continues rescue breathing at a rate of 10–12 breaths per minute
   - If a pulse is absent, Rescuer 2 finds hand position and performs five chest compressions at a rate of 100 per minute
4. After every five compressions, Rescuer 1 performs one rescue breath (1.5–2 seconds each). Rescuer 2 pauses so air can fill the lungs.
5. Perform 20 cycles of five compressions to one ventilation then reassess the pulse:
   - If there is a pulse, reassess breathing and treat accordingly
   - If there is no pulse, continue with five compressions to one ventilation. Reassess every few minutes

Circulation

Table 7.1	Adult CPR		
Adult CPR	**One-rescuer CPR**	**Two-rescuer CPR**	
Compression	15 compressions	5 compressions	
Ventilations	2 ventilations	1 ventilation	
Rescue breathing	10–12 per minute 1.5–2 seconds each		
Compression rate	100 per minute		
Number of initial cycles	4 cycles	20 cycles	
Depth of compressions	4.0–5.0 cm		

First Responder Alert

Make sure your hands are not placed over the xiphoid process while performing chest compressions. If compressions are performed over the xiphoid process, that piece of bone could break off and damage internal organs.

Review Questions

Cardiopulmonary Resuscitation and Techniques of Adult CPR

1. List the following steps of adult CPR in order:
   A. Assess responsiveness
   B. Assess circulation
   C. Assess breathing
   D. Call EMS
   E. Open airway

2. You should perform rescue breathing at 10–12 breaths per minute only on patients with no pulse. True or False?

3. Compressions should be done at a rate of _____ per minute in the adult patient.

4. For a non-trauma situation, the patient's airway should be opened with a _____ manoeuvre.

1. A, D, E, C, B; 2. False, patients with a pulse, but not breathing should have rescue breathing performed; 3. 100; 4. Head-tilt, chin-lift

TECHNIQUES OF INFANT AND CHILD CPR

Many of the techniques used in infant and child CPR are similar to those used in adult CPR, and where this is the case, the adult section will be referenced. As with adult CPR, infant and child CPR follows a step-by-step assessment process.

Steps of infant and child CPR

Step 1: Assess responsiveness
The rescuer must first assess responsiveness. Tap on the infant or child's shoulder or shout his or her name.

If the patient is unresponsive, a single rescuer should shout for help and then administer CPR for 1 minute before activating EMS. Infants and children suffer cardiac arrest primarily as a result of respiratory problems, unlike adults, in whom cardiac arrest usually results from a cardiac problem. Because of this, infants and children benefit from the immediate treatment of opening the airway, providing oxygen and circulating the oxygen to the tissues. If a second rescuer is available, he or she should contact EMS while the first rescuer continues the assessment.

Step 2: 'Ac' is for airway with cervical spine control
Maintaining an open airway is one of the most important aspects of infant and child CPR because the primary reason for cardiac arrest is respiratory arrest. The airway must be opened as soon as possible (**Fig 7.11**).

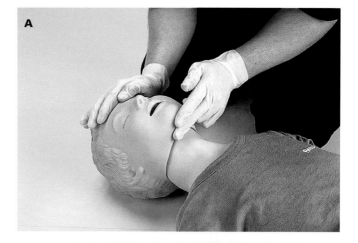

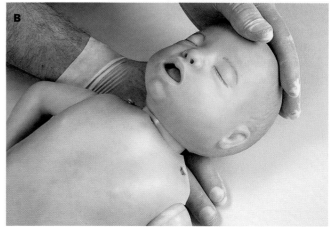

Fig. 7.11 (a) and **(b)** After assessing responsiveness, open the airway.

In a medical situation, open the airway with a head-tilt, chin-lift manoeuvre. The technique for infants and children is the same as for the adult who has not suffered trauma. The rescuer gently tilts the head back to the neutral position. Be careful not to put pressure on the fleshy part of the neck.

If you suspect that the patient has traumatic injuries, open the patient's airway using the jaw thrust without head tilt. The procedure is the same as the adult jaw thrust.

Step 3: 'B' is for breathing

Once the airway is open, the rescuer assesses the patient's breathing in the same manner that was used for the adult (**Fig. 7.12**). If the patient is breathing inadequately, perform rescue breathing.

Rescue breathing can be performed by mouth-to-mouth ventilations, mouth-to-barrier device ventilations or mouth-to-mouth ventilations (**Fig. 7.13**). If a mask is available, it should be used if it fits properly. However, do not delay treatment to find a mask. If the patient is under 1 year old, the rescuer should places his or her mouth over the mouth and nose of the patient to create a seal. If the patient is over 1 year old, the rescuer places his or her mouth over the patient's mouth and creates a seal that way. Use the index finger and thumb

of the hand on the forehead to pinch the nose closed. Administer slow rescue breaths (1–1.5 seconds per breath), attempting up to five rescue breaths to achieve two effective ventilations, and observe the rise and fall of the patient's chest with each breath. The volume of air should be enough to make the patient's chest rise. For the infant and child, the rate of rescue breathing is one breath every 3 seconds (20 breaths per minute).

Step 4: 'C' is for circulation

After assessing airway and breathing, the rescuer assesses the circulation.

For patients under 1 year old, the pulse is checked in the brachial artery of the upper arm (**Fig. 7.14**). The rescuer should place his or her thumb on the outside of the arm between the elbow and the shoulder, and then press the index and middle finger on the inside of the arm to palpate the pulse. If the infant has a pulse but is not breathing, perform rescue breathing at a rate of 20 breaths per minute (once every 3 seconds). For children over the age of 1 year, check the pulse in the carotid artery of the neck (**Fig. 7.15**). If the pulse is present, the rescuer provides rescue breathing at a rate of 20 breaths per minute (once every 3 seconds). After giving 20 breaths (that is, after about 1 minute), activate the EMS system.

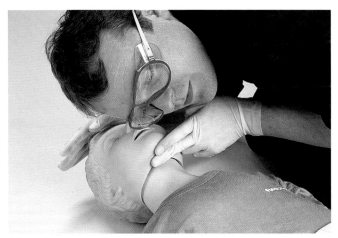

Fig. 7.12 Assess for breathing by looking, listening and feeling for respiration.

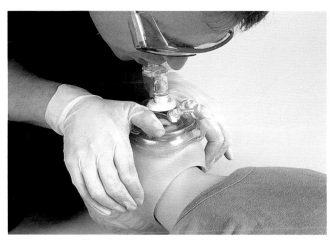

Fig. 7.13 Ventilate the patient if not breathing on his or her own.

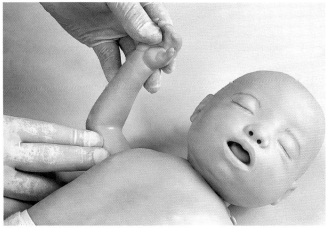

Fig. 7.14 Assess circulation in the infant by palpating the brachial artery.

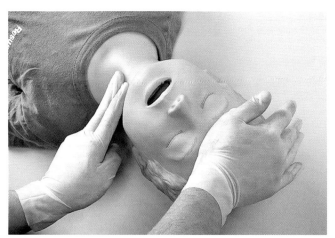

Fig. 7.15 Assess circulation in the child by palpating the carotid artery.

Circulation

Hand position for chest compression in the infant

If the infant does not have a pulse, place the infant on to a firm surface. Keep one hand on the patient's head to maintain a head tilt. Place the index finger of the other hand across the nipples of the patient. The next two fingers are placed beside the index finger. Lift the index finger from the chest; compressions are done with the middle and ring fingers (**Fig. 7.16**). Avoid compressing over the xiphoid process. Compress about one-third of the depth of the chest. Perform at least 100 compressions per minute for an infant.

Pause after five compressions to give one ventilation. Perform 20 cycles (that is, about 1 minute) and reassess

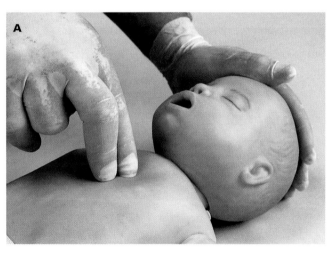

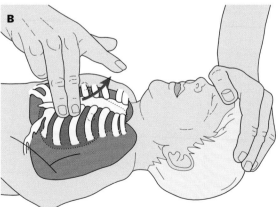

Fig. 7.16 (a) and **(b)** Correct finger position for chest compressions for an infant.

the patient. If you are alone, activate EMS at this time. If the patient's breathing and pulse return, place the infant in the recovery position. If only the pulse returns, continue with rescue breathing. If the pulse does not return or if it is less than 60 beats per minute, continue with compressions and ventilations and reassess every few minutes. **Box 7.6** lists the steps of infant CPR.

Hand position for chest compression in the child

If the patient does not have a pulse, provide chest compressions. Perform compressions for the child (aged over 1 year) on a firm, flat surface. Place your closest hand on the patient's forehead to maintain the head tilt throughout the CPR sequence. With the other hand, locate the margin of the rib cage and trace to the sternum, as in adult CPR. Visualise the location of the xiphoid process and place the heel of the hand above that area on the sternum (**Fig. 7.17**). The chest is compressed to about one-third of its depth with one hand.

The compressions should be smooth and the fingers should not lie on the chest. This hand should remain on the chest so that placement does not have to be found again.

The compressions are done at a rate of 100 per minute. At the end of every fifth compression, pause to perform one rescue breath (lasting 1–1.5 seconds).

Box 7.6	**Steps of Infant CPR**

1. Assess responsiveness
2. Open the airway using the head-tilt, chin-lift for medical patients or the jaw thrust for trauma patients
3. Assess breathing:
   - If the patient is breathing, place him or her in the recovery position
   - If the patient is not breathing, administer two rescue breaths (1 to 1.5 seconds each)
4. Assess circulation using the brachial artery:
   - If the patient has a pulse, continue rescue breathing at a rate of 20 per minute (every 3 seconds)
   - If the patient does not have a pulse, perform chest compressions at a rate of at least 100 per minute
5. Perform 20 cycles (about 1 minute) of five compressions to one ventilation and then reassess the patient
   - If the patient has regained pulse and breathing, place him or her in the recovery position.
   - If the patient has regained a pulse, but not breathing, continue with rescue breathing at a rate of 20 per minute
   - If the patient has not regained a pulse, continue with cycles of five compressions to one ventilation and reassess the patient every few minutes
6. If only one rescuer is present, activate EMS after the initial 20 cycles of CPR

Perform 20 cycles of five compressions to one ventilation and then reassess the patient. If you are a lone rescuer, the ambulance service should be contacted at this time. **Box 7.7** lists the steps of child CPR.

If the child is over the age of about 8 years, it may be necessary to use the 'adult' two-handed method of chest compression to achieve an adequate depth of compression, and the ratio changes to 15 chest compressions to two ventilations.

If the patient regains breathing and a pulse, place him or her in the recovery position. If the patient regains a pulse but is not breathing, continue with rescue breathing. If the patient does not have a pulse and is not breathing continue with CPR and reassess every few minutes.

In older children, CPR may be performed with two rescuers. One rescuer will ventilate the patient and the other will perform chest compressions, the same as in adult two-rescuer CPR. Two-rescuer CPR is not performed on infants because they are too small for the two rescuers to work together without interfering with each other; therefore one-rescuer CPR is performed. Refer to **Table 7.2** for a summary of infant and child CPR.

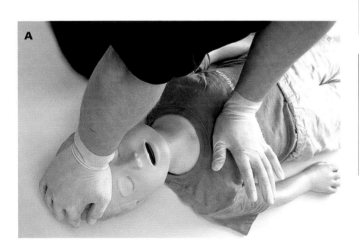

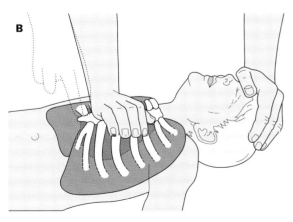

Fig. 7.17 (a) and **(b)** Correct hand position for chest compressions on a child.

Box 7.7	**Steps of Child CPR**

1. Assess responsiveness
2. Open the airway using the head-tilt, chin-lift for medical patients or the jaw thrust for trauma patients
3. Assess breathing
   - If the patient is breathing, place him or her in the recovery position
   - If the patient is not breathing, administer two rescue breaths (1–1.5 seconds)
4. Assess circulation, using the carotid artery:
   - If the patient has a pulse, continue with rescue breathing at a rate of 20 per minute
   - If the patient does not have a pulse, perform chest compression at a rate of 100 per minute
5. Perform 20 cycles (about 1 minute) of five compressions to one ventilation and then reassess the patient
   - If the patient has regained a pulse and is breathing, place him or her in the recovery position
   - If the patient has regained a pulse, but not breathing, continue with rescue breathing
   - If the patient has not regained a pulse, continue with cycles of five compressions to one ventilation and reassess every few minutes
6. If only one rescuer is present, activate EMS after the initial 20 cycles of CPR

First Responder Alert

If only one rescuer is present, activate EMS after performing CPR for 20 cycles (about 1 minute) in the infant or child patient.

Table 7.2	**Summary of Infant and Child CPR**	
	Infant	**Child**
Age	Under 1 year	1–8 years
Breathing	1–1.5 seconds each: rate 20/minute	
Pulse	Brachial artery	Carotid artery
Compressions	Two fingers on sternum; rate at least 100/minute	Heel of hand on sternum; rate 100/minute
Ratio	5 compressions : 1 ventilation	
Compression depth	1.5–2.5 cm	2.5–4.0 cm

Circulation

INTERACTING WITH THE PATIENT'S FAMILY AND FRIENDS

The responsibilities of the First Responder are not limited to care of the patient. The family members and friends of the patient may be experiencing extreme anxiety and fear about the situation. The First Responder should interact with understanding and empathy towards the family. First Responders must not offer diagnosis or advanced level treatment suggestions, but they can offer reassurance and a caring attitude.

CHAPTER SUMMARY

Review of the circulatory system

The circulatory system functions to deliver oxygen and nutrients to the tissues of the body and to remove waste products. The heart has four chambers: two atria and two ventricles. Arteries carry blood away from the heart and veins carry blood to the heart. Capillaries connect arteries to veins. Blood is the fluid portion of the circulatory system and it carries oxygen to the tissues and carbon dioxide away from the tissues.

When the left ventricle contracts, it sends a wave of blood through the arteries and a pulse can be felt. You can palpate the pulse anywhere that an artery passes near the skin surface and over a bone. When a patient has no pulse, he or she is in cardiac arrest. Organ damage will begin very quickly. External chest compression are combined with artificial ventilations to oxygenate the blood and circulate it; this is called cardiopulmonary resuscitation (CPR).

Cardiopulmonary resuscitation

CPR cannot sustain life indefinitely and is only effective for a short time. The effectiveness of delivering oxygen to the tissues decreases the longer CPR is performed. The chain of survival consists of: early access, early basic life support (BLS), early defibrillation and early advanced life support (ALS).

Techniques of adult CPR

CPR is indicated when the patient is not breathing and does not have a pulse. The performance of CPR is done in several steps of assessment and intervention – the 'AcBCs of CPR'. These steps consist of:
- assessing responsiveness and activating EMS;
- opening and monitoring the airway, and stabilising the spine;
- monitoring breathing and providing artificial respirations;
- assessing the circulation and providing chest compressions; and
- reassessing and monitoring the patient.

Adult CPR can be performed by one or two rescuers. If the adult patient has suffered cardiac arrest as a result of trauma or near-drowning, a single rescuer should remember to activate EMS after administering 1 minute of CPR.

Techniques of infant and child CPR

You should begin the assessment, open the airway, stabilise the spine and assess breathing the same as you would for an adult patient. If the patient is not breathing, deliver rescue breaths, then assess the carotid pulse in the child or the brachial pulse in the infant. Perform chest compressions on the lower half of the sternum with two fingers on the infant, with one hand on the child. Remember to activate EMS after 1 minute of CPR in infants and children.

Interacting with the patient's family and friends

Although the primary responsibility of the First Responder is the patient, the family and friends of the patient may also need comfort and reassurance.

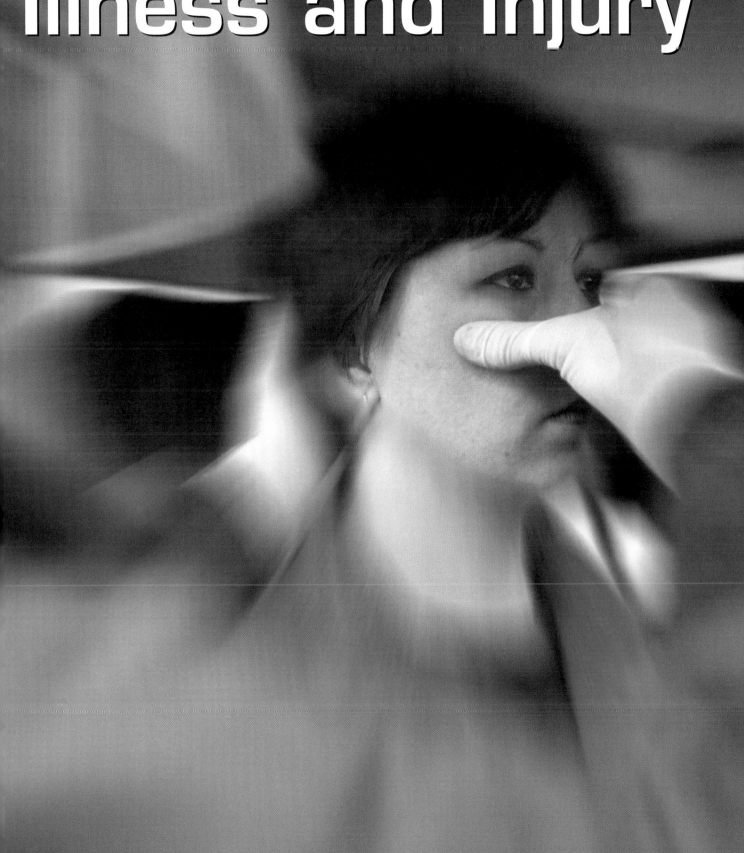

Division Five:
Illness and Injury

Chapter Eight

Medical Emergencies

I.   General medical complaints

II.   Specific medical complaints
    A. Altered mental status
    B. Fitting
    C. Exposure to cold
    D. Near-drowning
    E. Exposure to heat

III. Behavioural emergencies
    A. Behavioural changes

Key terms

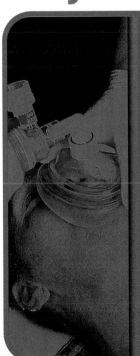

Altered mental status
> An ailment resulting in a patient's increased or decreased awareness, which can range from hyperactivity to unconsciousness.

Behaviour
> The manner in which a person acts or performs.

Convulsions
> Jerky, violent muscle contractions.

Drowning
> Death due to suffocation by immersion in water.

Fitting
> A type of impaired consciousness that may be characterised by convulsions or other sudden changes in responsiveness.

Hyperthermia
> A rise in the body temperature.

Hypothermia
> A drop in the body temperature.

Impaired consciousness
> A form of altered mental status in which there is a sudden or gradual decrease in a patient's level of responsiveness.

Near-drowning
> Initial survival following immersion in water.

Objectives

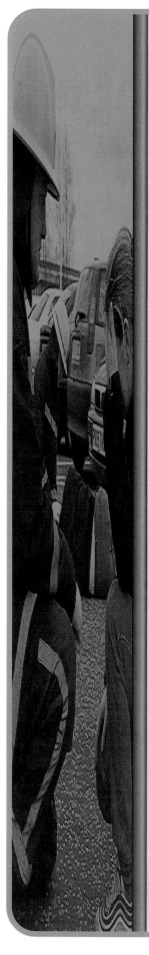

On completion of this chapter you will be able to meet the following objectives:

Cognitive objectives
1. Identify a patient who presents with a general medical complaint.
2. Explain the steps in providing emergency medical care to a patient with a general medical complaint.
3. Identify a patient who presents with a specific medical complaint of altered mental status.
4. Explain the steps in providing emergency medical care to a patient with altered mental status.
5. Identify a patient who presents with a specific medical complaint of fitting.
6. Explain the steps in providing emergency medical care to a patient who is fitting.
7. Identify a patient who presents with a specific medical complaint of exposure to cold.
8. Explain the steps in providing emergency medical care to a patient with an exposure to cold.
9. Identify a patient who presents with a specific medical complaint of near-drowning.
10. Explain the steps in providing emergency medical care to a near-drowning patient.
11. Identify a patient who presents with a specific medical complaint of exposure to heat.
12. Explain the steps in providing emergency medical care to a patient with an exposure of heat.
13. Identify a patient who presents with a specific medical complaint of behavioural change.
14. Explain the steps in providing emergency medical care to a patient with a behavioural change.
15. Identify a patient who presents with a specific complaint of a psychological crisis.
16. Explain the steps in providing emergency medical care to a patient with a psychological crisis.

Affective objectives
17. Attend to the feelings of a patient and the patient's family when dealing with a patient with a general medical complaint.
18. Attend to the feelings of a patient and the patient's family when dealing with a patient with a specific medical complaint.

19. Explain the rationale for modifying your behaviour towards a patient with a behavioural emergency.
20. Place the interests of a patient with a general medical complaint as the foremost consideration when making any and all patient care decisions.
21. Communicate empathically with a patient with a general medical complaint, as well as with family members and friends of the patient.
22. Demonstrate a caring attitude towards patients with a specific medical complaint who request emergency medical services.
23. Place the interests of a patient with a specific medical complaint as the foremost consideration when making any and all patient care decisions.
24. Communicate empathically with patients with a specific medical complaint, as well as with family members and friends of the patient.
25. Demonstrate a caring attitude towards patients with a behavioural problem who request emergency medical services.
26. Place the interests of a patient with a behavioural problem as the foremost consideration when making any patient care decision.
27. Communicate empathically with a patient with a behavioural problem, as well as with family members and friends of the patient.

Psychomotor objectives
28. Demonstrate the steps in providing emergency medical care to a patient with a general medical complaint.
29. Demonstrate the steps in providing emergency medical care to a patient with altered mental status.
30. Demonstrate the steps in providing emergency medical care to a patient who is fitting.
31. Demonstrate the steps in providing emergency medical care to a patient with an exposure to cold.
32. Demonstrate the steps in providing emergency medical care to a near-drowning patient.
33. Demonstrate the steps in providing emergency medical care to a patient with an exposure to heat.
34. Demonstrate the steps in providing emergency medical care to a patient with a behavioural change.

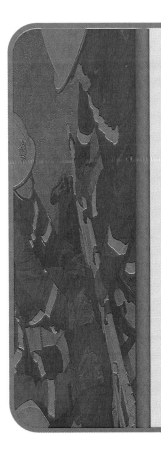

First response

GEORGE AND PAUL were attending a call to a car fire when their officer-in-charge detailed them to check out a report of a 64-year-old woman with shortness of breath, in a nearby house. On the way, George admitted to Paul that he never really liked those medical emergencies. "I know what to do if they are in cardiac arrest," he confessed, "but I never know what to say to these patients." Paul smiled and said, "I used to feel the same way, then I realised that just being there and acting professionally is the key; it makes the patient and the family feel so much better if you are just compassionate."

The patient was dripping with sweat as she huffed and puffed to catch her breath. Her husband was very distraught as he watched his wife struggle to breathe. George watched as Paul took control of the situation. He was calm, reassuring, kind and polite. He held the woman's hand and he looked her in the eye and said, "Everything is under control. The ambulance will be here in about 5 minutes and they will get you to the hospital in no time." You could see the tension melt off her husband's face when Paul turned to him and said with a smile, "She'll be all right; we'll look after her until the ambulance arrives."

Paul took an AMPLE history, and he was giving the ambulance crew a quick update when George realised that Paul was right – you don't have to be doing CPR or clearing an airway to make a difference.

Some of the patients that you attend as a First Responder will have called for help because of medical problems. There are, however, many causes of medical problems. Fortunately, as a First Responder you will not have to diagnose what is wrong with the patient. You will gather information and provide care based on your assessment findings. One of the most important roles that you will play in these cases is the ability to provide comfort and reassurance to the patient and family. These situations are very scary to the public. Your calm, professional and competent demeanour will provide great support in these moments of crisis.

This chapter covers some of the major medical situations you will encounter. The most common situation will be the patient who has a general medical complaint. The patient is usually awake and your role is to assess the patient, gather information about the patient's history and make the patient and family comfortable. Altered mental status and fitting are also common problems, and here your main role will be to perform an assessment and manage the patient's airway. Although environmental problems (exposure to heat and cold) and behavioural emergencies are less common, there are specific actions you should take in these cases. Therefore, considerable attention is paid to them in this chapter.

GENERAL MEDICAL COMPLAINTS

Until now, this book has focused on the treatment of patients with severe, immediately life-threatening conditions. Cases of airway obstruction or cardiac or respiratory arrest are highly critical events that require rapid intervention. However, they represent only a few of the situations that you will encounter as a First Responder. Many patients you see will be responsive, and can tell you about their chief complaint and any associated signs and symptoms (**Box 8.1**).

Some of these complaints may be the result of very serious medical conditions. Determining the exact cause of these symptoms can be extremely difficult. Fortunately, you do not need to determine the cause of a patient's medical problems in order to help. As a First Responder, you will assess each patient to determine the chief complaint as well as other associated signs and symptoms. You will then provide emergency care based on those findings.

As always, your priority is to assure your own safety. Be sure to complete a scene assessment before approaching the patient. Do not enter a scene that is not safe. The first step in assessing any patient is to complete the primary assessment to determine if there are any immediate threats to live. You should next perform a

	Common Signs and Symptoms in Patients with General Medical Complaints
Box 8.1	

- Pain (chest, abdominal, back, head, etc.)
- Shortness of breath
- Headache/dizziness
- Disorientation
- Nausea and vomiting

Medical emergencies

physical examination that is appropriate for the patient and gather information for the AMPLE history. You should also continually assess the patient for changes in his or her condition with the secondary assessment.

Some First Responders are uncomfortable when caring for patients with general medical complaints. These patients are typically responsive and may be very anxious. It is easy to feel that you are not helping since the patient does not need to have immediate threats to life managed. It is very important to appreciate how much you are helping by being caring and understanding. The most important thing that you can do for patients with general medical complaints and no life-threatening problems is to provide comfort, to calm them and to reassure them that help is on the way and that you are going to get them to hospital quickly.

You should talk to the patient and family and gather as much of the AMPLE history as you can. This will decrease the time that ambulance personnel will need to spend at the scene and help you feel confident that you are helping the patient. By approaching the patient with a general medical complaint calmly, professionally and with compassion, you can provide great comfort and support in a highly stressful situation (**Fig. 8.1**). **Box 8.2** lists the steps a First Responder should take when caring for a patient with a general medical complaint.

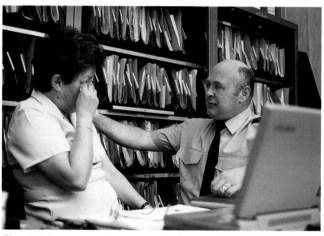

Fig. 8.1 By approaching the patient calmly, professionally and with compassion, you can provide great comfort and support in a stressful situation.

Box 8.2	**Role of the First Responder – General Medical Complaint**

Complete First Responder assessment
• Scene assessment
• Primary assessment
• Physical examination
• AMPLE History
• Secondary Assessment
Comfort, calm and reassure the patient and family
Provide a brief report to arriving EMS personnel

First Responder Alert

If the patient is conscious and has general medical complaints, you do not need to determine the exact cause of their illness. Provide care based on the patient's signs and symptoms.

SPECIFIC MEDICAL COMPLAINTS

There are a few specific medical complaints and situations that require special attention by the First Responder. These are less common than general medical complaints, but require a specific approach. You should treat the patient based on the assessment findings and not worry about the cause of the problem. In all cases, pay particular attention to the airway and maintain a safe environment for the patient.

Altered mental status

Altered mental status is an ailment resulting in a patient's increased or decreased awareness, which can range from hyperactivity to unconsciousness.

Impaired consciousness is a form of altered mental status in which there is a sudden or gradual decrease in the patient's level of responsiveness. This may range from the patient being slightly disoriented to one who seems asleep and cannot be woken up. Overall, the more unresponsive the patient is, the more critical the situation. Keep in mind, however, that even minor disorientation can signal a serious medical problem and should be considered a true emergency. A patient may suffer an altered mental status in which an increased awareness is later followed by impaired consciousness.

Common causes of altered mental status

There are many reasons why a patient may have altered mental status (**Box 8.3**). Impaired consciousness may last for any amount of time, from only a few seconds to many years. Remember that determining the cause is not important. You will support the patient, control the airway and maintain a safe scene while awaiting additional resources. Gather information about the AMPLE history, and calm and reassure the patient and family members.

The role of the First Responder

For a patient with altered mental status, you should complete the First Responder assessment, including the scene assessment, primary assessment, physical examination and secondary assessment. If the patient is unable to answer questions, you should obtain the AMPLE history from a family member, friend or bystander.

Keep in mind that the last sense a patient loses is hearing. Talking to the patient is important even if he or she is not responding to you. Always assume that the patient can hear you and provide comfort and reassurance.

Patients with impaired consciousness are at a very high risk of airway problems. Depending on the severity of the impaired consciousness, the airway may be open or the patient may need airway management and artificial ventilation. Maintain the airway and support ventilation as discussed in Chapter 5 ('The airway'). Be sure to have suction equipment immediately available.

All uninjured patients with impaired consciousness who are breathing adequately should be placed in the recovery position (**Fig. 8.2**). If the patient is gurgling or snoring with each breath, the tongue or fluids may be obstructing the airway; therefore, you should suction their airway immediately and consider the use of an oral or nasal airway.

Remember to reassess the airway of a patient with impaired consciousness frequently. Do not become distracted and forget the basic principles of airway management and patient assessment. Perform ongoing assessments at least every 5 minutes. **Box 8.4** summarises the steps of caring for a patient with altered mental status.

Fitting

Fitting is a type of altered mental status. There are many types of fitting, but the most dramatic form is characterised by jerky, violent muscle contractions called convulsions. The onset is typically sudden and is usually related to malfunctions of the nervous system. During the convulsions, patients are usually unresponsive, sometimes stop breathing and may vomit.

There are other forms of fitting, which can range from an episode in which the patient just seems to stare ahead blankly to convulsions affecting the entire body.

Although it can be dramatic, fitting alone is rarely a life-threatening emergency. The biggest dangers of fitting are that the patient will be injured during a fall or during the convulsions themselves, or that the patient will develop an airway obstruction. The length of fitting may vary tremendously, but it usually lasts less than 5 minutes. The longer the fitting, the greater the chances of complications, such as vomiting or inadequate respiration.

Common causes of fitting

Many conditions can cause fitting. Be aware, though, that the cause may remain unknown. Spending time trying to decide the cause of the fitting is not important. **Box 8.5** lists some common causes of fitting.

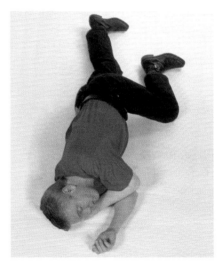

Fig. 8.2 All uninjured patients with an altered mental status should be placed in the recovery position and monitored.

Box 8.3	**Common Causes of Altered Mental Status**

- Fever
- Infections
- Poisonings (including drugs and alcohol)
- Low blood sugar
- Insulin reactions
- Head injury
- Decreased levels of oxygen to the brain
- Psychiatric reactions

Box 8.4	**Role of the First Responder – Altered Mental Status**

Complete First Responder assessment
- Scene assessment
- Primary assessment
- Physical examination
- AMPLE history
- Secondary assessment

Ensure airway patency
- Uninjured patient – place in recovery position
- Injured or possibly injured patient – consider the use of airway adjuncts and have suction available

Comfort, calm and reassure the patient and family

Box 8.5	**Common Causes of Fitting**

- Chronic medical conditions (such as epilepsy)
- Fever
- Infection
- Poisoning (including drugs and alcohol)
- Low blood sugar
- Head injury
- Decreased levels of oxygen
- Brain tumours
- Complications of pregnancy

Immediately after fitting, a patient may seem asleep and unresponsive. The brain has suffered a massive discharge of energy, and the body is recovering for a short time after the fitting. After the patient regains responsiveness, they may be agitated or combative. Although fitting is often a frightening event for bystanders, chronic fitting patients may be familiar with what occurs. They may refuse to let you help them after they become responsive. Fitting is especially frightening for the patient, family and bystanders when it occurs for the first time or unexpectedly.

The role of the First Responder

Although the patient may be actively fitting, you should still try to perform a First Responder assessment. As always, scene safety is important. Move objects away from the patient so he does not injure himself during convulsions. If the fitting patient is on a hard surface, try to keep the head from striking the ground or place padding on the floor to avoid serious head injuries. Generally, fitting itself is not particularly dangerous, but the patient can be seriously injured during the contractions. You should never attempt to restrain a fitting patient. Once you have made the scene safe for yourself and the patient, perform a primary assessment, physical examination, AMPLE history and secondary assessment.

The most dangerous part of fitting is the fact that the patient's airway may become obstructed. Therefore, you must pay very close attention to the airway of a fitting patient. Often the patient will have significant oral secretions. The patient should be placed in the recovery position as soon as possible. A patient with bluish skin is not breathing adequately and must be ventilated as soon as possible. The most effective technique is mouth-to-mask ventilation. This can be difficult, but it is critical to the survival of the patient. Never place anything into the mouth of a fitting patient. Since these patients often vomit, you should have suction equipment nearby. Remember that fitting can be very alarming to family and bystanders and embarrassing for patients. Provide comfort and reassurance while waiting for additional resources. During the convulsions, the patient may salivate, vomit and lose control of the bladder and bowels. If possible, you should attempt to protect the patient's modesty by asking bystanders to leave the area.

Since fitting usually lasts only a few minutes, you may be the only witness. Pay careful attention to what the patient is doing during the fitting. This information can help the receiving facility determine the cause of the fitting. You should report any findings or observations to the ambulance personnel.

Box 8.6 summarises the role of the First Responder for a fitting patient.

Exposure to cold

In any locality you may encounter a patient who has been exposed to a cold environment. Even in the tropics, prolonged immersion in water or exposure to night temperatures can cause the body temperature to drop. There are two results of exposure to cold:

- generalised cold injuries, in which the patient's body temperature drops; and
- localised cold injuries, in which a specific body part is affected.

A patient may have both generalised and local cold emergencies.

Generalised cold emergencies

Generalised cold emergencies occur when there is a drop in the temperature of the internal organs of the body, a condition known as hypothermia. The most common cause of generalised hypothermia is exposure

Box 8.6	**Role of the First Responder – Fitting**

Protect the patient from harming him- or herself

Complete First Responder assessment
- Scene assessment
- Primary assessment
- Physical examination
- AMPLE history
- Secondary assessment

Assure airway patency
- Place in recovery position
- Have suction available
- Ventilate the patient if necessary

Protect the patient's modesty

Comfort, calm and reassure the patient and family

to a cold environment. The temperature does not need to be extraordinarily cold for hypothermia to occur. In fact, the most dangerous temperatures are from 5–10°C, because people often underestimate the danger of hypothermia and do not dress warmly enough. Other common factors that contribute to hypothermia include exposure to water, ice and snow.

Alcohol is a complicating factor in many hypothermic patients. Alcohol affects judgement and decision making, and it often causes a patient not to seek shelter from the cold. Alcohol also causes blood vessels in the extremities to dilate, actually increasing heat loss, even though the patient may feel warm.

The old and the young are very susceptible to hypothermia. As people get older, they lose insulating fat and the body may not respond as efficiently to an increased need for heat production. Young people have a large surface area for their small size and very little fat for insulation. Pre-existing medical conditions also increase the likelihood of generalised cold emergencies.

Box 8.7 lists major contributing factors for generalised hypothermia.

Signs and symptoms of a generalised cold emergency

You should consider the possibility of hypothermia whenever the patient has obviously been exposed to the cold. Remember, even in relatively warm conditions hypothermia is possible. Hypothermia occurs in a progression, beginning with a slight drop in body temperature. The early signs and symptoms of hypothermia are very subtle and include shivering and loss of sensation. As the hypothermia becomes more profound, the signs and symptoms become more dramatic and include dizziness and memory loss.

Hypothermia may be less obvious in patients with underlying medical conditions, patients who have suffered from overdose or poisoning and patients who have spent a long time in a cool environment, such as a house with inadequate heating.

Cool skin in the extremities is not a reliable sign of hypothermia. To determine the patient's internal temperature, place the back of your hand under the patient's clothing against the abdomen. Cool abdominal skin is a sign of a generalised cold emergency.

When the body temperature drops, a normal response is to increase heat production by shivering.

Shivering is an effective method of generating body heat, but it is not always present in hypothermic patients. Usually the body stops shivering as the body temperature drops below 32°C. These patients may have a stiff or rigid posture. Children, infants and many elderly patients have small muscle mass that cannot generate very much heat by shivering.

The most important sign of hypothermia is a decrease in the mental status and motor function of the patient. In hypothermic patients, the level of responsiveness indicates the degree of hypothermia. Hypothermia affects the patient's level of responsiveness and ability to make rational decisions. Hypothermic patients may appear to be intoxicated or confused, and they may exhibit poor judgement. Some hypothermic patients become so confused that they remove their clothing in extremely cold weather! **Box 8.8** summarises the signs and symptoms of hypothermia.

The role of the First Responder

Complete a First Responder assessment, including scene assessment, primary assessment, physical examination, AMPLE history and secondary assessment. If you suspect that the patient may be hypothermic, you should prevent further heat loss. There is a major difference between rewarming a patient and preventing heat loss. Rewarming some hypothermic patients could cause life-threatening changes in the heart rhythm. You should focus your attention on preventing further heat loss and allow the body to warm itself. The patient should be rewarmed in the hospital under more controlled conditions.

To prevent heat loss, remove the patient from the cold environment. You should remove all wet clothing and cover the patient with a warm blanket. Contrary to popular belief, you should not permit the patient to eat or drink. Coffee, tea, chocolate, cigarettes and other stimulants can worsen the condition. Do not massage the patient's extremities or allow them to exert

Box 8.7	**Major Contributing Factors for Generalised Hypothermia**

- Cold environment
- Age (very young and the elderly)
- Medical conditions
- Alcohol, poisoning
- Illegal drugs
- Prescription or over-the-counter drugs

Box 8.8	**Signs and Symptoms of Hypothermia**

Cool/cold abdominal skin temperature
Shivering
Decreased mental status and motor function
- Poor coordination
- Memory disturbance/confusion
- Reduced or loss of touch sensation
- Mood changes
- Less communicative
- Dizziness
- Speech difficulty
Stiff or rigid posture
Muscular rigidity
Poor judgement
Complaints of joint/muscle stiffness

themselves or walk. Movement of the extremities can cause cold and stagnant blood to return to the heart and cause dangerous changes in the heart rhythm. Handle the patient extremely gently.

Unresponsive hypothermic patients may have a very slow and weak heart beat and may seem to be dead. Check for a pulse for at least 30–45 seconds to confirm that the patient is pulseless. If there is any pulse at all, do not begin chest compressions.

If the patient has no pulse, begin CPR immediately. Patients can survive long periods of cardiac arrest if they are cold. If the patient is in a cold environment or in cold water and has been in cardiac arrest for less than 60 minutes, begin CPR. **Box 8.9** provides a summary of the treatment for a patient with generalised hypothermia.

Local cold emergencies

The generalised cooling of the body is a danger to life, but local cooling can present a danger to the extremities and other body tissues. Local cold injuries result from the freezing or near-freezing of a body part. Local cold injuries occur in a gradual progression: the deeper the freezing occurs, the more damage that will

Box 8.9	**Role of the First Responder – Generalised Hypothermia**

Complete First Responder assessment
• Scene assessment
• Primary assessment
• Physical examination
• AMPLE history
• Secondary assessment

Ensure airway patency – place in the recovery position if patient has decreased level of responsiveness

Prevent further heat loss
• Remove the patient from the cold environment
• Remove wet clothing and cover the patient with warm blankets

Comfort, calm and reassure the patient and family

result. Local cold injuries are most common in the fingers, toes, ears, nose and face. These injuries are often called frostbite.

Signs and symptoms of local cold injuries

The signs and symptoms of local cold injuries causing early or superficial injury include (**Fig. 8.3**):
• pale skin that does not return to normal colour;
• loss of feeling and sensation in the injured area;
• skin that remains soft; and
• a tingling sensation when rewarmed.

The signs and symptoms of local cold injuries causing late or deep damage include (**Fig. 8.4**):
• white or waxy skin;
• firm or frozen feeling when you palpate the area;
• swelling and blisters;
• loss of sensation in the injured area; and
• skin that appears flushed with purple, pale, mottled or cyanotic areas after the injury has thawed or partially thawed.

The role of the First Responder

Rewarming of local cold injuries is extremely painful and best performed in the hospital where the patient can be given medication for the pain. The role of the First Responder is to complete the First Responder assessment, including a scene assessment, primary assessment, physical examination and secondary assessment. In many cases, the patient will be concerned about permanent damage. Continue to provide comfort and calm the patient while you wait for additional resources.

First, remove the patient from the cold environment. Protect the cold extremity from further injury. Because the tissues in the cold extremity are susceptible to additional injury, prevent unnecessary contact with that extremity. The patient often cannot feel pain, so protecting the extremity is important. Remove wet or restrictive clothing and all jewellery to improve blood

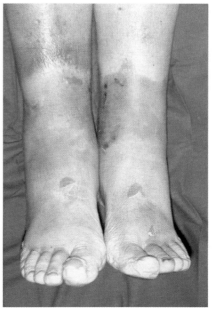

Fig. 8.4 Deep local cold injury.

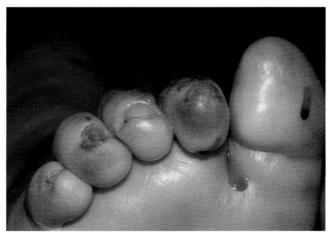

Fig. 8.3 Superficial local cold injury.

flow to the area. Manually stabilise the extremity, and cover the injury with clean, dry clothing or a dressing. There are several actions to avoid:

- do not re-expose the area to the cold;
- do not break blisters;
- do not rub or massage the area;
- do not apply heat or rewarm the area; and
- do not allow the patient to walk on an affected extremity.

As the patient's internal temperature drops, the level of responsiveness decreases. If the patient has any impaired consciousness, he or she should be placed in the recovery position. **Box 8.10** lists the steps a First Responder should take when caring for a patient with a local cold injury.

Near-drowning

Drowning normally occurs when a small amount of water enters the lungs and prevents the inhalation of air. Drowning may also be caused by spasm of the larynx and consequent lack of oxygen. Extreme, sudden lowering of body temperature may result in immediate cardiac arrest.

There are over 5000 cases of near-drowning in the UK each year. A near-drowning patient who is unconscious is unable to protect the airway and so inhales water. Profound lack of oxygen will develop. A near-drowning patient may swallow water, which will be in his or her stomach. This water may gush from the mouth after rescue.

A patient who has been in cold water is also likely to suffer hypothermia. The body's normal reaction to hypothermia is to divert blood from the extremities to the core. While in water the body is effectively weightless, with the lower limbs under more pressure than the trunk. As time passes this will further reduce the amount of blood in the lower limbs and increase the blood diverted to the core. The body will react to the increased volume of fluid in the core by excreting fluid, and the patient will feel the need to urinate.

The overall effects of being immersed can increase the time that a patient can survive hypothermia. However, during and after rescue, the patient's condition may become critical. As the patient is removed from the water, the release of pressure on the lower limbs will allow blood vessels to dilate. This and the renewed effects of gravity will result in blood flow from the core to the lower limbs, and the cold blood in the limbs will be released into the body's core. There will be less fluid

Box 8.10	**Role of the First Responder – Local Cold Injury**

Complete First Responder assessment
- Scene assessment
- Primary assessment
- Physical examination
- AMPLE history
- Secondary assessment

Ensure airway patency – place in the recovery position if patient has decreased level of responsiveness

Remove the patient from the cold environment

Protect the injured area
- Remove wet or restrictive clothing
- Cover with dry, clean clothing or dressings
- Manually stabilise the injured extremity

Comfort, calm and reassure the patient and family

in the body than when first immersed and these combined effects will cause the patient's blood pressure and core temperature to drop; the patient may suffer heart failure. Water entering the lungs causes irritation. A patient's air passages may begin to swell several hours after rescue and there may be increasing fluid accumulating in the lungs, leading to severe hypoxia.

The role of the First Responder

The role of the first responder is to complete the First Responder assessment, including scene assessment, primary assessment, physical examination and secondary assessment. In many cases the patient's condition may deteriorate after rescue. The First Responder should continue to provide treatment while waiting for additional resources.

The patient should be removed from the water in a horizontal position (**Fig. 8.5**). This will reduce the effects of gravity on the flow of blood to the lower limbs. If the patient is unconscious the head should be slightly lower than the trunk; this reduces the risk of

First Responder Alert

Do not attempt to force water from the stomach of a near-drowning casualty. It may result in the stomach contents being inhaled.

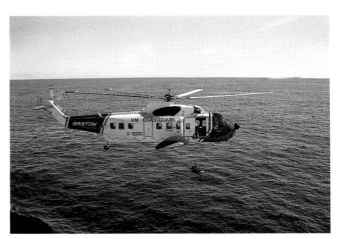

Fig. 8.5 An air–sea rescue helicopter winching a near-drowning patient on board in a horizontal position.

vomiting and will allow water from the stomach to drain from the mouth.

Check the patient's airway and breathing and be prepared to resuscitate if necessary. The effects of water in the lungs and the effects of cold may increase resistance to artificial ventilation and chest compression. It may be necessary to resuscitate at a slower rate than normal. You should check for a pulse for at least 30–45 seconds to confirm that a patient is pulseless. Defibrillation may also be more difficult in severely hypothermic patients.

Ensure airway patency. Place the patient in the recovery position and, if possible, keep the patient's head slightly lower than the trunk. The patient may vomit and water from the stomach may block the airway, and therefore suction should be immediately available. Do not attempt to force water from the stomach.

Treat the patient for hypothermia. Comfort, calm and reassure the patient and family.

All near-drowning patients should be assessed and treated in a hospital, even if they seem to have recovered fully. Water may have irritated the lungs and could cause swelling in the air passages several hours later. Patients who have undergone prolonged CPR can recover fully after 60 minutes of immersion; this is particularly likely in children and severely hypothermic patients.

Box 8.11 summarises the role of the First Responder when caring for near-drowning patients.

Exposure to heat

The body is able to warm itself more effectively in the cold than to cool itself in the heat. Delicate brain tissue is extremely sensitive to high body temperatures; therefore, heat injuries can be a severe threat to life. Hyperthermia is a progression of events that occur as the patient's body temperature rises. The terms heat exhaustion and heat stroke have been used to describe the condition of generalised hyperthermia.

The body eliminates excess heat by sweating and increasing blood flow to the extremities, where heat can be lost from the skin. During exercise or vigorous activity, a person can lose more than 1 litre of sweat per hour! Heat emergencies occur most often when the environment is hot and humid. In these circumstances, the body cannot effectively evaporate sweat or radiate heat to the environment.

The elderly are predisposed to heat emergencies because they have less effective temperature regulation, may be on medications that affect their ability to eliminate heat and may not be able to get away from a hot environment. Infants and new-born babies also have less effective control of their body temperature. Infants are not able to obtain drinking water or remove clothing on their own. Pre-existing medical conditions can also predispose an individual to heat injuries. **Box 8.12** lists factors that increase the risk of heat injuries.

Signs and symptoms of exposure to heat

Most healthy patients can easily tolerate a small rise in body temperature. If the patient's temperature continues to rise, however, the signs and symptoms of a generalised heat emergency develop.

As in cold emergencies, impaired consciousness is an important finding in the assessment of a hyperthermic patient. As body temperature rises, the patient becomes disorientated and confused. If the temperature continues to rise, the patient becomes unresponsive.

The signs and symptoms of heat emergencies are:
- muscle cramps;
- weakness or exhaustion;
- dizziness or fainting;
- rapid, pounding heart beat; and
- impaired consciousness, ranging from disorientation to unresponsiveness.

The role of the First Responder

First, you should complete the First Responder assessment, including the scene assessment, primary assessment, physical examination and secondary assessment. Continue to calm and reassure the patient while waiting for additional resources. You should remove the patient from the heat and place him or

Box 8.11	**Role of the First Responder – Near-Drowning**

Complete First Responder assessment
- Scene assessment
- Primary assessment
- Physical examination
- AMPLE history
- Secondary assessment

Remove the patient from the water in a horizontal position

Resuscitate the patient if necessary

Assure airway patency
- Place in the recovery position with the head slightly lower than the trunk
- Have suction available
- Treat the patient for hypothermia
- Ensure all near-drowning patients are transferred to hospital for reassessment
- Comfort, calm and reassure the patient and family

Box 8.12	**Factors Increasing the Risk of Heat Injuries**

- High heat and humidity
- Exercise and activity
- Age (very old, very young)
- Pre-existing illness and/or condition
- Drugs/medications

her in a cool environment (for example, in the shade). Cooling the patient by fanning may be effective. However, fanning is not effective if the patient is still in a humid environment. As the patient's internal temperature rises, the level of responsiveness decreases. If the patient has impaired consciousness, he or she should be placed in the recovery position. **Box 8.13** summarises the role of the First Responder when caring for patients exposed to heat

BEHAVIOURAL EMERGENCIES

First Responders may encounter situations involving behavioural emergencies, ranging from reactions to stress to severe mental illness. Some behavioural emergencies result from psychological problems, but many are caused by the use of mind-altering substances such as alcohol, illegal drugs or prescription medications. Other behavioural emergencies result from a traumatic injury or acute illness.

You must be familiar with behavioural emergencies and know how to handle these delicate situations. Sometimes First Responders approach an apparently safe scene, but then discover that the patient represents a danger to the rescuer. In this case, it is acceptable for First Responders to leave the patient and request assistance from the police.

Behaviour is the manner in which a person acts or performs. All the physical and mental activities of a person are behaviours. Humans behave differently for various reasons. For example, one person may be frightened of something that another person finds humorous. A behavioural emergency results when a person exhibits abnormal behaviour that results in potential harm to himself or others (**Fig. 8.6**).

A behavioural emergency is a situation in which a patient exhibits behaviour that is unacceptable or intolerable to the patient, family members or the community. This behaviour might be the result of extreme emotion or mental illness and can lead to acts of violence. Abnormal behaviour can also be caused

Box 8.13	**Role of the First Responder – Exposure to Heat**

Complete First Responder assessment
• Scene assessment
• Primary assessment
• Physical examination
• AMPLE history
• Secondary assessment

Ensure airway patency – place the patient in the recovery position if he or she has decreased level of responsiveness
• Cool the patient
• Remove the patient from the hot environment
• Cool by fanning
• Comfort, calm and reassure the patient and family

Specific Medical Complaints

1. Why is it NOT important for the First Responder to determine the cause of altered mental status or fits?
2. How should you manage the airway of an uninjured patient with an altered mental status?
3. The jerky, violent muscle contractions of a patient having a fit are called _____.
4. What are the two most dangerous complications of a fit?
_____
_____
5. List the six signs or symptoms of generalised hypothermia.
_____
_____
_____
_____
_____
_____
6. You should check the pulse of a hypothermic patient for _____–_____ seconds before starting CPR.
7. What are the three ways that a First Responder should prevent heat loss in a hypothermic patient?
8. What is the definition of a local cold injury?
9. How should a near-drowning patient be removed from the water.
10. Why should all near-drowning patients be transferred to hospital.
11. List three factors that increase the risk of heat injuries.
_____
_____
_____
12. How should you cool a patient who has been exposed to heat?
A. Immerse them in cold water
B. Cover them with rubbing alcohol
C. Give them cold liquids to drink
D. Remove them from the heat and fan them

1. The First Responder will provide care based on the assessment finding, not the cause of the problem; 2. Place the patient in the recovery position; 3. Convulsions; 4. Airway obstruction and injury during a fall or convulsions; 5. Cool or cold abdominal skin temperature, shivering, decreased mental status and motor function, poor coordination, memory disturbances/confusion, reduced or loss of touch sensation, mood changes, less communicative, dizziness, speech difficulty, stiff or rigid posture, muscular rigidity, poor judgement, complaints of joint/muscle stiffness; 6. 30–45 seconds; 7. Remove the patient from the cold environment, remove wet clothing, cover with warm blankets; 8. The freezing or near freezing of a body part; 9. In a horizontal position; 10. To allow assessment and exclude swelling of the air passage; 11. High heat and humidity, exercise and activity, age (very old, very young), pre-existing illness and/or condition, drugs/medications; 12. D

by traumatic injuries or acute illness, such as lack of oxygen or low blood sugar.

Behavioural changes

Many situational stresses, medical illnesses and legal or illegal drugs – including alcohol – may alter a person's behaviour. Patients with diabetes who have low blood sugar may have a change in behaviour, such as aggressiveness, restlessness or anxiety, if they do not stay on a proper diet. Lack of oxygen and inadequate blood flow to the brain are other causes of altered mental status that may result in a behavioural emergency. Behavioural emergencies may also result from head trauma or other trauma with blood loss.

Exposure to excessive cold or heat may also produce a reaction in the body which changes a person's behaviour. People exposed to a very stressful situation may temporarily panic. Other changes in behaviour may result from acute mental illness and long-term psychiatric illness.

People experiencing a psychological crisis or bizarre thinking or behaviour may panic easily as a result of very little stress, or they may become agitated with no apparent or obvious provocation. These patients may be a danger to themselves or to others. They can become violent very easily, and their behaviour can change quickly and unpredictably. Treat these patients gently and without sudden moves or actions to prevent scaring and agitating them. Patients in psychological crises may engage in self-destructive or suicidal behaviour.

The role of the First Responder

As with any patient, care begins with the First Responder assessment. Even if the patient is displaying bizarre behaviour, you still need to assess him or her. When performing the scene assessment, be careful to examine the patient's environment. The primary assessment, physical examination, and secondary assessment should begin after you are sure the scene is safe for you to enter. The situation may be unsafe, or the patient may have an object that could be used as a weapon. The way of assessing potentially violent situations will be discussed later in this section.

Providing calm reassurance to the patient who is experiencing a behavioural emergency is particularly important. Often, a professional demeanour and empathic approach can significantly defuse a stressful situation. In general, if you are not in danger, do not leave the patient alone. If you think that the patient represents a hazard to him- or herself or others, ensure that police assistance is part of the response. In some cases, you may have to involve the police and the patient may have to be transported against his or her will.

Assessing behavioural emergency patients

Experienced First Responders have developed a variety of techniques to help them communicate and assess the patient who is experiencing a behavioural emergency.

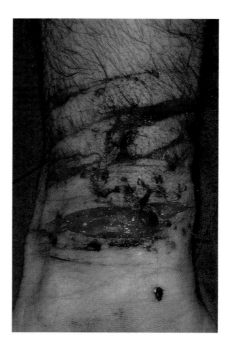

Fig. 8.6 A behavioural emergency resulted in these self-inflicted wounds.

Using these techniques will help you to calm the patient and make your assessment safer and more complete. You should usually avoid physical contact with the patient and not get so close that the patient will perceive you as a threat.

You should use your own judgement, but it is acceptable to delay or skip the physical examination if you believe that physical contact with the patient may escalate the situation or place you in danger. Do not let the patient get between you and the nearest exit route (**Fig. 8.7**). Stay near doors or exits if possible. If the scene becomes unsafe and cannot be secured after you have entered and begun care, exit as quickly as possible. See Chapter 6 ('Patient assessment') for more detailed information regarding scene safety.

Be sure to introduce yourself and any other strangers to the patient. Explain to the patient why you are there, especially if the patient is not the one who called for help. Assess the patient for illness or injury to the best of your ability, but do not let the physical examination upset the patient or place you in danger. If there is a medical problem, perform the appropriate interventions while explaining everything to the patient. When you speak to the patient or ask questions, use a calm, reassuring voice. Be sure to avoid becoming judgemental, and allow the patient to explain what happened.

Limit your questions to those that affect your care as you determine if there is a medical problem that needs treatment. Too much prying may provoke aggressive behaviour. Ask basic questions to assess the patient, such as, "What is your name?" "Are you hurt?" and "Would you like me to help you with your problem?" Usually the answers to simple questions such as these can help you determine the psychological status of the patient.

When the patient responds, show that you are listening by rephrasing or repeating what he or she

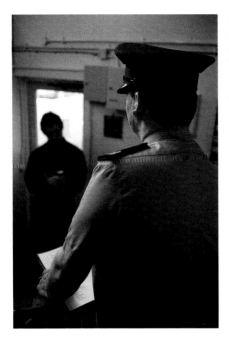

Fig. 8.7 Do not allow any participant in a dispute to position him or herself between you and the door or exit route.

has said. Sometimes a patient will tell you how he or she is feeling (angry, frustrated, anxious, depressed, etc.). You should acknowledge these feelings without judgement. Everybody has different responses to extreme events, and a person's feelings are not right or wrong. Always treat the patient with respect and dignity. Occasionally a patient will have disturbed or bizarre thinking. Do not agree with the patient, but avoid getting into arguments. You can respond in a non-confrontational, non-judgemental way, such as, "I believe that you hear voices, but I do not hear them."

Observe the patient's appearance, activity and speech, and check for orientation for time, person and place. If you suspect a drug overdose, collect the drugs or medications found at the scene and give them to the ambulance personnel.

Predicting the potential for violence

One of the most important assessment skills you must develop as a First Responder is the ability to predict the potential of a patient becoming violent. This begins in the scene assessment, and must continue throughout your interaction with the patient.

Contact the police if the patient was or is displaying destructive behaviour towards him- or herself or others. You should also request assistance from the police if you feel threatened or sense that the situation may get out of control. **Box 8.14** lists the signs of potential violence.

Calming the patient

Try to calm the patient by acknowledging that he or she is upset and emphasising that you are there to help. Do not leave the patient alone unless you are in danger. Ask all questions calmly and reassuringly, and do not be judgemental towards the patient. Repeat the patient's answers to show that you are listening. Recognise how the patient feels, but do not challenge or argue with him or her. Encourage the patient to tell

you what is troubling him or her.

During questioning, remain a comfortable distance away from the patient, use good eye contact and do not make sudden movements. You should avoid any unnecessary physical contact. The patient may misinterpret this as a threatening gesture, or as a violation of personal space.

Sit at the same level or lower than the patient. Standing over the patient and talking down to him or her may be threatening. It is imperative that you remain calm. Respond honestly to any questions. Never lie about what you are going to do or what will happen to the patient. Avoid threatening, challenging or arguing with any disturbed patient. Do not play along with visual or auditory delusions. You may be able to use family members or friends to help you calm or communicate with the patient. You should be prepared to stay at the scene for as long as necessary to gain the patient's co-operation.

If possible, have witnesses present at all times. Some patients have accused First Responders of sexual misconduct. The presence of First Responders of the same sex as the patient is beneficial.

Box 8.15 contains a summary of the role of the First Responder when dealing with a behavioural emergency patient.

Box 8.14	**Signs of a Potentially Violent Patient**

- History of aggression – check with the family and bystanders if the patient has a history of aggression, combativeness or violent behaviour
- Posture – stands or sits in a position that threatens themselves or others
- Gestures – fists clenched
- Holding objects that can be used as a striking weapon or thrown
- Muscle tension and rigidity
- Yelling
- Verbally threatens to harm self or others
- Use of profanity
- Moves towards care giver
- Carries heavy or threatening objects
- Quick and irregular movements

Box 8.15	Role of the First Responder – Behavioural Emergencies

Complete First Responder assessment
- Scene assesment
- Primary assessment
- Physical examination
- AMPLE history
- Secondary assessment

Ensure airway patency

Comfort, calm and reassure the patient and family

Consult with medical direction and police

CHAPTER SUMMARY

General medical complaints

General medical complaints represent many of the situations you will encounter as a First Responder. The patient may have a variety of signs or symptoms. It is important to provide care to the patient based on the assessment findings and not to attempt to determine the cause of the illness. The main role of the First Responder in treating the patient with general medical complaints is to perform a First Responder assessment, including an AMPLE history, and to calm and reassure the patient and the patient's family.

Specific medical complaints

There are five medical complaints that require specific actions of the First Responder. Altered mental status resulting in impaired consciousness requires that the First Responder pays particular attention to the airway, performs an assessment to determine life threats and gathers an AMPLE history. The roles of the First Responder in treating fitting are to ensure that the patient does not suffer injury during convulsions and to maintain the airway. The First Responder should care for generalised and local cold injuries by assessing the patient and preventing further heat loss. The First Responder should rescue a near-drowning patient so that the patient is in the horizontal position. Such patients may recover even after prolonged CPR. All near-drowning patients should be transferred to hospital. Patients exposed to heat should be assessed, removed from the hot environment and cooled by fanning.

Review Questions

Behavioural Emergencies

1. For a patient who is anxious or upset, the First Responder should try to _____ the patient and not leave them alone.

2. Treat the patient with _____, but do not agree with _____ thinking.

3. Contact _____ if a situation becomes out of control or you need help.

4. Involve family and friends when gathering the _____ of a patient.

5. List at least six signs of a potentially violent patient.
   _____
   _____
   _____
   _____
   _____

6. A _____ must always be present when a First Responder is caring for a patient with a behavioural emergency.

1. Calm; 2. Respect; disturbed or abnormal; 3. Law enforcement; 4. AMPLE history; 5. History of aggression, combativeness or violent behaviour, threatening position, fists clenched, holding objects that can be used as a striking weapon or that can be thrown, muscle tension and rigidity, shouting, verbally threatens to harm self or others, use of profanity, moves towards care giver, carries heavy or threatening objects, quick and irregular movements; 6. Witness

Behavioural emergencies

Any call can become a behavioural emergency. Behaviour is the manner in which a person acts or performs, including all physical and mental activity. A behavioural emergency is a situation in which a person exhibits abnormal or unacceptable behaviour that is intolerable to the person, family or community. Change in behaviour may result from mental illness, situational stress, alcohol, drugs, medical illness or trauma. Be very cautious when dealing with a behavioural emergency. Emotionally disturbed patients often refuse treatment. Patients may accuse the First Responder of assault or sexual harassment. Always try to have a witness and not to be alone with the patient. If you think that the patient represents a hazard to him- or herself or others, request police assistance.

Chapter Nine

Bleeding and soft tissue injuries (wounds)

I. **Shock**
    A   Signs and symptoms of shock
    B. Role of the First Responder
    C. Treatment of shock

II. **Bleeding**
    A. External bleeding
    B. Internal bleeding
    C. Role of the First Responder

III. **Specific injuries**
    A. Types of injuries
    B. Role of the First Responder
    C. Special considerations

IV. **Burns**
    A. Depth of burns
    B. Role of the First Responder
    C. Special considerations

V. **Dressing and bandaging**

Key terms

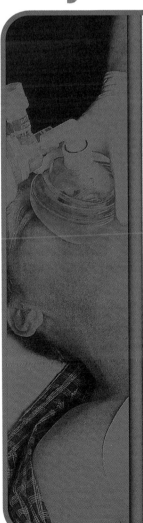

AcBC A mnemonic for the initial protocol to be adopted by the First Responder when performing the primary assessment; it stands for 'Airway with cervical spinal control, Breathing and Circulation'.

Abrasion
An open injury involving the outermost layer(s) of skin.

Amputation
The detachment of an extremity or part of an extremity.

Bandage
A non-sterile cloth used to cover a dressing and secure it in place.

Bleeding
The loss of blood, either externally or internally, because of a wound, injury or illness.

Burn An injury to surface body tissue and, in some cases, underlying tissue caused by a significant change in heat to the affected area.

Contusion
A wound caused by the rupturing of blood cells under the skin surface, often resulting in a bruise; the skin is not broken.

Dressing
A sterile cloth used to cover open injuries in order to protect them from further infection, stem fluid loss and assist healing.

Evisceration
An open injury in which the internal organs are protruding.

Gunshot wound
A wound caused by a bullet or similar projectile entering the body.

Incision
A clean cut that bleeds freely, caused by a sharp edge.

Laceration
A wound that usually occurs from the tearing or ripping of tissue.

Occlusive dressing
An airtight dressing, such as a petroleum gauze, that is placed over a wound and sealed.

Puncture wound
A wound caused by a pointed object piercing the skin; though apparently small it often conceals underlying damage.

Shock
Inadequate oxygenation of the body tissues and inadequate organ perfusion caused by an abnormality in the cardiovascular system.

Objectives

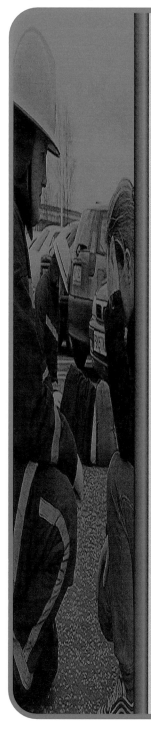

On completion of this chapter you will be able to meet the following objectives:

Cognitive objectives

1. Differentiate between arterial, venous, and capillary bleeding.
2. State the steps in the emergency medical care for external bleeding.
3. Establish the relationship between body substance isolation and bleeding.
4. List the signs of internal bleeding.
5. List the steps in the emergency medical care of the patient with signs and symptoms of internal bleeding.
6. Establish the relationship between body substance isolation (BSI) and soft tissue injuries.
7. State the types of open soft tissue injuries.
8. Describe the emergency medical care of the casualty with a soft tissue injury.
9. Discuss the emergency medical care considerations for a casualty with a penetrating chest injury.
10. State the emergency medical care considerations for a casualty with an open wound to the abdomen.
11. Describe the emergency medical care for a casualty with an impaled object.
12. State the emergency medical care for an amputation.
13. Describe the emergency medical care for burns.
14. List the functions of dressing and bandaging.

Affective objectives

15. Explain the rationale for body substance isolation when dealing with bleeding and soft tissue injuries.
16. Attend to the feelings of the casualty with a soft tissue injury or bleeding.
17. Demonstrate a caring attitude towards casualties with a soft tissue injury or bleeding who request emergency medical services.
18. Place the interests of the casualty with a soft tissue injury or bleeding as the foremost consideration when making any and all patient care decisions.
19. Communicate empathically with casualties with a soft tissue injury or bleeding, as well as with family members and friends of the patient.

Psychomotor objectives

20. Demonstrate direct pressure as a method of emergency medical care for external bleeding.
21. Demonstrate the use of diffuse pressure as a method of emergency care for external bleeding.
22. Demonstrate the use of pressure points as a method of emergency medical care for external bleeding.
23. Demonstrate the care of the patient exhibiting signs and symptoms of internal bleeding.
24. Demonstrate the steps in the emergency medical care of open soft tissue injuries.
25. Demonstrate the steps in the emergency medical care of a casualty with an open chest wound.
26. Demonstrate the steps in the emergency medical care of a casualty with open abdominal wounds.
27. Demonstrate the steps in the emergency medical care of a casualty with an impaled object.
28. Demonstrate the steps in the emergency medical care of a casualty with an amputation.
29. Demonstrate the steps in the emergency medical care of an amputated part.

First response

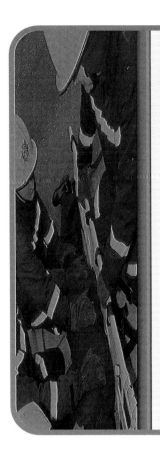

MIKE AND IAN were crew members on the emergency rescue tender when it received a call to a two-car, head-on collision. Arriving at the scene first, their officer-in-charge assessed the situation – two cars, heavy damage, no fire or liquid hazards. One person was lying on the ground outside one of the vehicles and another person was still sitting behind the steering wheel of the other. The officer-in-charge detailed Ian to assess the driver in the car and Mike to assess the casualty lying on the ground.

Mike assessed the casualty's airway, breathing and pulse. He found the airway and breathing to be adequate, but the casualty's pulse was rapid and weak. Mike directed another crew member to stabilise the casualty's head and neck. The casualty was responsive to verbal stimuli but not oriented to what had happened. Mike noticed a large tear in the casualty's trousers with blood oozing from a wound. After taking appropriate universal precautions, he quickly retrieved dressings and bandages from the appliance and placed them over the wound, with pressure to control the bleeding. He reassured the casualty that an ambulance was on its way and covered him with a blanket to keep him warm. Mike continued to monitor the casualty's airway and breathing until the ambulance arrived.

Mike recognised the early signs of hypoperfusion in this casualty and quickly controlled the bleeding, monitored the airway and prevented further heat loss with a blanket. When the ambulance arrived, they thanked the fire-fighters and transported the casualty rapidly to the hospital.

SHOCK

The function of the circulatory system is to distribute blood to all the parts of the body, so that the oxygen and nutrients it carries can pass through, or perfuse, the tissues. When the system fails and insufficient oxygen reaches the tissues, the medical condition known as shock or hypoperfusion will develop.

The three main factors involved in achieving normal perfusion are:
1. An intact working pump (that is a healthy heart);
2. An intact vascular system (that is arteries and veins of the right diameter through which blood can flow to the capillaries);
3. An adequate circulating volume of blood.

Any alteration in the body's ability to deliver blood to all of the organs is detrimental. Cell death and organ failure can result from a disruption of blood flow. When patients bleed profusely, they lose blood from within the cardiovascular system. This loss of blood volume decreases perfusion to the many body tissues. This situation of widespread hypoperfusion is called shock.

Shock results when the cardiovascular system cannot adequately deliver oxygenated blood to the body's vital organs. Shock causes delicate tissues to be damaged from a lack of oxygen and a build-up of waste products, and it is a life-threatening condition. Hypoperfusion easily damages the brain, heart, lungs and kidneys. The key to effective management of shock is to recognise the early signs and symptoms of shock and to ensure that the patient is transported to the hospital before late shock develops.

This condition of inadequate tissue oxygenation is also known as tissue hypoxia.

There are four main causes to consider:
- hypovolaemic shock;
- cardiogenic shock;
- neurogenic shock; and
- anaphylactic shock.

Hypovolaemic shock
This is the most common cause of shock in the severely injured casualty. It is caused by a loss of body fluid, either internally or externally. It may be due to:
- blood loss from external or internal haemorrhage;
- plasma loss from burns;
- electrolyte loss from gastrointestinal infections (caused by diarrhoea and vomiting); or
- water loss from heat stroke or vomiting in infants and young children.

This loss of body fluid results in inadequate tissue perfusion, leading to specific cellular and metabolic responses and thus creating a vicious cycle of events.

Cardiogenic shock
Cardiogenic shock occurs when the heart is unable to pump adequate circulating volumes of blood. It may be due to heart failure or to direct cardiac damage following trauma.

The clinical presentation is similar to that of a myocardial infarction but the central venous pressure is elevated because of pump failure. This elevation in the venous pressure can be detected by distended neck veins. The pulse may be irregular or slow.

Bleeding and soft tissue injuries (wounds)

Neurogenic shock

Neurogenic shock is caused by injury or insult to the nervous system. It is characterised by a decrease in peripheral resistance, resulting in the pooling of blood within the vascular spaces owing to the loss of sympathetic nervous control, and leading to peripheral vasodilatation. Causes of neurogenic shock include:

- spinal injury;
- fainting; and
- certain drugs.

Patients may have a slow pulse and warm, dry skin.

Anaphylactic shock

Sometimes referred to as 'allergic shock', anaphylactic shock is caused by a hypersensitivity reaction to a substance that the individual has previously been exposed to. The antigen–antibody reaction releases large quantities of histamine, which causes widespread capillary and arteriolar dilatation. The capillaries also become increasingly permeable. This results in sudden loss of fluids into the tissues (oedema).

Signs and symptoms include:

- bronchospasm;
- skin rash;
- tachycardia;
- respiratory wheeze
- tightness of the chest;
- generalised oedema; and
- altered level of consciousness.

Psychogenic shock

Another use of the term 'shock' relates to 'psychogenic shock', but this is not related to a deficiency in the cardiovascular system. At a time of sudden emotional stress or overload, a person's built-in defence mechanisms activate a method of coping with the turmoil that is being experienced. The result may range from a feeling of nausea and revulsion to complete cut-off from the situation (fainting). As the name suggests, the condition emanates from the mind rather than the physical being.

Signs and symptoms of shock

The main symptoms and signs of shock (**Fig. 9.1** and **Box 9.1**) relate to the redistribution of the circulation.

At first, a flow of adrenaline causes the following symptoms and signs:

- a rapid pulse;
- pale, grey skin, especially inside the lips;
- delayed capillary refill, in which a fingernail or

earlobe, if pressed, blanches but does not regain its colour immediately; and

- sweating with cold, clammy skin because the sweat does not evaporate.

The last three points above are known as 'peripheral shutdown', because the body is concentrating the remaining blood supply to the vital organs.

As shock develops further, the following signs and symptoms may arise:

- weakness and giddiness;
- nausea and possibly vomiting;
- thirst;
- rapid, shallow breathing; and
- an irregular pulse at first; later the pulse at the wrist may disappear, indicating that fluid loss is probably equal to half the blood volume and that the patient has reached the uncompensated stage of shock (late shock).

It is important to note that not all of the above signs may be present.

As the oxygen supply to the brain weakens, the following signs and symptoms may develop:

- restlessness, anxiety and even aggression;
- yawning and gasping for air;
- loss of consciousness; and
- cardiac arrest.

Role of the First Responder

The First Responder should always consider the possibility of 'shock' when dealing with any patient. Taking steps to avoid developing the stage of uncompensated shock will greatly enhance a patient's recovery.

If this is not possible, your aims should be:

- to recognise the severity of shock;
- to treat any obvious cause;

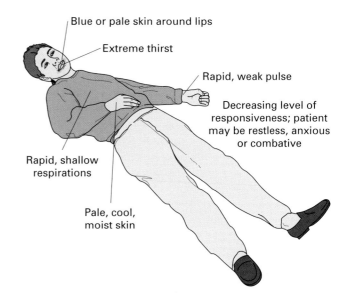

Blue or pale skin around lips

Extreme thirst

Rapid, weak pulse

Decreasing level of responsiveness; patient may be restless, anxious or combative

Rapid, shallow respirations

Pale, cool, moist skin

Fig. 9.1 Signs and symptoms of shock.

Box 9.1	**Signs and Symptoms of Shock**

- Mental status changes, including restlessness or anxiety
- Pale, cool and moist skin
- Rapid, weak pulse
- Low blood pressure
- Rapid, shallow respirations
- Extreme thirst

- to improve the blood supply to the brain, heart and lungs;
- to administer high-flow oxygen, in order to increase the delivery of oxygenated blood to the vital organs, thus slowing down the onset of shock; and
- to try to stabilise the patient until the arrival of the ambulance service.

Do not allow the patient to move unnecessarily or to eat, drink or smoke. If he or she complains of thirst, moisten the lips with water. Do not leave the patient unattended and reassure constantly.

Treatment of shock

The treatment of shock can be summarised as follows:
1. Treat any cause of shock that you can, such as external bleeding.
2. If the patient is not trapped (for example, in a vehicle) and it is possible to lie the patient down, do so, keeping the head low.
3. Begin oxygen therapy as soon as possible, using the highest percentage of oxygen available.
4. If the casualty's injuries allow, raise and support the legs. Be careful if you suspect a leg fracture or, most importantly, a spinal injury.
5. Loosen tight clothing, braces, straps or belts to reduce constriction at the neck, chest and waist.
6. Insulate the patient from cold, from both above and below, even in warm weather.
7. Check and record breathing, pulse and level of response. Be prepared to resuscitate if necessary.

Complete an ongoing assessment every 5 minutes until Emergency medical services (EMS) arrive. Comfort and reassure the patient that an ambulance is on the way. **Box 9.2** summarises the emergency care of patients who have the signs and symptoms of shock.

Remember that all cases of shock have a cause, and that there is no use in treating shock without treating the cause. If you cannot treat it get someone who can.

BLEEDING

Before beginning care for any patient, the First Responder must be aware of the risk of infectious disease from contact with blood or other body fluids. When treating a casualty with obvious external

Box 9.2	**Emergency Treatment of Patients with Signs and Symptoms of Shock**

- Maintain airway/ventilation
- Stabilise the spine if necessary
- Prevent further blood loss
- Keep the patient calm and place them in a position of comfort
- Keep the patient warm
- Do not give food or drink
- Provide care for specific injuries

Review Questions

Shock (Hypoperfusion)
1. List three signs and symptoms of shock.
   _____
   _____
   _____

2. Which of the following is true?
   A. Patients in shock often have slow, strong pulses.
   B. Patients in shock often become very warm and must be cooled.
   C. Pale, cool, moist skin results from poor blood flow to the skin.
   D. Blood flow is diverted away from the brain in patients in shock.

3. List three reasons why a patient may be in shock.

1. Mental status changes; pale, cool or moist skin; rapid, weak pulse; low blood pressure; rapid, shallow respirations; extreme thirst; 2. C; 3. Blood loss, abnormal blood vessel dilation, inability of the heart to pump effectively

---

bleeding, take appropriate universal precautions before you approach the casualty. Several infectious diseases are transmitted by blood, so protect yourself. Because blood can spurt or splash, you should wear gloves, eye protection and a mask. Gowns may be worn in situations where there is a lot of blood. Hand washing after each incident is essential, since it also helps to decrease the possibility of diseases spreading. Refer to Chapter 2 ('The well-being of the First Responder') for a detailed discussion of universal precautions.

The First Responder should also be aware of the body's response to bleeding. The body normally responds to bleeding by contracting the affected blood vessels and through clotting. A serious injury with active bleeding may prevent effective clotting from occurring. Uncontrolled bleeding with significant blood loss can lead to shock and possibly to death.

Bleeding may be external or internal. Both types can result in blood loss severe enough to result in shock and subsequent death. You can estimate the severity of the blood loss based on the patient's signs and symptoms. For external bleeding, you should also try to estimate how much blood the casualty has lost by looking around the scene. Soiled dressings can also give a useful indication of quantity of blood loss.

External bleeding

External bleeding can come from three sources: arteries, veins or capillaries. Each type of bleeding has a slightly different presentation (**Fig. 9.2**).

Arterial bleeding

Blood in the arteries is under high pressure. External arterial bleeding is characterised by large amounts of bright-red, oxygen-rich blood spurting from the injury. Arterial bleeding is the most difficult to stop because of the high arterial pressure, though the spurting may also diminish as the casualty's blood pressure drops because of the blood loss. You must act quickly to reduce significant bleeding from an artery.

Venous bleeding

In contrast to arterial bleeding, venous blood is dark red and poor in oxygen; and flows in a steady stream from the injury. Venous bleeding may be profuse and dangerous, but it is usually easier to control because it is under much lower pressure than arterial bleeding.

Capillary bleeding

Capillary bleeding is usually dark red and oozes from the injury. Capillary bleeding is the least dangerous type of bleeding and normally clots by itself. The most common form of capillary bleeding occurs when the top layers of skin are scraped away, as in a graze or abrasion.

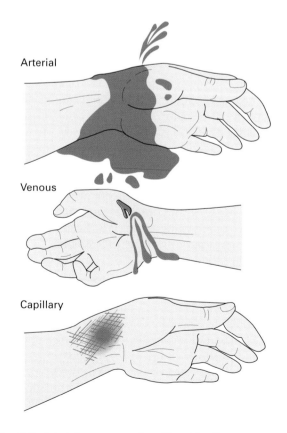

Fig. 9.2 Arterial, venous and capillary bleeding.

Bleeding control techniques

Before assessing or caring for the patient, you should always take appropriate universal precautions. Perform the scene assessment before entering the scene to begin care. Complete the initial assessment and the physical examination for each patient as needed. Make sure that the patient has an open airway and is breathing adequately, then control any bleeding.

Fingertip pressure – Most major bleeding originates from damage to one main artery or a large vein. The most effective method of controlling this type of bleeding is fingertip pressure. To apply, use the flat part of your fingertip to press directly on the bleeding point. Ideally, do this with sterile gauze. If you do not have immediate access to gauze, simply apply pressure with your gloved finger. If more than one site of bleeding is found, apply additional pressure. **Figure 9.3** illustrates the technique for fingertip pressure.

Hand pressure – If the injury is large or the bleeding is not coming from one spot, more diffuse pressure is required. Hand pressure works by decreasing the blood flow through the arteries and veins leading to the injury. To apply hand pressure, place sterile gauze pads on the injury and apply pressure with your entire hand. If blood soaks through the dressings, do not remove them, but simply place more dressings on top, up to a maximum of three. For gaping wounds with severe bleeding, pack the injury with sterile gauze. **Figure 9.4** illustrates the technique for hand pressure.

When an extremity is injured, there are two additional techniques used as needed when fingertip or hand pressure alone does not stop the bleeding: extremity elevation and the use of pressure points.

Extremity elevation – If there is no pain, swelling or deformity, you should elevate the extremity as a matter of course. Elevation above the level of the heart will decrease blood flow and help to slow all three types of

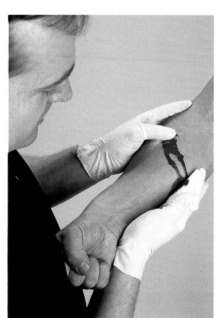

Fig. 9.3 Find exactly where the bleeding is coming from. (This is often one major vessel.) Apply pressure to this point with a gloved thumb and continue until you can apply a dressing that will keep pressure on the injury.

bleeding. Never move an extremity that is painful, swollen or deformed, because there may be skeletal injuries present and this would aggravate the injury. **Figure 9.5** illustrates the technique for elevating the extremity.

Use of pressure points – Another technique to decrease bleeding is the use of pressure points (**Fig. 9.6**). If the injury is to the arm, the pressure point is

the brachial artery. If the injury is to the leg, the pressure point is the femoral artery. Pressing on the pressure point decreases blood flow to the extremity (**Fig. 9.7**). Because no extremity is supplied by a single artery, and because venous bleeding is usually also present along with arterial bleeding, a pressure point will slow bleeding but will rarely stop it. **Figure 9.8** illustrates the technique for controlling bleeding with a pressure point. Generally, pressure points are not held

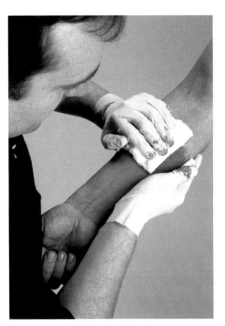

Fig. 9.4 Apply hand pressure with a gloved hand and absorbent dressing. If blood soaks through the dressing, place more dressings on top. Continue to apply manual pressure until you apply a dressing that will keep pressure on the injury.

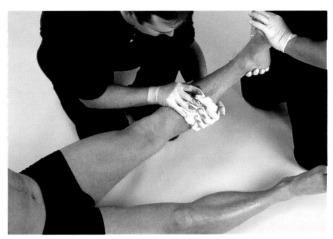

Fig. 9.5 Attempt to control bleeding by direct pressure. Check the entire extremity for other injuries; if there are signs or symptoms of skeletal injuries, do not elevate the extremity until it is splinted. Elevate the extremity above the level of the heart to slow external bleeding.

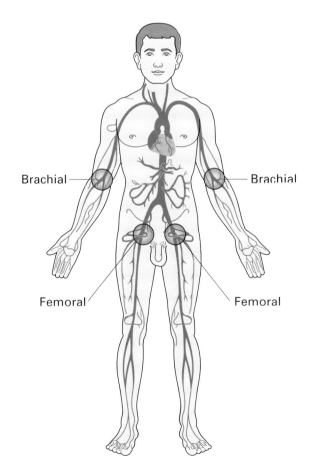

Fig. 9.6 Pressure on the arteries can be used to control bleeding in the extremities.

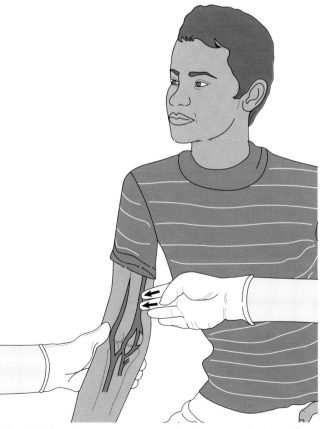

Fig. 9.7 Pressing on a pressure point decreases the blood flow to the extremity.

Bleeding and soft tissue injuries (wounds)

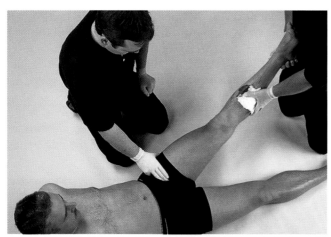

Fig. 9.8 Attempt to stop the bleeding with direct pressure and elevation if possible. Apply manual pressure to the brachial artery or the femoral artery to decrease bleeding in the extremity. Continue to apply pressure while transporting the casualty, because release may cause bleeding to resume.

for more than 10 minutes. After 10 minutes, release the pressure sufficiently long enough to reperfuse the limb and then apply pressure again.

A combination of direct pressure, elevation, and pressure points will stop almost all bleeding. After you control the bleeding, complete ongoing assessments every 5 minutes. Monitor the patient's airway, breathing, and circulation, and reassess bleeding control measures. Comfort the patient and reassure him or her that an ambulance is on the way.

Internal bleeding

Although external bleeding is dramatic and obvious, internal bleeding can be deceptive. Injured or damaged internal organs or painful, swollen, deformed extremities can lead to extensive bleeding that is concealed. Not only is internal bleeding more difficult to recognise, but it is much more difficult to stop. Severe internal blood loss can quickly result in profound shock and even death.

A patient can lose huge quantities of blood into cavities of the body, such as the chest, abdomen, pelvis and the upper legs. Often, there is no external indication of the bleeding. Any patient who has the signs and symptoms of shock should be assumed to have internal bleeding, be treated for shock, and transported immediately.

Signs and symptoms of internal bleeding
The signs and symptoms of internal bleeding include discoloured, tender, swollen or hard tissue, such as a large bruise. Increased respiratory rate and pulse rate, along with pale, cool skin, suggest shock and internal bleeding. Nausea, vomiting, thirst, cyanosis and changes in mental status may also indicate internal blood loss.

Box 9.3 lists the signs and symptoms of internal bleeding.

Role of the First Responder

The First Responder should complete a scene assessment before entering the scene. Perform an initial assessment on all patients and a physical examination and ongoing assessment as needed. If additional EMS resources are en route, comfort, calm and reassure the patient while waiting.

As always, be sure to follow universal precautions in all cases of bleeding. Ensure that the patient has a patent airway and provide artificial ventilation if necessary. Manage any external bleeding and reassure the patient. Keep the patient calm. If spinal immobilisation is not necessary, the patient may be placed in a position of comfort. Keep the patient warm by placing a blanket over him or her. If the patient has signs and symptoms of shock, treat appropriately.

Above all, if the patient has signs and symptoms of internal bleeding, they need immediate transport! Internal bleeding is extremely difficult to control and must be evaluated in hospital. Little can be done in the field to stop the bleeding, so the First Responder must rapidly assess, recognise the signs and symptoms of internal bleeding, and ensure rapid transport. **Box 9.4** summarises the management of internal bleeding.

SPECIFIC INJURIES

First Responders will encounter patients with many types of soft tissue injuries. These injuries are frequently painful and may look more serious than they actually are. Trauma to soft tissues may cause closed or open injuries. In a closed injury, the skin

Box 9.3	**Signs and Symptoms of Internal Bleeding**

- Signs and symptoms of shock, including increased respiratory and pulse rates, pale, cool skin and changes in mental status
- Discoloured, tender, swollen or hard tissue
- Nausea and vomiting
- Thirst
- Mental status changes

Box 9.4	**The Management of Internal Bleeding**

- Follow universal precautions
- Maintain an open airway and provide artificial ventilation
- Manage external bleeding
- Keep the patient calm and reassure them
- Place in position of comfort if not immobilised
- Keep the patient warm and treat for shock

remains intact and there is no external bleeding. Open injuries cause a break in the skin and there is usually external bleeding.

Types of injuries

Soft tissue injuries, or wounds, usually fall into one of six categories. However, the principles of bleeding control do not alter and the chances of developing shock must not be forgotten.

The six types of injuries are:
- contusion wounds;
- lacerations;
- incision wounds;
- puncture wounds;
- abrasions; and
- gunshot wounds.

Contusion wounds

In contusion wounds, blood vessels under the skin are ruptured but the surface is not broken. The blood leaks into the tissue surrounding the ruptured vessels, resulting in a bruise.

Lacerations

Lacerations usually result from the tearing or ripping of tissue. Bleeding is not so perfuse as it is with an

incision, but tissue damage contamination is more likely.

Incision wounds

An incision wound is a clean cut caused by a sharp edge. Incision wounds bleed freely. The deeper the cut, the greater is the chance of damage to underlying tendons and larger blood vessels.

Puncture wounds

Puncture wounds are caused by pointed objects such as nails piercing the skin. An apparently small puncture wound, with little bleeding, may have penetrated deeply and caused damage to underlying tissue and organs. The risk of contamination is high and increases with the depth of penetration.

Abrasions

An abrasion is an open injury that occurs when shearing or scraping forces damage the outermost layer of skin. Abrasions are painful but rarely life-threatening. The injury is superficial and causes very little, if any, oozing of blood (**Fig. 9.9**). Owing to the large area of the wound and the possibility of particles being embedded in it, there is a high risk of contamination.

Gunshot wounds

A gunshot wound is caused by a bullet or other projectile entering the body. The wound may be larger at the exit point than at the entry point. Serious internal injury may occur owing to the erratic path that the projectile may have taken.

Role of the First Responder

The role of the First Responder includes performing a scene assessment and then an initial patient assessment. Care for any life-threatening conditions first, such as an airway obstruction or difficulty in

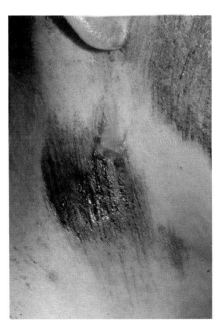

Fig. 9.9 An abrasion of the neck containing ingrained road dirt.

Review Questions

Bleeding

1. Place the correct type of bleeding beside the following descriptions (arterial, venous, capillary):
   _____ Blood oozes from the wound
   _____ Blood is bright red
   _____ Blood flows as a steady stream
   _____ Blood spurts from the wound
   _____ Blood often clots spontaneously

2. Place the following steps of bleeding control in order:
   A. Pressure points
   B. Fingertip pressure
   C. Elevation

3. Which of the following statements is correct regarding the management of internal bleeding?
   A. The patient should be kept cool so that the blood flows slower.
   B. Direct pressure should be placed over the injury site.
   C. The patient should be kept calm and treated for shock.
   D. Gloves do not need to be worn because there is no external bleeding.

4. If bleeding continues through the dressing while providing diffuse pressure, the dressing should be removed and then replaced with another clean one. True or False?

1. Capillary, arterial, venous, arterial, capillary; 2. B, C, A; 3. C; 4. False, the new dressing should be placed over the used one

Bleeding and soft tissue injuries (wounds)

breathing. Soft tissue injuries often involve bleeding, so be sure to take appropriate universal precautions. Provide care for the soft tissue injuries as described in **Principle 9.1**.

Complete ongoing assessment every 5 minutes. Comfort and calm the patient, and provide reassurance that an ambulance is on the way.

Special considerations

Some injuries require special considerations for emergency medical care. Examples of special injuries include:

- penetrating chest injuries;
- injuries due to impaled objects;
- eviscerations;
- amputations;
- crush injuries; and
- injuries resulting from a blast.

Penetrating chest injuries

For penetrating chest injuries, apply an occlusive dressing to the wound. An occlusive dressing keeps air out of a wound. The dressing is placed over the wound and sealed only on three sides. Leaving one side open will allow the air inside the chest to escape but will prevent more air from entering through the wound (**Fig. 9.10**). If no spinal injury is suspected, the casualty may assume a position of comfort, ideally with the injured side of the chest slightly lower than the other side in order to allow fluids to drain away from the good side.

Be especially aware of signs and symptoms of damage to the heart and respiratory organs.

Injuries due to impaled objects

Any object that is still in the wound when you reach the patient is an impaled object. The care you give depends on the site of the object. Impaled objects are typically left in place, since removal of the object may cause uncontrollable bleeding. You may remove an object through the cheek if it could interfere with the

Principle 9.1	**Emergency Medical Care for Patients with Soft Tissue Injury**

1. Follow universal precautions
2. Ensure an open airway. Provide artificial ventilation if the patient is not breathing adequately
3. Treat for shock
4. Manage the injury by exposing the wound. Control the bleeding and reduce contamination by placing a dry sterile dressing over the wound and bandaging it in place (refer to the steps for dressing and bandaging later in this chapter.) For serious bleeding, refer to the bleeding control techniques described previously.

airway. After removing the object, dress the cheek on both sides. You may also remove an object that would interfere with chest compressions in cardiopulmonary resuscitation (CPR) or with transportation. Objects in other sites should be left in place and stabilised there, including an object in the cheek that does not pose a threat to the airway or an object in the chest that does not interfere with chest compressions. If you can cut off or shorten the protruding portion of the object, stabilise it and cut or break that portion off rather than removing the whole object and risking further damage. Secure the object in place following the technique illustrated in **Figure 9.11**.

Do not remove objects lodged in the eye, ear, or nose. Stabilise the object and transport the casualty. You should stabilise and bandage an impaled object in the eye. Place a protective covering, such as a cone or a cup, over the injured eye and the protruding object. Also cover the other eye, because both eyes move together. Covering the uninjured eye will help minimise the movement of the injured eye. Remember that the casualty now has temporary blindness and should be treated appropriately.

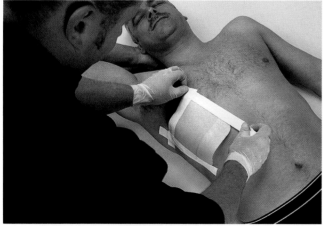

Fig. 9.10 For an open chest wound, use an occlusive dressing taped on three sides, leaving one side open to allow air inside the chest to escape, but to prevent more air from entering. The packaging can be taped over the gauze to secure the dressing.

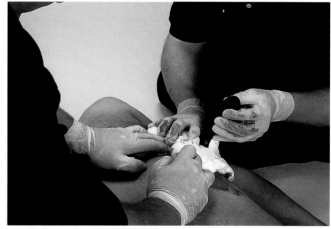

Fig. 9.11 Care for casualties with an impaled object. Follow universal precautions. Manually secure the object in place. Expose the wound area and control bleeding. Secure the dressing in place with tape or bandages.

Eviscerations

An evisceration is an open injury in which the organs are protruding through the wound, exposed to the outside environment (**Fig. 9.12**). Do not attempt to replace the protruding organs. **Figure 9.13** illustrates the technique for caring for an evisceration.

Open abdominal wounds should be treated as follows:

1. Carry out primary survey AcBCs.
2. Anticipate that the casualty may vomit.
3. Give nothing by mouth.
4. Give the highest flow of oxygen therapy available.
5. Control external sources of bleeding where possible.
6. If possible, lie the casualty on his or her back with the legs flexed (this reduces the pain by relaxing the abdominal muscles).
7. Do not touch the exposed organs or try to relocate them; cover them with moist, lint-free dressing or cling film to maintain the warmth of the exposed organs.
8. Do not remove any impaled objects. Stabilise them by using bulky dressings, blankets, or tunics.
9. If the casualty coughs or vomits, support his or her abdomen by gently applying pressure to the dressing covering the wound.

Amputations

An amputation is the loss of an extremity or part of an extremity. An amputation of an extremity requires special considerations. There may be massive bleeding from the amputation site, but the bleeding is sometimes limited.

Treat any bleeding using the appropriate bleeding control techniques, treat for shock, and endeavour to keep the casualty calm. Not only does the casualty require emergency medical care, but the amputated part (if salvageable) also requires appropriate care to prevent damage and ensure the success of reattachment. Refer to **Principle 9.2** for the care of a casualty who has sustained a traumatic amputation.

Principle 9.2	**Care for Patients with an Amputation**

1. Follow universal precautions
2. Control the bleeding, place sterile dressings over the wound and secure them in place
3. Take special care to locate and preserve the amputated part. Place the part in a plastic bag. Place that bag in a larger bag and into a container of ice and water. Do not use ice alone and do not use dry ice. Keep the part cool, but do not freeze it
4. Make sure the amputated part is transported to the hospital with the patient

Crush injuries

Crush injuries most commonly occur when a casualty is trapped in or by machinery or collapsed structures or trapped in a vehicle as a result of a road traffic accident. The dangers associated with prolonged crushing are threefold.

First, prolonged crushing of the muscles and organs of the respiratory and circulatory systems may result in the casualty becoming dangerously hypoxic or indeed may lead to respiratory failure and finally death.

Secondly, once the source of the entrapment has been removed the sudden release of pressure allows blood and tissue fluids to flow again into the areas below the crush. This then leads to shock because, as the blood and fluids flow rapidly into the areas below the crush, the casualty's blood pressure will suddenly drop as the heart tries to compensate for this sudden increase in the demands being placed upon it.

Thirdly, toxic substances that have built up in the muscles as a result of the damage will be released suddenly into the circulatory system and may cause kidney failure. This process is known as crush syndrome; it is extremely dangerous and may even be fatal.

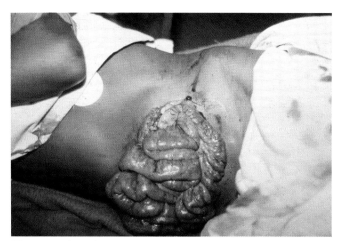

Fig. 9.12 An evisceration injury.

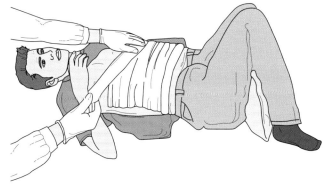

Fig. 9.13 Care of casualties with an evisceration. Follow universal precautions. Do not touch or try to replace the exposed organs in the body. Cut clothing away from the injured area. Cover the organs with a thick, moist dressing and secure it in place.

Bleeding and soft tissue injuries (wounds)

To protect a casualty against the effects of crush syndrome a general rule with regards to the length of time the casualty has been trapped is applied. Any casualty who has been trapped for longer than 10 minutes must not be released unless there is an immediate threat to life (such as respiratory distress) or if they are trapped in an area with the possibility of further injury or harm.

A casualty who has been crushed for less than 10 minutes should be treated as follows:
1. Carry out a primary survey of AcBCs while other rescuers release the casualty.
2. Treat for shock, raise the legs if the injury allows, keep the casualty warm, and give the the highest flow of oxygen therapy available.
3. Control any external bleeding and dress any wounds.
4. Secure and immobilise any suspected fractures.
5. Carry out a secondary survey. On the arrival of EMS, pass on the history and details of the duration of the entrapment and the time of the release.

A casualty who has been crushed for more than 10 minutes should be treated as follows:
1. Carry out a primary survey of AcBCs.
2. If the casualty's breathing is seriously impaired, the object may have to be raised, rammed, or spread off the casualty enough to allow them to breath.
3. Control any external bleeding.
4. Check the pulse points below the crush level to ascertain the severity of the constriction on the vascular system.
5. On the arrival of the EMS, liaise with them as to the best possible method of safely removing the source of the entrapment.
6. Before the fire-fighters release the casualty, EMS personnel will, if appropriate, set up intravenous infusions and administer pain relief. Fire-fighters, on the instructions of the EMS personnel, will very slowly release the crushing object. The reason for this is to allow intravenous fluids to maintain the required levels of circulating fluid volume within the body in order to prevent the sudden loss of blood pressure at the time of release from the entrapment.

Injuries resulting from a blast

There are incidents where emergency first aid will have to be given to casualties who may have suffered injuries caused by explosions. Although these incidents are rare they can happen in any type of premises, from industrial to residential. The degree and type of injury that a casualty may suffer can be classified as being due to one or more of:
• the primary shock wave;
• the secondary injury; and
• the tertiary injury.

The primary shock wave – The shock wave causes injury and burns to the lungs, the gastrointestinal organs, and the ears. The effects of the shock wave may cause death without leaving any external signs of trauma on the casualty's body.

The secondary injury – Flying glass and falling debris produced by the actual explosion causes this type of injury. The severity of the injury will range from minor lacerations to crush injuries or even death.

The tertiary injury – These injuries are caused by the casualty being thrown by the force of blast and the consequent impact with other objects.

Emergency first aid treatment for blast injuries

Ensuring scene safety and your own safety is absolutely paramount.
1. Carry out the primary survey (the AcBCs).
2. Open and maintain the airway (remembering the possibility of C spine injury).
3. As the respiratory organs may have been damaged administer the highest flow oxygen available.
4. If the casualty's breathing rate is below 10 breaths per minute consider applying assisted ventilations.
5. Assist the casualty's damaged or impaired circulatory system by controlling external bleeding, and immobilise any fractures.
6. Begin the secondary survey and continue until the EMS take over. Thereafter assist as required.

Review Questions

Specific Injuries

1. Fill in the blank with the appropriate soft tissue injury (abrasion, laceration, penetration):
   _____ Only the outermost layer of skin is damaged
   _____ An example would be a stab wound
   _____ Very little or no external or internal bleeding
   _____ Caused by a forceful impact with a sharp object and bleeding can be severe
   _____ Usually caused by a sharp-pointed object with little external bleeding, but possible severe internal bleeding

2. To prevent further contamination of soft tissue injuries the First Responder should place a sterile _____ over the wound.

3. List the steps for managing an impaled object in order:
   A. Expose the wound area
   B. Use bulky dressing to secure the object
   C. Manually stabilise the object
   D. Control bleeding

4. The care of a casualty with an amputation includes care of the amputated part by placing the part in plastic and freezing it. True or False?

1. Abrasion, penetration, abrasion, laceration, penetration; 2. Dressing; 3. C, A, D, B; 4. False, never freeze an amputated part, place it in a plastic bag on ice and water.

BURNS

Depth of burns

Burns are another type of soft tissue injury and are classified by depth. A burn is classified as being:
- superficial (**Fig. 9.14a**);
- partial thickness (**Fig. 9.14a**); or
- full thickness (**Fig. 9.14b**).

This has superseded the old classification of first-, second-, and third-degree burns. Superficial burns are normally classed as slight, whereas partial and full-thickness burns are classed as severe. This can vary however with the type of burn.

The skin consists of three main layers, each of which may be effected by a burn. In simplest terms they are:
- the epidermis (the top surface);
- the dermis; and
- the subcutaneous tissue.

Table 9.1 shows which layer(s) are involved and how this is recognised.

Full-thickness burns are often combined with partial-thickness and superficial burns, with the less severe burns emanating away from the centre of the injury like a 'bull's-eye' target).

Treatment for a burn will be dictated by:
- the cause of the burn;
- the extent of the burn; and
- the location of the burn.

Cause of the burn

Thermal burns – Thermal burns are caused by direct contact with flames, hot surfaces, extreme cold, or heated gases.

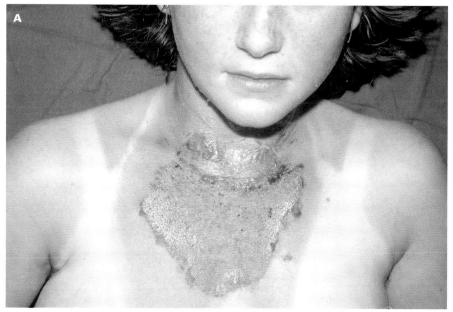
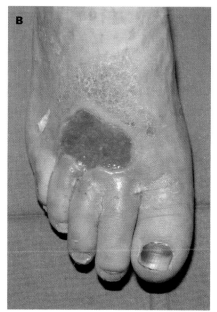

Fig. 9.14 (a) Partial-thickness and superficial burns in the same patient. **(b)** A full- thickness burn.

Table 9.1	**Burns**		
Type	**Superficial**	**Partial thickness**	**Full thickness**
Layer(s) involved	Epidermis and part of dermis	Epidermis	Epidermis, dermis, and subcutaneous tissue
Signs and symptom	Redness and pain. Slight tenderness. Oedema. Blanching on pressure	Redness and mottling with pain. Blisters. Blanching on pressure	Leathery and charred appearance Pearly grey in colour. Burnt smell. Painless or limited pain. No blanching
Estimated healing time	7–10 days (following appropriate treatment)	10–21 days (following appropriate treatment)	Hospital intervention required

Bleeding and soft tissue injuries (wounds)

Chemical burns – Chemical burns are caused by contact with corrosive acid or alkali in solid, liquid, or gaseous form.

Electrical burns – Electrical currents generate heat that can burn skin and the underlying tissues. The source of electricity may be the domestic supply, lightning, or, in extreme cases, a build-up of static charge.

Friction burns – Friction burns are caused by two surfaces rubbing together (for instance, burns to a hand from sliding down a rope).

Radiation burns – Radiation burns may occur rapidly or over a period of time, for example sunburn, or be the result of over-exposure to X-rays or radioactive substances.

Burns from hot liquid and steam – Known as scalds, these are 'wet' burns.

Cold burns – Cold burns may result from contact with metals in freezing conditions. Freezing agents such as liquid nitrogen can also cause cold burns.

Extent of the burn
The area of the burn is given as a percentage of the total skin area (**Figs 9.15** and **9.16**). It is calculated either by taking the size of the palm of the casualty's hand to be 1% or by using the 'rule of nines'.

Wallace's rules of nines – The extent of the burns can be measured by the 'rule of nines'. This system assigns a percentage value to each part of the body that represents 9% or a multiple of 9%. For example, a full arm is 9% and a full leg is 18%; a burn involving a whole arm and a whole leg would therefore amount to 27% of the body surface area. The palm surface of the casualty's hand represents approximately 1% of his or her body surface area. Estimation of the extent of the burn differs considerably for children (for example, the head of an infant or young child represents a greater proportion of the body surface area and the lower extremities a lesser proportion than in adults).

Take extra care and precaution when dealing with an infant or child with a burn. They are at a greater risk than adults for shock (hypoperfusion), airway problems, and hypothermia. Make sure you cover the casualty to maintain adequate body temperature.

Location of the burn
The part of the body that is directly affected by a burn may have a considerable bearing on the overall effect on the casualty. For example, a burn to the lower leg will cause relatively few problems, however, a similar burn to the face is likely to be fatal.

Role of the First Responder

The First Responder should perform a scene assessment before providing emergency medical care. All patients should receive an initial assessment and physical examination. Take appropriate universal precautions. Remove the cause of burning, and ensure that the casualty's AcBCs are maintained or carry out CPR as appropriate.

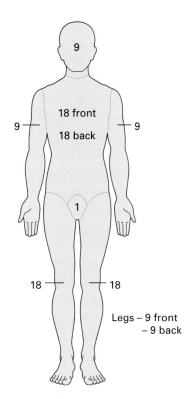

Fig. 9.15 Wallace's rule of nines assigns a percentage value to the surface area of the body that represents 9% or a multiple of 9%.

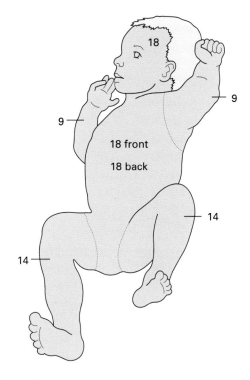

Fig. 9.16 In infants, estimates of the surface area differ considerably. For example, the head is proportionally much bigger.

144

Because the airway of a patient who has inhaled hot air may swell at any time, you must continually monitor the airway for difficulty in breathing or blockage. Be prepared to ventilate the patient.

General rules for treatment

The general rules for the treatment of burns are relatively simple, but they form a good basis on which to work following the primary (AcBC) survey:

1. Reduce the spread of damaging heat in the tissues by immersion in or under cool or cold water. Running water is best. Continue cooling for at least 10 minutes or until the pain ceases. However, if the extent of the burn is over 10% do not immerse in water since this may cause hypothermia or increased shock.
2. Administer oxygen.
3. Be aware of and treat for shock.
4. Remove rings or jewellery at or near the burnt area.
5. Remove boots, shoes or potentially constrictive items at or near the burnt area.
6. Remove dry clothing only if it is affected and not adhering to the injury.
7. Remove all clothing that is wet and hot in case of a scalding.
8. Do not attempt to remove tar or other similar molten substances that are adhering to the skin surface.
9. Do not apply lotions, oils, creams, or home-made remedies.
10. Do not burst any blister or disturb the surface of the wound unnecessarily.
11. Without applying pressure, lightly cover the injury with a sterile dressing (of non-fluffy material) and dampen the dressing to prevent it sticking to the injury.
12. Ensure that the casualty does not eat or drink anything.

Perform ongoing assessments every 5 minutes, and comfort and reassure the patient.

Special considerations

Chemical burn

Chemical burns are a type of burn that are caused not by heat or fire but by a chemical reaction. Take appropriate precautions for protection against any hazardous material. Make sure the scene is safe. An industrial facility should have information on all chemicals that are used at the site. This documentation describes the first-aid care for that particular chemical. If the chemical's container is at the scene, check the label for instructions for managing contact burns.

Flush the area of the burn with copious amounts of water for at least 20 minutes, but continue for as long as necessary to both cool the skin and remove the chemical. Remove all contaminated clothing as soon as possible (remember many chemicals give off vapours, so the contamination may spread further than the burnt

area). Ensure chemical information (name, brand, concentration, etc.) is passed to EMS. Apply a neutralising agent if one is readily available but do not waste time looking for it.

Electrical burns

Electrical burns results from exposure to an electrical source. Do not attempt to remove patients from the source unless you have been educated in how to do so. Do not touch patients until they have been removed from the electrical source. Electrical burns are very deceptive injuries. Usually the damage on the skin from an electrical burn is very minimal, but the damage inside the body may be devastating.

With an electrical burn there will be the possibility of both an entry wound and an exit wound owing to the current earthing itself (**Fig. 9.17**). (For example, if the casualty's hand came into contact with the source of electricity, the exit wound would normally be the heel of the foot.)

As the current passes through the body it can cause muscles to spasm violently and this can cause fractures. The most serious effect of these muscular spasms is to stop the heart.

Emergency first aid for a casualty with electrical burns can be summarised as follows:
1. Remove the casualty from or isolate the supply.
2. Carry out the primary survey (the AcBCs).
3. Carry out the secondary survey, with special attention to entrance and exit wounds and distal limb pulses both before and after any fractures have been immobilised.
4. Keep the casualty warm and oxygenated.
5. Monitor the casualty's level of consciousness and feel the carotid pulse frequently; casualties with electrical burns may suddenly sustain cardiac arrest.

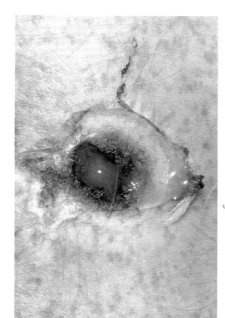

Fig. 9.17 Entrance wound of an electrical burn.

Bleeding and soft tissue injuries (wounds)

First Responder Alert

Do not use any type of ointment, lotion, or antiseptic on a burned area, and do not break any blisters that have formed.

Cold burns

Do not apply a lot of heat rapidly to the affected area. The aim is to restore the area to 'normal' temperature, so tepid water is normally sufficient. Once the area has been returned to normal temperature, treat as for any other burn.

Inhalation injury

Any casualty who has sustained burns to the face or who has inhaled super-heated products of combustion will, without doubt, have a serious airway problem. Laryngeal oedema (swelling, blistering in the larynx) can develop within minutes and completely close off the airway. The lungs may also have sustained damage as a result of the inhalation of heated products.

The symptoms and signs of inhalation injury can be summarised as follows:
- burns to the face or neck;
- singed nasal hairs;
- stridor (noisy breathing similar to snoring); and
- a hard cough, spitting up soot.

Inhalation injury is a major cause of death in burns victims. Recognise the potential for airway problems. In addition to normal first-aid measures, the administration of high-flow oxygen is essential. Consider the use of cold compresses applied to the outside of the throat and neck to assist in reducing swelling. If a cold compress is applied do not exert any pressure on the windpipe as this will only aggravate the injury. Monitor continuously and closely, handing over to EMS as soon as possible.

The determination of a critical burn

Any of the following burns is considered critical:
- burns to the neck and face, which may complicate the respiratory system;
- burns of any degree involving more than 30% of the body surface;
- full-thickness (third-degree) burns of more than 10% of the body surface;
- nearly all burns to the face, hands, feet or genitalia;
- full-thickness burns caused by acid or electricity; and
- burns sustained together with fractures or major soft tissue injuries.

Also, bear in mind that any full-thickness burn requires medical treatment, as does any burn covering more than 10% of the body surface area.

Infection

All burns carry a very high risk of infection, which in turn affects healing and recovery. Endeavour to keep all dressings to burns sterile and the injury clean and free of contamination. Do not touch the dressing unnecessarily.

Burns should be covered as quickly as possible and this can be done using a sterile burns dressing, a gel-impregnated burns dressing, a non-fluffy sterile dressing or a clean sheet of cling film wrap. Do not apply cling film all the way around a limb.

DRESSING AND BANDAGING

To manage soft tissue injuries, you will use dressings and bandages. Dressings are made of sterile material and protect the wound from further contamination and infection. The dressing is used to stop bleeding and prevent further damage to the wound. The bandage is the material that secures the dressing in place.

Dressings come in many shapes and sizes (**Fig. 9.18**). There are universal dressings, dressings classified according to size (such as 2 × 2, 4 × 4, 5 × 9, etc.), and adhesive and occlusive types of dressings. An occlusive dressing is made of non-porous material to prevent the entry of any air and it usually contains an ointment that seals the dressing; a piece of plastic wrap or foil can be used as a seal. A dressing of the appropriate size should be used to cover the wound completely, with about 2.5 cm extra on each side. All dressings should be sterile.

Bandages are used to secure dressings in place. Bandages do not have to be sterile and should be chosen according on the size of the injury and the type of dressing used (**Fig. 9.19**). Some bandages are self-adherent and sticky. Others are not self-adherent

---

Review Questions

Burns

1. Match the following descriptions to the type of burn (superficial, partial-thickness, full-thickness):
   _____ Involves the outermost and middle layers of skin. Has deep intense pain and blisters.
   _____ Involves only the outermost layer of skin and has redness and swelling at the site.
   _____ Involves all layers of skin and some skin may be charred.

2. First Responders should apply a lotion or ointment to a casualty's burns to ease the pain. True or false?

3. Although electrical burns produce extensive external damage, there is rarely any hidden internal damage. True or False?

1. Partial-thickness, superficial, full-thickness; 2. False; 3. False

---

and require the use of adhesive tape placed directly over the bandage with some pressure to help control bleeding.

Gauze rolls may be wrapped around the dressing and the injured extremity. A triangular bandage may also be used in this manner. **Principle 9.3** summarises the steps for dressing and bandaging soft tissue injuries.

Some examples of how to dress and bandage specific injured areas are given here.

Forehead – If there is no accompanying skull injury, place a dressing over the wound and wrap the bandage around the head to secure the dressing (**Fig. 9.20**).

Shoulder – Wrap the bandage around the armpit and shoulder (**Fig. 9.21**).

Hip – Secure the dressing by wrapping the bandage around the body and round the leg on the injured side (**Fig. 9.22**).

Principle 9.3	**Dressing and Bandaging**

1. Follow universal precautions
2. Expose the injured area
3. Place a sterile dressing over the entire injury
4. Maintain pressure to control bleeding
5. Use a bandage to secure the dressing in place with some pressure
6. If the dressing becomes saturated with blood, add another dressing over it and secure in place

Hand – Wrap the bandage around the hand and the wrist in a figure-of-eight pattern (**Fig. 9.23**).

Joint (elbow or knee) – Wrap the bandage around the extremity to secure the dressing. Attempt to stabilise the extremity in the position in which it was found (**Fig. 9.24**).

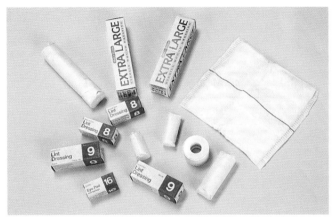

Fig. 9.18 Different sizes of dressings are used for different sizes of soft tissue injuries including large universal dressings and gauze. Tape and bandages secure dressings in place.

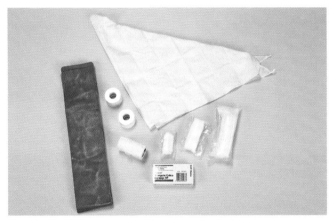

Fig. 9.19 Different types of bandages include adhesive tape, triangular bandages, gauze rolls, self-adherent bandages, and a rigid splint.

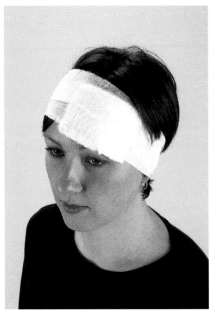

Fig. 9.20 Wrap the bandage around the head to secure the dressing.

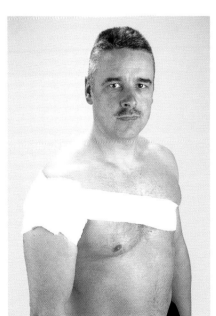

Fig. 9.21 For an injured shoulder, wrap the bandage around the armpit and shoulder to secure the dressing.

Bleeding and soft tissue injuries (wounds)

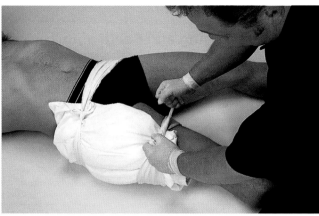

Fig. 9.22 To bandage a hip wound, secure the dressing with bandages wrapped around the waist and leg.

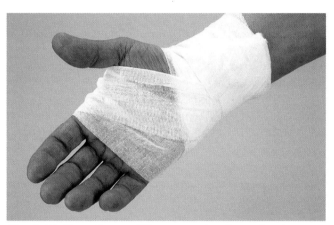

Fig. 9.23 Use a 'figure of 8' pattern to bandage a hand wound.

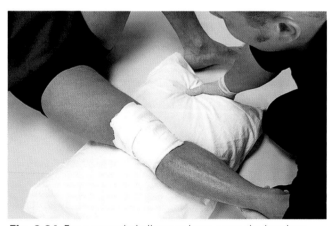

Fig. 9.24 For a wounded elbow or knee, wrap the bandage around the extremity to secure the dressing. Support the joint and secure it in the position found.

CHAPTER SUMMARY

Shock

Shock (or hypoperfusion) results when the cardiovascular system cannot adequately deliver oxygenated blood to the body's vital organs. Shock can be the result of a failure of the heart to provide oxygenated blood, abnormal dilation of the vessels, or loss of blood volume. Signs and symptoms of shock

---

include extreme thirst; restlessness; anxiety; a rapid and weak pulse; rapid and shallow respirations; changes in the mental status; and pale, cool, moist skin.

Bleeding

The First Responder must be aware of the risk of infectious disease from contact with blood or other body fluids. Assessment of the severity of the blood loss must be based on the patient's signs and symptoms. Internal and external bleeding can result in severe blood loss with resultant shock and subsequent death.

Arterial bleeding is under high pressure, and the blood is bright red and spurts from the wound. It can be difficult to control. Venous bleeding is under low pressure, and the blood is dark red and flows steadily from the wound. Capillary blood is dark red and oozes slowly from the wound.

Techniques for controlling external bleeding are direct pressure and elevation, occasionally accompanied by the use of pressure points.

Specific injuries

Wounds are categorised into six types: contusion wounds, lacerations, incision wounds, puncture wounds, abrasions and gunshot wounds. Each type presents particular complications but the principles of bleeding control remain the same.

Other specific injuries require special consideration by the First Responder. An open chest injury requires the application of an occlusive dressing to the injury. An impaled object must be stabilised, the bleeding must be controlled and a bulky dressing applied. An evisceration involves a protruding organ and should be covered with a thick, moist dressing. A casualty with an amputation must be cared for, along with the amputated part. The part should be placed in plastic and then into ice and water.

First Responders will on occasions have to deal with crush injuries (crush syndrome). If treating a casualty with crush injuries within the first 10 minutes, the crushing object should be released. If release takes longer than 10 minutes close liaison between agencies prior to release is essential in order to achieve a successful outcome.

Casualties caught in a blast may suffer from the primary shock wave, a secondary injury, or tertiary injury. Each requires the skilled application of First Responder skills.

Burns

Burns are classified according to their depth. A superficial burn involves only the outermost layer of skin and will be red and painful. A partial-thickness burn involves the outermost and middle layers of skin and will be red with pain and blisters. A full-thickness burn extends through all the layers of the skin and will look like the partial thickness burn along with some charred skin.

The severity of the burn is determined by its extent (the 'rule of nines') and its location. All burns require treatment to stop the burning process, limit the effect of the injury and inhibit contamination.

Chemical burns should usually be flushed with water. Electrical burns often produce severe internal damage with little external damage.

Dressing and bandaging

Dressings are used to stop bleeding, protect the wound and prevent further contamination. Dressings come in various styles and sizes, and are sterile. Bandages also come in various types and are used to hold the dressings on to the wound with pressure, but they may not be sterile.

Chapter Ten

Injuries to muscles and bones

I. **Review of the musculoskeletal system**
    A. The skeletal system
    B. The muscular system

II. **Injuries to bones and joints**
    A. Mechanism of injury
    B. Bone and joint injuries
    C. Role of the First Responder

III. **Injuries to the spine**
    A. Mechanism of injury
    B. Assessment of a casualty with suspected spinal injury
    C. Signs and symptoms of potential spinal trauma
    D. Management of spinal injuries
    E. Role of the First Responder

IV. **Injuries to the brain and skull**
    A. Head injuries
    B. Role of the First Responder

Key terms

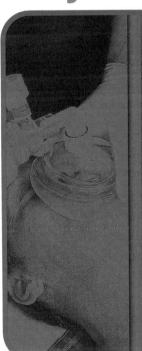

AcBC A mnemonic for the initial protocol to be adopted by the First Responder when performing the primary assessment; it stands for 'Airway with cervical spinal control, Breathing and Circulation'.

Cardiac muscle
The muscle found only in the heart.

Closed injury
An injury that does not produce a break in the continuity of the skin.

Direct injury
The result of force applied to a part of the body.

Indirect injury
The injury affecting an area that results from a force applied to another part of the body.

Involuntary muscle
Smooth muscle found in the digestive tract, blood vessels and bronchi. Involuntary muscle is not under the individual's conscious control.

Open injury
An injury that produces a break in the continuity of the skin.

Twisting injury
The result of a force applied to the body in a twisting motion.

Voluntary muscle
Muscle that is attached to bone. Voluntary muscle is under the individual's direct control.

Objectives

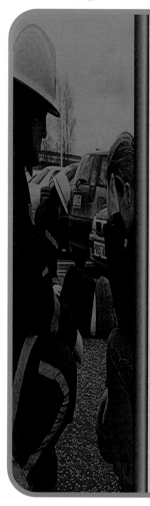

On completion of this chapter you will be able to meet the following objectives:

Cognitive objectives
1. Describe the function of the musculoskeletal system.
2. Differentiate between an open and a closed painful, swollen, deformed extremity.
3. List the emergency medical care for a patient with a painful, swollen, deformed extremity.
4. Relate mechanism of injury to potential injuries of the head and spine.
5. State the signs and symptoms of a potential spine injury.
6. Describe the method of determining if a responsive patient may have a spine injury.
7. List the signs and symptoms of injury to the head.
8. Describe the emergency medical care for injuries to the head.

Affective objectives
9. Explain the rationale for the feeling of patients who have the need for immobilization of the painful, swollen, deformed extremity.

10. Demonstrate a caring attitude towards casualties with a musculoskeletal injury who request emergency medical services.
11. Place the interests of the casualty with musculoskeletal injury as the foremost consideration when making any and all casualty care decisions.
12. Communicate empathically with casualties with a musculoskeletal injury, as well as with family members and friends of the casualties.

Psychomotor objectives
13. Demonstrate the emergency medical care of a patient with a painful, swollen, deformed extremity.
14. Demonstrate opening the airway in a casualty with suspected spinal cord injury.
15. Demonstrate evaluating a responsive casualty with a suspected spinal cord injury.
16. Demonstrate stabilisation of the cervical spine.

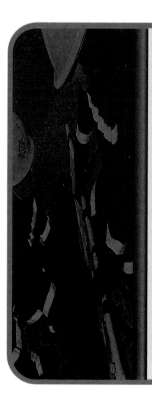

First response

"TWO PUMP FIRE at 29 Glenarm Avenue, Glasgow!" As John and Bill responded in the pump to the fire, control called them with an update: "One person has jumped from a third-storey window on to the front lawn, bystander report. EMS contacted." As First Responders, John and Bill were prepared for the emergencies that came with the job of fire-fighting.

As they entered the scene, they looked around for any hazards. Finding none, they approached the casualty as the other appliance responding assessed the fire. John immediately initiated manual immobilisation of the casualty's head and Bill began asking the responsive casualty what had happened and if there were any other victims. The casualty stated that he had jumped from the window when he realised he could not get out of the house. Bill assessed the casualty's airway and pulse. The casualty said he felt some tingling in both hands but that he couldn't move his feet. Both responders kept the casualty calm by talking and asking questions, but they did not allow him to move.

After EMS personnel arrived and fully immobilised the casualty to the spine board, John could release manual immobilisation of the casualty's neck. John and Bill turned towards the house to help fight the fire.

REVIEW OF THE MUSCULOSKELETAL SYSTEM

The following sections briefly review the musculoskeletal system. For more detailed information, see Chapter 3 ('The human body').

The skeletal system

The skeletal system, together with the muscular system, helps provide body shape, protect internal organs and assist in body movement. The skeletal system consists of the bones of the skull, the face, the spinal column and thorax, the pelvis, the lower extremities and the upper extremities. The skull houses and protects the brain. The thorax is made up of the ribs and the breastbone (sternum). The lower end of the breastbone extends into the xiphoid process, which is the landmark for finding the position for chest compressions during cardiopulmonary resuscitation (CPR). The lower extremities consists of the upper leg (femur), the knee cap (patella), the lower leg (tibia and fibula), the ankle, the feet, and the toes. The shoulder is part of the upper arm, and consists of the collar-bone (clavicle) and shoulder blade (scapula). The upper extremities consists of the shoulder, the upper arm (humerus), the forearm (radius and ulna), the wrist, the hand and the fingers.

Muscles and bones, together with other connective tissue, allow for body movement. Extremities move at the joints where bones are connected to other bones. The skeletal system is illustrated in detail in **Figure 10.1**.

The muscular system

No movement in the body could occur without muscles. Every physical activity, from riding a bike to turning the pages of this book, occurs with the contraction of muscles. Muscles, together with the skeletal system, give the body shape, protect internal organs and assist movement. There are three different types of muscle (**Fig. 10.2**).

Voluntary muscles – Voluntary muscles are attached to bones. These muscles form the major muscle mass of the body and are controlled by the nervous system and brain. They can be contracted and relaxed at will and are responsible for movement. Voluntary muscles are also called skeletal muscles.

Involuntary muscles – Involuntary muscles are found in the walls of the hollow structures of the gastrointestinal tract and urinary system, as well as in the walls of the blood vessels and bronchi. Involuntary muscles control the flow of blood, body fluids and other substances through these structures, and there is generally no conscious control of these muscles. Involuntary muscles are also called smooth muscles.

Cardiac muscle – Cardiac muscle exists only in the heart. Cardiac muscle has the unique ability to contract

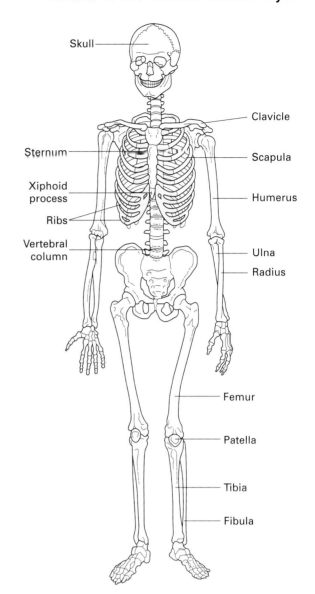

Fig. 10.1 The skeletal system.

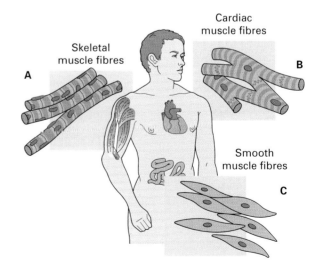

Fig. 10.2 The three types of muscles are **(a)** voluntary (skeletal), **(b)** cardiac and **(c)** involuntary (smooth).

on its own through its in-built automaticity. Cardiac muscle is involuntary muscle that has its own supply of blood from the coronary arteries. This muscle can tolerate only short interruptions of blood supply.

INJURIES TO BONES AND JOINTS

Various injuries to bones and joints are described in the following sections. In order to care properly for casualties who have bone or joint injuries, you must understand the mechanism of injury. First Responders should maintain a high index of suspicion for casualties who have sustained a serious mechanism of injury.

Mechanism of injury

The mechanism of injury can help you determine the potential severity of the injury. The mechanism of injury is the force that acts upon the body to produce an injury. Musculoskeletal injuries are the result of a force applied to an area of the body. The modern fire-fighter is increasingly called on to attend a wide variety of road traffic accidents in which his or her specialised skills and equipment are applied in the stabilisation and extrication of the trapped occupants from the wreckage of vehicles. Improving your ability to 'read' the wreckage of a vehicle and appreciate the energy

changes involved in deforming a vehicle will improve your ability to determine the injuries that the occupants are likely to have suffered.

In the majority of cases it is most important to assess a casualty's injuries before treating and moving him or her. A knowledge of what to look for enables the rescuer to approach the problem in a confident, controlled and informed manner. Understanding patterns of injury is often a blend of common sense and simple mechanics.

Direct injuries – Some injuries result from a direct force (**Fig. 10.3a**). A direct injury is the result of a force applied to the body. An example of a direct injury might be one caused by a baseball bat swung into a person's arm. The arm's injury results from direct contact with the baseball bat.

Indirect injuries – Other injuries are caused by indirect forces (**Fig. 10.3b**). An indirect injury is an injury caused by a force applied to another part of the body. An example of indirect injury might be a motor vehicle collision in which a casualty's knees are thrown forwards into the dashboard – the knees are directly injured from contact with the dashboard, but the hips and pelvis are indirectly injured because the knees are pushed backwards with a great force that reaches the hips and pelvis.

Twisting injuries – Some injuries are caused by twisting forces (**Fig. 10.3c**). If an extremity becomes pulled and twisted, a twisting injury may result from that force. For instance, a wrestler who becomes entangled in an opponent's hold may have his or her body pulled and twisted. This force may produce an injury to the muscles and bones that are twisted.

Always consider the force that caused the injury. It takes a much greater force to injure the thigh, for example, than it takes to injure the forearm. This is because the bone is much larger and more dense and is protected by larger muscles. Gather as much information as possible about the mechanism of injury, and include this in your report to EMS personnel.

Use of Polaroid cameras at operational incidents

Some fire brigades now carry cameras that can develop the film immediately. Photographs of the wreckage of road traffic accidents can then be forwarded with the casualty to the hospital to enable the medical staff to analyse the damage to the vehicles and thereby ascertain the likely injuries to the casualty.

For more information on the mechanism of injury, refer to Chapter 6 ('Patient assessment').

Bone and joint injuries

Musculoskeletal injuries are either open or closed. An open injury involves a break in the continuity of the skin and usually produces some external bleeding (**Fig. 10.4**). A closed injury does not involve a break in the

---

Review Questions

Review of the Musculoskeletal System

1. The _____ is used to determine the correct hand position for chest compressions during CPR.

2. Which of the following statements is correct?
   A. The musculoskeletal system provides for body shape and movement, but does not protect internal organs.
   B. The musculoskeletal system provides protection for internal organs only.
   C. The musculoskeletal system provides for body shape and movement, along with protecting internal organs.
   D. The musculoskeletal system provides protection from germs and gives the body shape.

3. The skull houses and protects the _____.

4. Place the correct type of muscle in each blank (voluntary, involuntary, cardiac):
   _____ Attached to bones
   _____ Found in the heart
   _____ Can tolerate only very short interruptions of the blood supply
   _____ Found in the gastrointestinal tract and urinary system
   _____ Can be contracted by the will of the individual

5. Where bones attach to bones to provide movement is called a _____.

1. Xiphoid process; 2. C; 3. Brain; 4. Voluntary, cardiac, cardiac, involuntary, voluntary; 5. Joint

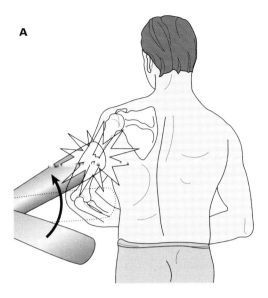

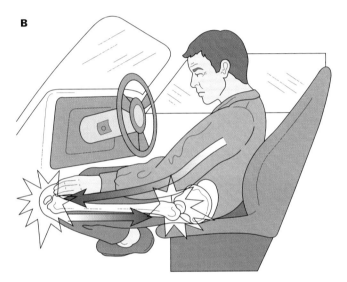

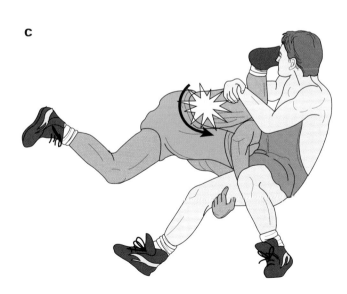

skin or external bleeding, although it may produce internal bleeding (**Fig. 10.5**).

There are several signs and symptoms that are characteristic of bone or joint injuries. The area of injury may have some deformity or angulation and may be painful to move and tender to the touch. If the bone ends are separated, you may hear or feel some grating during the examination, caused by the bone ends rubbing together. Do not purposely seek this sign, and do not try to repeat it if you note it during the assessment. Grating bone ends together produces intense pain and potentially further injury. The area of injury may be swollen, appearing larger than the same area on the other side of the body, and it may be bruised and discoloured. In an open bone injury, the bone ends that are injured may be protruding through the skin and exposed to the outside environment. With a joint injury, the joint may be locked in position and immovable. **Box 10.1** summarises the signs and symptoms of a bone or joint injury.

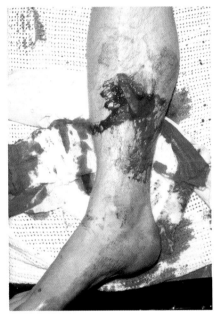

Fig. 10.4 An open injury of the lower leg with protruding bone ends.

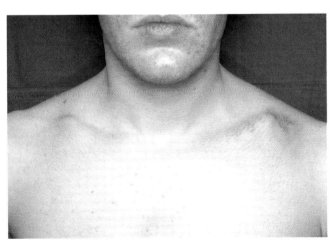

Fig. 10.5 A collar-bone injury with obvious deformity.

Fig. 10.3 **(a)** A direct injury. **(b)** An indirect injury. **(c)** A twisting injury.

Box 10.1	**Signs and Symptoms of a Bone or Joint Injury**

- Deformity or angulation
- Pain and tenderness
- Grating
- Swelling
- Bruising (discolouration)
- Exposed bone ends (open injury)
- Joint locked into position

Role of the First Responder

A First Responder's emergency medical care for a casualty with bone or joint injuries always includes taking appropriate universal precautions before examining the casualty. Even a closed injury that is not bleeding may become an open injury because of movement or pressure. Perform a scene assessment, and make sure the scene is safe before you approach the patient.

Perform a primary assessment. Bone and joint injuries are often obvious and eye-catching, but control of the airway, breathing and circulation always take priority. Make sure the casualty has a clear airway and is breathing adequately. Control any major bleeding or life-threatening situations using methods such as direct pressure, described in Chapter 9 ('Bleeding and soft tissue injuries'). If you suspect that the casualty may also have spinal injuries, stabilise the head in a neutral position and do not allow the casualty to move until he or she can be immobilised. Do not forcibly restrain the casualty's cervical spine.

If the injury is to an extremity, allow the casualty to remain in a position of comfort after any threats to life have been controlled. Apply a cold pack to an extremity that is painful, swollen and deformed in order to reduce pain and swelling. Manually stabilise the extremity until additional EMS resources arrive with immobilisation equipment. See **Principle 10.1** and **Figure 10.6** for the steps for manual immobilisation of an extremity.

Do not allow the casualty to move the extremity until it can be immobilised with a splint. Splinting

Principle 10.1	**Manual Stabilisation of an Extremity**

1. Support above and below an injury
2. Cover open wounds with a sterile dressing
3. Pad to prevent pressure and discomfort to the casualty
4. When in doubt, manually stabilise the injury
5. Do not intentionally replace any protruding bones

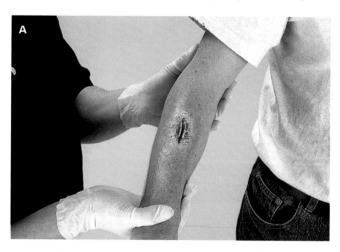
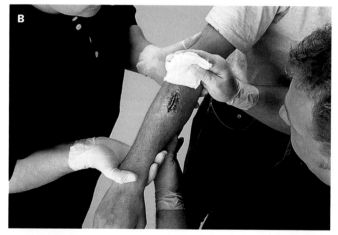
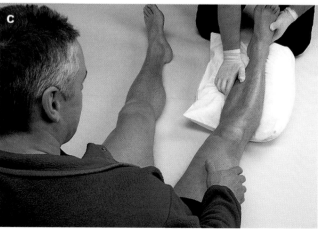
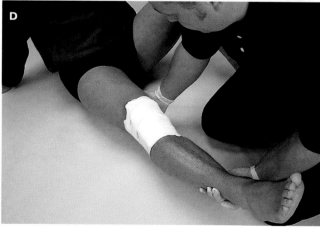

Fig. 10.6 **(a)** Support above and below an injury. **(b)** Cover open wounds with a sterile dressing. **(c)** Pad to prevent pressure and discomfort to the casualty. **(d)** When in doubt, manually stabilise the injury.

extremities is within the scope of practice for some First Responders. If you are responsible for splinting injuries in your system, refer to Appendix E ('Principles and techniques of splinting').

INJURIES TO THE SPINE

It is most important to realise the dangers of potential spinal injuries in order to prevent a simple vertebral fracture becoming a case of permanent quadriplegia. For this reason, you need to be aware of the mechanisms of injury that may result in spinal injury.

Mechanism of injury

In general, spinal injuries must be suspected in all casualties in the following circumstances (**Box 10.2**):
- a road traffic accident over 25 miles per hour;
- a fall or jump from a height of two or three times the casualty's body height or more;
- any accident resulting in impact or crush injuries and involving entrapment;
- any accident resulting in the casualty's losing consciousness;
- any traumatic injury above the collar-bone;
- near-drowning accidents; and
- anyone complaining of mid-line neck pain.

As a rule carry out the AcBCs (Airway with cervical spinal control, Breathing and Circulation; see Chapter 6, 'Patient assessment') and if in any doubt treat all casualties as if they have spinal injuries. Immobilise the casualty accordingly.

Assessment of a casualty with suspected spinal injury

Primary survey
Begin with the AcBCs. Do not tilt the head when opening the airway – use the jaw thrust without head tilt technique; see Chapter 5, 'The Airway'. Once the AcBCs have been assessed and dealt with, begin the secondary survey to obtain more information.

Secondary survey
History – When did the accident occur? The time of accident is of great importance to medical staff, since the chance of restoring lost functions decreases as the time since the injury increases.

Mechanism of injury – Determine the mechanism of injury by asking the casualty, questioning witnesses and examining damage to any vehicle involved.

Consciousness – If the casualty is conscious, question him or her to determine the location of any pain, numbness or tingling. Ask if the limbs feel weak or heavy.

Breathing – Determine if the casualty is experiencing any difficulty in breathing owing to paralysis of the

Box 10.2 — Significant Mechanisms of Injury
- Motor vehicle crashes
- Pedestrian–vehicle collisions
- Falls
- Blunt trauma
- Penetrating trauma to head, neck or torso
- Motorcycle crashes
- Hangings
- Springboard or platform diving accidents

Box 10.3 — Important Questions for Responsive Trauma Patients
- What happened?
- Where does it hurt?
- Does your neck or back hurt?
- Can you move your hands and feet?
- Where am I touching you now (while touching fingers and toes)

intercostal chest muscles. If so, consider assisted ventilation using a suitable method.

The general appearance and position of the casualty should be noted when carrying out the survey. Do not attempt to change the casualty's position unless the casualty is in immediate danger or it is absolutely necessary to maintain an airway.

Injuries to muscles and bones

Signs and symptoms of potential spinal trauma

The signs and symptoms of potential spinal trauma are as follows:

- slow pulse (bradycardia – a classic sign);
- abdominal breathing, owing to paralysis of the intercostal muscles;
- loss of power in the limbs;
- numbness, tingling or loss of sensation;
- warm, dry skin and low blood pressure;
- muscle spasm;
- deformity of the spine;
- bruising, swelling and tenderness over the spine;
- priapism (prolonged penile erection); and
- abnormal position of the arms (for instance, the arms folded over the chest with clawed fingers, or the 'hands-up' position).

There may be no signs and symptoms at all, but this does not rule out the possibility of spinal trauma. Persons who have been involved in an incident with a significant mechanism of injury should always be managed as if they have suffered a spinal injury.

Management of spinal injuries

Spinal injuries, although extremely serious, are not in themselves life threatening. However airway obstruction, cardiac arrest and profuse bleeding will result in death unless rapid treatment is given. The first priority in treating a casualty with spinal injury is the sequential assessment of the AcBCs.

Airway with cervical spinal control

Employ the jaw-thrust chin-lift technique, taking care not to tilt the head. If the casualty is unconscious and slumped against the steering wheel of a vehicle, and if the airway is compromised, the casualty should be manoeuvred to the neutral position.

The head should be manually immobilised both before and after a cervical collar has been sized and fitted as well as while it is being fitted.

Breathing

If the casualty has suffered paralysis of the intercostal muscles, you may need to assist the casualty by giving oxygen therapy. If the casualty is unconscious, automatic resuscitation may be used. Care should be taken to ensure that only the chest inflates. If air is allowed to inflate the abdomen this may cause gastric distension. The expansion of the abdomen would restrict the volume of the lungs and lead to inadequate ventilation of the casualty.

Role of the First Responder

The role of the First Responder is as follows:
1. Ensure scene safety and your personal safety.
2. Establish a clear airway.
3. Maintain manual in-line stabilisation of the cervical spine at all times (**Fig. 10.7**).

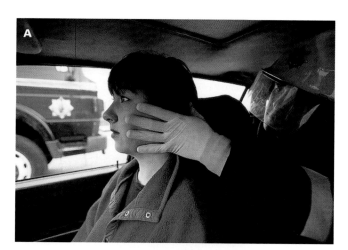

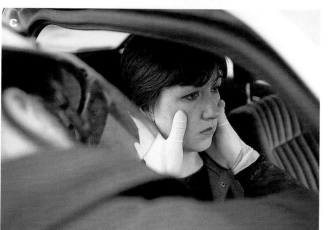

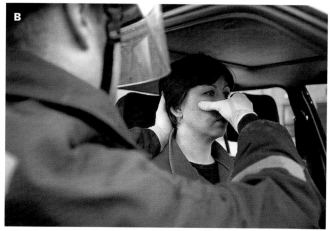

Fig. 10.7 Three different methods of cervical spine manual immobilisation. (**a**) Rear hold; (**b**) side hold; (**c**) frontal hold. Do not obstruct the airway when performing these holds.

First Responder Alert

The ability to walk, move the extremities, feel sensation or the absence of pain does NOT rule out a spinal injury.

---

4. Apply a rigid collar when appropriate.
5. Give high-concentration oxygen.
6. Control any external bleeding.
7. Always move the casualty in neutral alignment (that is, with the casualty's ears in line with his or her shoulders), and always transfer the casualty on to a spine board with head immobilisers, if available. Where suitable head immobilisers are not available, you should improvise (for example, roll up towels and place them on either side of the casualty's head, and tape the head to the board).

Be careful when using suction on casualties who have suffered spinal trauma, since this may cause vagal stimulation, which leads to slowed pulse rate and potentially to cardiac arrest.

INJURIES TO THE BRAIN AND SKULL

Many injuries involving the spine also involve the brain and skull. Any patient with suspected brain and skull injuries should be suspected of having a spinal injury.

Head injuries

Injuries to the head may be closed or open. Both closed and open injuries may present with discolouration or swelling or a depression of the skull bones. Open injuries may, in addition, present with bleeding. Wounds to the scalp often look severe because many capillary beds are located there, and even a small cut can produce major bleeding. Control this bleeding with direct pressure.

An injury to the skull may damage brain tissue directly or may result in bleeding inside the skull. Internal bleeding causes increased pressure inside the skull, which can result in changes in mental status.

Role of the First Responder

The primary survey
Severe head injuries seldom occur in isolation, always check for other injuries.

The first priority in aiding a casualty is to ensure an adequate airway, especially if the casualty is unconscious. Remember that every head-injured casualty who is or has been unconscious has a suspected cervical spine injury. Establish the airway using the jaw thrust or chin lift technique.

Evaluate the casualty's breathing. Where the breathing is laboured consider assisted ventilation, for example when there are fewer than 10 breaths a minute. The primary survey is summarised in **Table 10.1**.

The secondary survey
You should obtain a history of the accident. Ascertain from the casualty or any witness the time that the injury occurred. This information is of great importance

to medical staff because it will assist them to make a more accurate assessment of whether the casualty's condition is improving or deteriorating.

The nature of the damage to any vehicle involved will also give valuable information in determining the possible injury to occupants – for instance, was the impact head on, side on, rear end shunt or rollover?

The interior of the vehicle may also show signs of damage owing to impact on it from a casualty's body – for instance, there may be windscreen damage, a bent steering wheel or damage to the dashboard. Ingress of vehicle bodywork to the passenger compartment should also be noted. All of these indications will assist medical staff in determining what injuries may have been sustained. Remember to use the instant camera, if one is available.

Note whether the casualty has lost consciousness at any time and, if so, note when and for how long. Also note whether the casualty has vomited at any time since the accident, and whether any seizures have

---

Table 10.1	**Head Injury**

Airway and C spine
Maintain a clear airway (for example, use the jaw thrust, suction and airway adjuncts as necessary). Ensure cervical spine in-line immobilisation

Breathing
Give high-concentration oxygen and monitor respiration, including visual check of the chest

Circulation
Apply direct pressure to any scalp wounds to prevent further blood loss, and monitor carotid pulse

Disability
Assess the level of consciousness

occurred. Both vomiting and seizures are signs of possible brain damage.

If the casualty is able to communicate, determine the chief complaint:
1. The location of pain.
2. Any feelings of numbness and tingling.
3. Any feelings of weakness or heaviness of limbs.
4. Any feelings of nausea or dizziness.
5. Any problems with vision.

Note if any of these symptoms have changed since the injury occurred.

Physical assessment

Ascertain the state of consciousness and perform a neurological assessment of the casualty:
1. Is the casualty able to speak?
2. Is the speech slurred or rambling?
3. Is stimulus required to keep the casualty awake (for example, gently pinching the skin on the back of the hand or speaking in a slightly raised voice?)

Note, however, that the most important single sign in the assessment of a head-injured casualty is the changing state of consciousness.

Vital signs

Check the carotid pulse frequently. Take notes and pass this information to the paramedics on their arrival. A slow bounding pulse can indicate that the pressure inside the skull is rising; this could be due to bleeding or swelling. A rapid, weak pulse is a sign of shock. In this case look for external haemorrhage or suspect internal haemorrhage.

Remember a head injury alone does not normally cause shock. If the casualty is in shock, there must be sources of bleeding elsewhere in the body.

Complications of head injury

The complications of head injury include fitting, which is common at the time of injury or shortly thereafter; and restlessness – be aware of hypoxia as a possible cause of this.

Signs and symptoms of head injury

A casualty is considered to have a potentially serious head injury if he or she exhibits any of the following:
• fluctuating or altered level of consciousness;
• unequal pupils;
• blood or cerebrospinal fluid leak from the ear or nose;
• continuous vomiting (a more serious sign in adults because it is to be expected in children with head injuries);
• visual disturbances;
• increase in the severity of a headache or an extraordinarily severe headache;
• development of weakness or numbness on one side;
• bilateral black eyes ('panda' eyes); and
• bruising behind the ear (Battle's sign) – this may take 24–48 hours to develop.

The AVPU scale and the Glasgow coma scale

Emergency care for a casualty with a head injury involves universal precautions, maintaining the airway and ventilation, performing initial assessment and manual spinal stabilisation. Closely monitor the patient's mental status, control bleeding and be prepared for changes in the casualty's condition (**Box 10.4**).

The most valuable contribution that a fire-fighter can make to the care of a head-injured casualty is to record the neurological signs, frequently and accurately, using the 'AVPU' scale (see Chapter 6, 'Patient Assessment'):

A = Alert (casualty is aware of surroundings);
V = Verbal (casualty responds only to voice commands);
P = Painful (casualty responds only to pain, for instance, he or she reacts when nipped);
U = Unresponsive (no reactions whatsoever).

The more complicated 'Glasgow' coma scale is summarised in **Table 10.2**. The Glasgow coma score equals the total from each of the three sections. For example, if a casualty opens his eyes to verbal

Box 10.4	**Emergency Medical Care for the Head-Injured Patient**

• Take universal precautions
• Perform initial assessment and provide manual stabilisation of the head
• Maintain an open airway and provide artificial ventilation if needed
• Control bleeding
• Monitor mental status

Table 10.2	**The Glasgow Coma Scale**

Eyes	
open spontaneously	4
open to verbal command	3
open to pain	2
no response	1
Best verbal response	
orientated and converses	5
confused	4
inappropriate words	3
incomprehensible sounds	2
no response	1
Best motor responses	
obeys verbal command	6
localises verbal command	5
flexion (withdrawal)	4
flexion (abnormal)	3
extension	2
no response	1

command, withdraws his hand on a slight pinch to skin, and is confused on questioning, his Glasgow coma scores are:

- eyes – a score of **3**
- best motor response – a score of **4**
- best verbal response – a score of **4**

Therefore, the Glasgow coma score is **11**.

The highest and healthiest Glasgow coma score a casualty can have is **15**; the lowest score is **3**. A patient with a Glasgow coma scale of **8** or less is defined as being in a coma.

The AVPU scale can be correlated with the Glasgow coma scale, as summarised in **Table 10.3**.

Table 10.3	The AVPU Scale Can Be Correlated With The Glasgow Coma Scale	
AVPU scale	**Glasgow coma score**	
Alert	15	
Verbal	9–14	
Pain	4–8	
Unresponsive	3	

Review Questions

Injuries to the Brain and Skull

1. Control bleeding of the head with _____.

2. Place the following steps for managing a head injury in order:
   A. Control bleeding
   B. Universal precautions
   C. Initial assessment with spinal stabilisation
   D. Maintain airway and provide artificial ventilations

3. The two types of head injuries are _____ and _____.

1. Direct pressure; 2. B, C, D, A; 3. Open, closed

CHAPTER SUMMARY

Review of the musculoskeletal system

The skeletal system helps provide body shape, protects internal organs and assists in body movement. Muscles and bones, together with other connective tissue, allow for body movement. Muscles give the body shape, protect internal organs and provide movement. Voluntary, or skeletal, muscles are attached to bones.

They can be contracted and relaxed at will and are responsible for movement. Involuntary, or smooth, muscles are found in the walls of the hollow structures of the gastrointestinal tract and urinary system, as well as in the walls of the blood vessels and bronchi. Cardiac muscle exists only in the heart.

Injuries to bones and joints

The mechanism of injury can help you determine the potential severity of the injury. Injuries can result from a direct force to an area of the body, an indirect force or a twisting force. Always consider the force that was involved in the cause of the injury.

Musculoskeletal injuries are either open or closed. Signs and symptoms of a bone or joint injury include deformity or angulation, pain and tenderness, grating, swelling, bruising (discolouration), exposed bone ends (open injury) and joints locked into position.

Emergency medical care for bone or joint injuries for the First Responder always includes taking appropriate universal precautions. Establish a patent airway and control any major bleeding or life-threatening situations. Allow the patient to remain in the position of comfort. Any extremity that is painful, swollen and deformed should have a cold pack applied to it to reduce pain and swelling. The extremity should be manually stabilised until additional EMS resources arrive.

Injuries to the spine

By considering factors such as the damage to a vehicle or the height of a fall, you can determine whether the mechanism of injury involved a significant force to the casualty's body. In most situations, the mechanism of injury can be determined as part of the scene assessment.

Signs and symptoms of a spinal injury include tenderness or pain (with or without movement); soft tissue injuries; numbness, weakness or tingling; loss of sensation, paralysis or respiratory impairment; and loss of bladder control.

To assess the responsive casualty, the First Responder should question the casualty to determine what happened and where the casualty is injured and to judge the casualty's mental status. To assess the unresponsive casualty, the bystanders and family members may have the information the First Responder requires. Complications in a spine-injured patient include inadequate breathing effort and paralysis.

Emergency care includes universal precautions; establishing and maintaining manual spinal stabilisation; establishing and maintaining airway and ventilation without moving the casualty; and assessing the pulse, motor function and sensation in the extremities.

Injuries to the brain and skull

Head injuries may be open or closed. Open head injuries may bleed profusely and look worse than they actually are because of the large number of blood vessels on the scalp.

161

Injuries to muscles and bones

Points to remember

1. Do not allow yourself to become distracted by the severity of the casualty's injuries. Always carry out the primary survey (AcBCs).
2. Every casualty with a head injury has a suspected cervical spine injury until proven otherwise. Immobilise the neck with manual in-line stabilisation and apply a rigid cervical collar.
3. The most important single sign in the assessment of a head-injured casualty is a changing state of consciousness.
4. Head injury in an adult does not itself cause hypovolaemic shock. If signs of shock are present, look for possible injury elsewhere.
5. The most common causes of death in patients with head injury are hypoxia (an inadequate supply of oxygen to the body tissues) and hypovolaemia due to injury elsewhere. To prevent hypoxia ensure an adequate airway and administer the highest percentage of oxygen available (usually 100% oxygen at 15 litres per minute via a non-rebreather mask fitted with a reservoir bag).

How to deal with head injuries

1. Maintain a clear airway ensuring cervical spine in-line immobilisation.
2. Give high concentration oxygen.
3. Maintain in-line spinal immobilisation and apply a cervical collar (it must be assumed that the force that rendered the casualty unconscious is significant enough to cause a cervical spine injury).
4. Control bleeding from scalp wounds.
5. Cover any leak of cerebrospinal fluid from ears with a gauze pad. Do not plug, allow the leaking fluid to flow.
6. Monitor vital signs and level of consciousness as a baseline and reassess frequently.
7. Maintain the casualty's body temperature.
8. The casualty should be transported with complete spinal immobilisation on a spinal board.

The most common cause of death in the unconscious head injury is hypoxia. To prevent this, remember the importance of maintaining a clear airway and the early administration of oxygen.

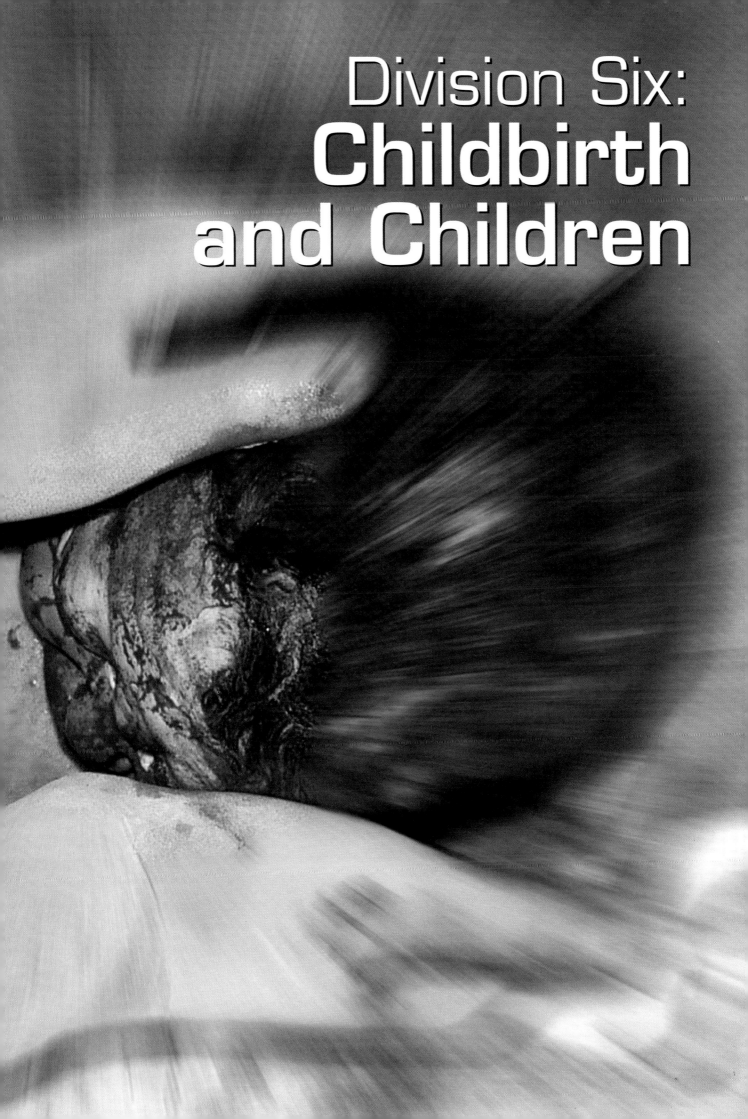

Division Six:
Childbirth and Children

Chapter Eleven
Childbirth

I. Reproductive anatomy and physiology

II. Labour
   A. First stage of labour
   B. Second stage of labour
   C. Third stage of labour
   D. Pre-delivery emergencies

III. Delivery

IV. Role of the First Responder
   A. Initial care of the newborn baby
   B. Post-delivery care of the mother

Key terms

Abortion
   The medical term for any delivery or removal of a human foetus before it can live on its own.

Amniotic sac
   The membrane forming a closed, fluid-filled sac around a developing foetus.

Birth canal
   The lower part of the uterus and the vagina.

Bloody show
   The expulsion of the mucus plug as the cervix dilates; the show is sometimes mixed with blood and often occurs at the beginning of labour.

Cervix
   The neck of the uterus.

Crowning
   The stage in which the head (or other presenting part) of the baby is seen at the vaginal opening.

Foetus
   An unborn, developing baby.

Miscarriage
   Spontaneous delivery of a human foetus before it is able to live on its own.

Perineum
   The area of skin between the vagina and anus.

Placenta
   The foetal and maternal organ through which the foetus absorbs oxygen and nutrients and excretes wastes; it is attached to the foetus via the umbilical cord.

Presenting part
   The part of the foetus that appears at the vaginal opening first.

Umbilical cord
   The cord that connects the placenta to the foetus.

Uterus
   The female reproductive organ in which a baby grows and develops.

Vagina
   The canal that leads from the uterus to the external opening in females.

Objectives

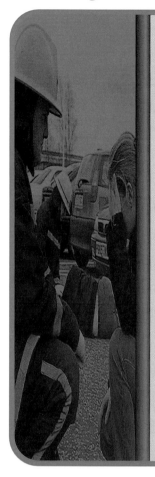

On completion of this chapter you will be able to meet the following objectives:

Cognitive objectives
1. Identify the following structures: birth canal, placenta, umbilical cord, amniotic sac.
2. Define the following terms: crowning, bloody show, labour, abortion.
3. State the indications of an imminent delivery.
4. State the steps in the pre-delivery preparation of the mother.
5. Establish the relationship between universal precautions and childbirth.
6. State the steps to assist in delivery.
8. Discuss the steps in delivery of the placenta.
9. List the steps in the emergency medical care of the mother post-delivery.
10. Discuss the steps in caring for a newborn.

Affective objectives
11. Explain the rationale for attending to the feelings of a patient in need of emergency care during childbirth.

12. Demonstrate a caring attitude towards patients during childbirth who request emergency medical services.
13. Place the interests of the patient during childbirth as the foremost consideration when making any and all patient care decisions.
14. Communicate empathically with patients during childbirth, as well as with family members and friends of the patient.

Psychomotor objectives
15. Demonstrate the steps to assist in the normal delivery.
16. Demonstrate the necessary care procedures of the foetus as the head appears.
17. Attend to the steps in the delivery of the placenta.
18. Demonstrate the post-delivery care of the mother.
19. Demonstrate the care of the newborn.

First response

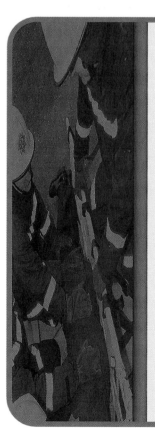

FIRST RESPONDERS Charlie and Sally were teaching infant CPR to a class of expectant mothers and fathers at the local YMCA. Halfway through the practice session, one of the women, further along in her pregnancy than most in the class, said she had been experiencing some contractions during the day and that her water had just broken. She said her contractions were now strong and regular. Because she was expecting her third baby, Charlie and Sally knew the delivery might occur soon. Charlie went to call for an ambulance while Sally assessed the patient.

Although Sally had never assisted with a delivery, she had been well educated in this area and knew what questions to ask. When she confirmed that the patient's waters had broken and that her contractions were about 2 minutes apart, Sally and Charlie prepared for delivery on the scene. The closest ambulance was about 45 minutes away, and the baby would probably not wait that long. Sally and Charlie, along with the patient and her husband, were a little nervous, but they knew that childbirth is a natural process and that it is rarely an emergency for the mother or the newborn baby.

The delivery went well. After the baby was born, the mother, father and healthy baby girl were all transported to the hospital for evaluation. Charlie and Sally had just participated in one of the most professionally rewarding calls a First Responder can experience.

Although most babies in the UK are born in hospital, this is not true world-wide. Most babies in the world are not born in any type of medical facility. Birth is a natural process and one that does not usually require any medical intervention.

When an ambulance is called for a woman in labour, there is usually enough time for the mother to be transported to hospital. In some cases, however, First Responders may arrive on the scene to find a woman who is so far into labour that there is not enough time to get to hospital before delivery. In situations when pre-hospital delivery is likely to occur, First Responders must be ready to assist the mother with the delivery.

This chapter discusses what First Responders need to understand to assist with a pre-hospital delivery, beginning with a description of the anatomy of the woman and the developing baby. Emergency medical care for pre-delivery emergencies is discussed, as well as the procedure for assisting with a normal delivery. Resuscitation of the newborn baby and post-delivery care of the mother are also discussed.

REPRODUCTIVE ANATOMY AND PHYSIOLOGY

The anatomy of the human female and the growing baby allow pregnancy and delivery to occur with few problems (**Fig. 11.1**). The mother's uterus, or womb, is the structure in which the baby grows and develops. The uterus is a muscular organ that eventually contracts and expels the foetus during childbirth. During pregnancy, the cervix (the neck of the uterus) contains a mucous plug. As the cervix dilates (widens) during labour to allow the foetus to pass through, the mucous plug becomes dislodged.

When the muscles of the uterus contract, the foetus is pushed into the birth canal, which consists of the lower part of the uterus and the vagina. The vagina is the canal that leads from the uterus to the external opening in females. The foetus is pushed through the birth canal into the outside world during childbirth. The perineum is the area of skin between the vagina and anus. This skin may tear as a result of the pressure exerted by the foetus during childbirth.

An unborn developing baby is called a foetus. The foetus is nourished through the placenta. The placenta attaches to the wall of the uterus and is composed of foetal and maternal tissue. It is attached to the baby via the umbilical cord. The placenta is an organ that develops during pregnancy. It is not present when a woman is not pregnant, and it is expelled from the body following childbirth. The placenta is also known as the afterbirth, because it is delivered after the baby is born. The placenta allows oxygen and nutrients to pass from the mother's bloodstream to the foetus. The placenta also allows carbon dioxide and waste products to pass from the foetus to the mother for elimination.

The transfer of material from the placenta to the foetus and back to the placenta is accomplished through the umbilical cord. The umbilical cord is an extension of the placenta and contains two arteries and one vein. Blood flows from the foetus to the placenta and back to the foetus. Maternal and foetal circulatory systems are independent of each other, and blood does not flow directly from mother to foetus.

The foetus is surrounded by a bag of fluid, which is called the amniotic sac. The amniotic sac contains 1–2 litres of liquid, called amniotic fluid. The amniotic fluid cushions the baby and helps protect it from injury. The amniotic sac generally ruptures before childbirth (often described by the patient as 'my water broke'). The amniotic fluid lubricates the birth canal during delivery. **Figure 11.2** illustrates the anatomical structures of pregnancy.

The foetus grows and develops for approximately 9 months, or 40 weeks. During pregnancy, the mother's uterus expands for the growing foetus (**Fig. 11.3**). Her blood volume increases along with the amount of blood travelling through her heart each minute and her heart rate. Her blood pressure decreases slightly and her digestion slows.

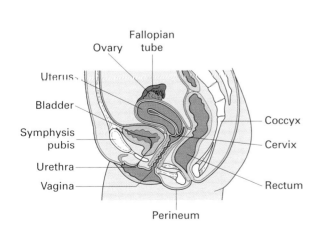

Fig. 11.1 The female reproductive system.

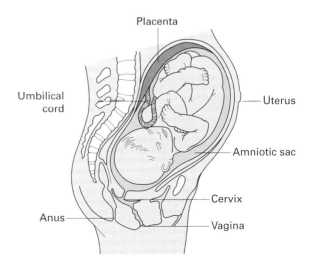

Fig. 11.2 The anatomical structures of pregnancy.

Childbirth

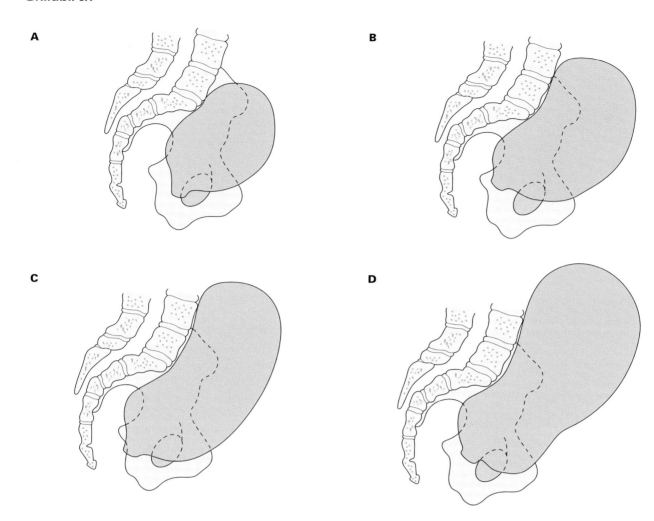

Fig. 11.3 The uterus enlarges and expands to encompass the growing infant. **(a)** At 20 weeks. **(b)** At 23 weeks. **(c)** At 27 weeks. **(d)** At 32 weeks.

Review Questions

Reproductive Anatomy and Physiology
Match the terms in the left column with their definitions in the right column.

1. Uterus
2. Cervix
3. Birth canal
4. Perineum
5. Foetus
6. Placenta
7. Amniotic sac
8. Umbilical cord

A. The passageway from the uterus through which the baby is born.
B. The organ where the baby develops.
C. The skin between the vagina and the anus.
D. The neck of the uterus.
E. The organ that allows nutrients to pass from mother to foetus and waste from foetus to mother.
F. The fluid-filled sac that cushions the foetus.
G. The connection from the placenta to the foetus.
H. The unborn developing baby.

1. B; 2. D; 3. A; 4. C; 5. H; 6. E; 7. F; 8. G

LABOUR

Labour is the process by which babies are born. Labour is generally divided into three stages, beginning with the first uterine contractions and ending when the placenta is delivered after childbirth (**Fig. 11.4**). Labour consists of contractions of the walls of the uterus that push the foetus through the cervix and into the birth canal.

First stage of labour

The first stage of labour begins with regular contractions of the uterus and continues until the foetus enters the birth canal. During this stage of labour, the cervix must dilate to allow the baby to pass into the birth canal. As the cervix dilates, mucus and blood may pass through the vagina. This mucus and blood, called the 'bloody show', is normal. Each contraction causes the cervix to become thinner and shorter in order to allow the head of the foetus to pass. Once the cervix dilates to approximately 10 cm, the head can pass through and the second stage of labour begins.

Second stage of labour

The second stage of labour begins when the foetus enters the birth canal and ends when the baby is born. Rhythmic contractions of the uterus push the foetus through the birth canal into the vaginal opening. Most babies are born with their head as the presenting part. The presenting part is the part that appears at the vaginal opening first. Crowning occurs when the head (or other presenting part) bulges against the vaginal opening. When you see crowning, delivery is imminent and you should be prepared for immediate delivery (**Fig. 11.5**).

Third stage of labour

In the third stage of labour, which starts after the baby is born, the placenta, umbilical cord and other tissues are delivered. The placenta detaches from the uterine wall and passes through the birth canal. This tissue is still connected to the foetus by the umbilical cord unless the cord has already been cut.

Labour pains occurring with each contraction are normal. Women generally experience pain when the uterus contracts and experience relief from pain as the contraction ends. A support person should be available to help the mother. The father, a friend or another First Responder should encourage her, help her to breathe regularly through the contractions and make her as comfortable as possible. The length of normal labour varies greatly among women, depending on the woman's age, previous deliveries and other individual factors and circumstances. The length of time a woman spends in labour generally decreases with each delivery.

Pre-delivery emergencies

A miscarriage is the delivery of the foetus before it can live independently of the mother. The medical term for this early delivery is abortion, but it is generally referred to as a miscarriage when it occurs spontaneously. The commonest time for a miscarriage is during the first 3 months of pregnancy. A woman experiencing a miscarriage generally has abdominal cramping, which may be severe. She may be bleeding and there may be noticeable vaginal discharge of clots and tissue. Any pads or towels that contain clots or tissue should be transported to the hospital with the patient. Be prepared to treat for shock early, particularly if the mother exhibits signs and symptoms of hypoperfusion. Along with medical care, emotional support is very important for the mother. Grief is normal and should be expected from both parents.

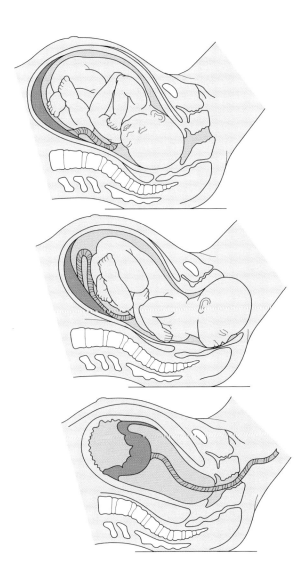

Fig. 11.4 The three stages of labour. **(a)** Contraction and dilation. **(b)** Baby moves through birth canal and is born. **(c)** Delivery of placenta.

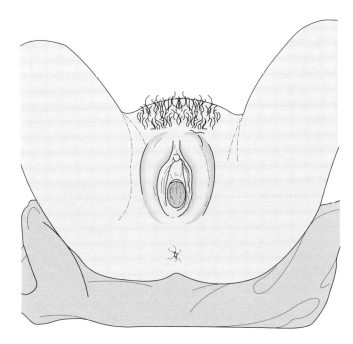

Fig. 11.5 Crowning occurs when the head or other presenting part bulges against the vaginal opening.

DELIVERY

Childbirth is not an emergency unless complicating factors are involved. In a normal delivery, your role as a First Responder is to provide support and assistance to the mother as she delivers her child and to provide care and, if necessary, resuscitation to the newborn baby.

In general, it is best to transport the expectant mother to the hospital unless delivery is anticipated within five minutes. When deciding whether to transport or to assist in delivery on the scene, the following questions will help in making that decision:
1. What is your due date?
2. Is there any bleeding or discharge?
3. Do you have the sensation of having a bowel movement with increasing pressure in the vaginal area?

If the patient answers yes to the second and third questions, examine for crowning. If crowning is present, prepare for delivery. If the decision is made to deliver on the scene, take the following precautions. Practising universal precautions is a must when you assist in childbirth. Blood and amniotic fluid should be expected and may splash. The mother may feel the need to go to the lavatory, but should not be allowed to use the toilet. The feeling of a bowel movement is common and is caused by the baby's head pressing against the walls of the rectum. The baby may deliver

while she is trying to have a bowel movement. Do not try to delay the delivery by measures such as holding the mother's legs together. These measures are ineffective and can harm the baby.

Once the decision has been made to assist in delivery on the scene, you must prepare for the delivery. While making these preparations, ask the mother if there is any chance of multiple births. Request more assistance if there is a possibility of two or more babies. Follow these steps for delivery:
1. Follow universal precautions.
2. Position the mother by having her lie with her knees flexed, drawn up and widely separated.
3. Elevate the buttocks with blankets or a pillow (**Fig. 11.6**).
4. Place absorbent, clean material such as towels or pads under the patient's buttocks. Place towels over her legs.
5. When the infant's head appears, place the palm of your hand on top of the delivering baby's head and exert very gentle pressure to prevent explosive delivery.
6. If the amniotic sac does not break or has not broken, tear it with your fingers and push it away from the infant's head and mouth.
7. As the infant's head is being delivered, determine whether the umbilical cord is around the infant's neck. If it is, attempt to slip the cord over the baby's head. If you are unable to do that, attempt to lessen pressure on the cord.
8. Once the head delivers, support the head as it rotates and suction the baby's mouth and then nostrils two or three times, using a mucus extractor. Do not place the mucus extractor in so far that it touches the back of the mouth and gags the baby (**Fig. 11.7**). If a mucus extractor is not available,

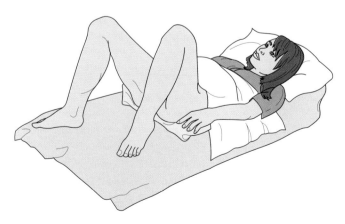

Fig. 11.6 Position the mother for delivery.

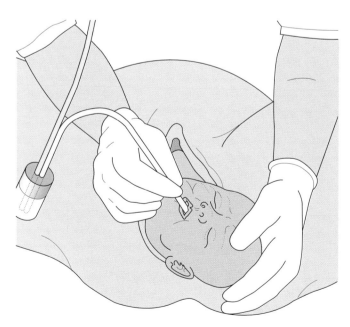

Fig. 11.7 After the infant's head is born, support the head and wipe the mouth and nose. Suction the baby's mouth and nose with a mucus extractor.

wipe the baby's mouth and then the nose with gauze.

9. As the torso and full body are delivered, support the infant with both hands. As the feet are delivered, grasp the feet. Do not pull on the infant.
10. Keep the infant level with the vagina.
11. When the umbilical cord stops pulsating, it should be tied with gauze between the mother and the newborn baby and the infant may be placed on the mother's abdomen.
12. Wipe blood and mucus from the baby's mouth and nose with sterile gauze; suction the mouth and nose again.
13. Dry the infant, wrap him in a warm blanket, and place him on the side with the head slightly lower than the trunk to aid the draining of fluid from the mouth and nose (**Fig. 11.8**).
14. Rub the baby's back or flick the soles of his feet to stimulate breathing.
15. Record the time of delivery.
16. If there is a chance for multiple births, prepare for the second delivery.
17. Observe for delivery of the placenta. This may take up to 30 minutes.
18. If the placenta is delivered, wrap it in a towel with three-quarters of the umbilical cord and place in a plastic bag. Keep the bag at the level of the infant.
19. Place a sterile pad over the vaginal opening, lower the mother's legs and help her hold them together.

There is no need to cut the cord in a normal delivery. Keep the infant warm and wait for additional ambulance or medical personnel, who will have the proper equipment to clamp and cut the cord. **Figure 11.9** shows a delivery from crowning up to the delivery of the shoulder.

Following delivery, vaginal bleeding of 300–500 ml of blood can be expected. This is usually well tolerated by the mother. It is important for First Responders to be aware of this so as not to cause undue psychological stress on themselves or on the mother. If the mother continues to bleed well beyond the expected amount, it will be necessary to massage the uterus. With the

fingers of one hand fully extended, place the palm of the hand on the lower abdomen above the pubic bone and continue to massage this area until the bleeding stops (**Fig. 11.10**).

If during delivery the head is not the presenting part, the delivery may be complicated. The First Responder should tell the mother not to push, and update responding ambulance and medical personnel about the situation. Calm and reassure the mother until additional ambulance and medical personnel arrive on scene.

ROLE OF THE FIRST RESPONDER
Initial care of the newborn baby

Immediately after birth, dry the baby and wrap him in a warm blanket with the head covered to preserve body heat. Position the infant on his side with the head slightly lower than the feet to aid fluid drainage from the mouth and nose; repeat suctioning as necessary.

Count the infant's respiratory rate. A normal respiratory rate for a newborn baby is greater than 40 breaths per minute with crying. Next, determine the pulse rate, either at the umbilical cord or the brachial artery. Normal pulse rates for a newborn baby are greater than 100 beats per minute. If the baby is not breathing, flick the soles of the feet or rub the infant's back to stimulate. If after one minute the baby does not begin breathing or continues to have difficulty (with persistent gasping or shallow or irregular breathing), or if the heart rate is less than 100 beats per minute, you will need to assist the infant's respiratory efforts and offer supplementary oxygen. This would include ensuring an open and patent airway, and possibly ventilating at a rate of 40 breaths per minute. Reassess the infant's respiratory efforts after one minute. Refer to Chapter 5 ('The airway') for a review of techniques of ventilation.

If the heart rate is less than 60 beats per minute, initiate chest compressions following guidelines for infant cardiopulmonary resuscitation (CPR). Chapter 7 ('Circulation') lists the steps for infant CPR.

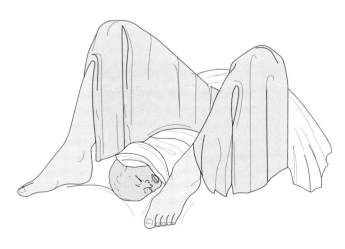

Fig. 11.8 Positioning for newborn infants.

Review Questions

Delivery

1. A _____ is the spontaneous delivery of the foetus before it is able to live outside the womb.
2. After the head delivers, you should check to see if the _____ is wrapped around the baby's neck.
3. The _____ usually delivers within 30 minutes of the baby and should be taken to the hospital to be checked for completeness.

1. Miscarriage; 2. Umbilical cord; 3. Placenta

Childbirth

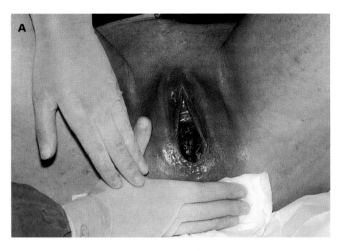

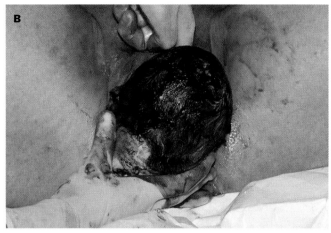

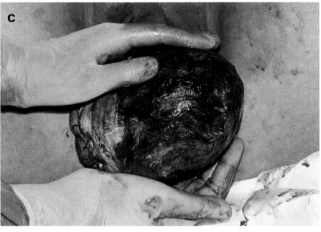

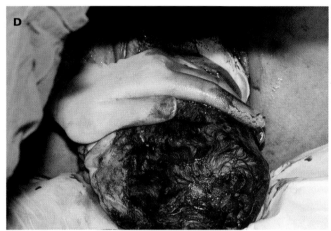

Fig. 11.9 The delivery process. **(a)** Crowning. **(b)** Check the neck for the presence of the umbilical cord. **(c)** Support the head as it rotates. **(d)** Guide the head downwards to deliver the shoulder. **(e)** The other shoulder is delivered.

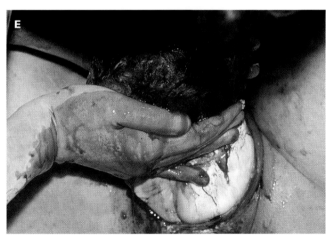

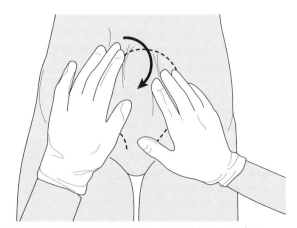

Fig. 11.10 Uterine massage to help control bleeding after delivery.

Post-delivery care of the mother

After initial care for the newborn baby, do not forget to address the mother's needs as a patient. It is important to keep contact with the mother throughout the process. Monitor the mother's respirations and pulse. Replace any blood-soaked sheets and blankets while waiting for transport to the hospital. Remember that delivery is an exhausting process for the mother also. Be attentive to her needs, both physical and psychological.

Review Questions

Role of the First Responder

1. Infants who have poor respiratory effort or slow heart beats may require _____ or _____.

2. If the newborn's heart rate is less than _____ beats per minute, begin CPR.

3. List two ways to stimulate a baby who is not breathing:

   _____

   _____

1. Ventilations, chest compressions; 2. 60; 3. Flick the soles of the feet, rub the back

CHAPTER SUMMARY

Reproductive anatomy and physiology

The foetus grows and develops in the mother's uterus. The foetus is attached to the placenta by the umbilical cord. The foetus is surrounded by a bag of fluid called the amniotic sac.

Labour

There are three stages of labour. During the first stage, contractions of the uterus cause the cervix to dilate. The baby enters the birth canal and is born during the second stage. The placenta delivers in the third stage of labour. A miscarriage is the spontaneous delivery of a foetus before it is able to survive on its own,

Delivery

If the mother feels the need to push, or if she has had any bleeding or discharge, you should evaluate her for crowning. If the baby is crowning, delivery will occur soon, and you should prepare to assist. Take universal precautions including gloves, eye wear, gown and mask. Prepare the mother for delivery and assist her.

Role of the First Responder

Dry the infant and wrap him to keep him warm. Position the infant on his side with the head lower than the feet. If the infant is not breathing on his own, you should stimulate him by rubbing the back or flicking the soles of the feet. Offer supplementary oxygen and ventilate the infant if necessary. If the heartbeat is less than 60 beats per minute, initiate chest compressions. Keep in contact with the mother while caring for the infant.

Chapter
Twelve
Infants and children

I. **The airway**
A. Anatomical and physiological concerns
B. Opening the airway
C. Suctioning
D. Using airway adjuncts

II. **Assessment**

III. **Common medical problems in infants and children**
A. Airway obstruction
B. Respiratory emergencies
C. Circulatory failure

D. Fits
E. Altered mental status
F. Sudden infant death syndrome (SIDS)

IV. **Trauma**
A. Head injury
B. Chest injury
C. Abdominal injury
D. Injury to an extremity

V. **Reactions to ill and injured infants and children**

Key terms

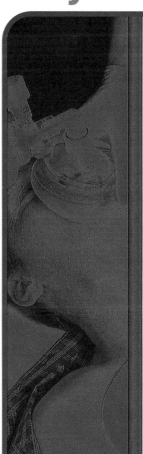

Child
Generally, a young person over the age of 1 year.

Crowing
A harsh noise heard on inspiration.

Grunting
A sound made when a patient in respiratory distress attempts to trap air to keep the alveoli open.

Infant
Generally, a young person under the age of 1 year.

Nasal flaring
An attempt by the infant in respiratory distress to increase the size of the airway by expanding the nostrils.

Neglect
The act of not giving attention to a child's essential needs.

Respiratory distress
A clinical condition in which the infant or child begins to increase the work of breathing.

Respiratory failure
A clinical condition in which the patient is continuing to work hard to breathe, the effort of breathing is increased and the patient's condition begins to deteriorate.

Retractions
The use of accessory muscles to increase the work of breathing, which appears as the sucking in of the muscles between the ribs and at the neck.

Stridor
An abnormal, high-pitched inspiratory sound, often indicating airway obstruction.

Sudden infant death syndrome (SIDS)
The sudden, unexplained death of an infant, generally between the ages of 1 month and 1 year, for which there is no discernible cause on autopsy.

Objectives

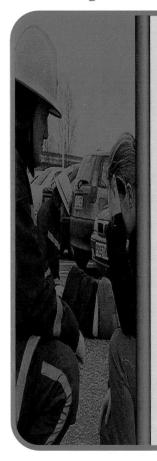

On completion of this chapter you will be able to meet the following objectives:

Cognitive objectives
1. Describe differences in anatomy and physiology of the infant, child and adult patient.
2. Describe assessment of the infant or child.
3. Indicate various causes of respiratory emergencies in infants and children.
4. Summarise emergency medical care strategies for respiratory distress and respiratory failure/arrest in infants and children.
5. List common causes of seizures in infants and children.
6. Describe management of seizures in infants and children.
7. Discuss emergency medical care of the infant and child trauma patient.
8. Recognize need for First Responder debriefing following a difficult infant or child transport.

Affective objectives
9. Attend to the feelings of the family when dealing with an ill or injured infant or child.
10. Understand the provider's own emotional response to caring for infants or children.
11. Demonstrate a caring attitude towards infants and children with illness or injury who require emergency medical services.
12. Place the interests of the infant or child with an illness or injury as the foremost consideration when making any and all patient care decisions.
13. Communicate empathically with infants and children with an illness or injury, as well as with family members and friends of the patient.

Psychomotor objectives
14. Demonstrate assessment of the infant and child.

First response

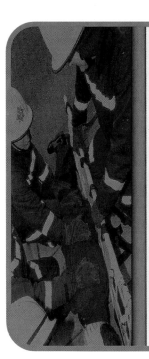

DENISE AND SANDRA were watching the nursery children play on the swings during playtime. Some of the teachers in the school had recently been trained as First Responders. As they were watching, a 5-year-old boy fell approximately 1.5 metres from a swing and landed on his left arm and side. Immediately, both Denise and Sandra felt the adrenaline starting to pump. They heard the little boy cry and ran towards him. The thought of caring for an injured child caused anxiety for both of them, but they knew that they had been well educated for this. They knew to start with the basics of airway, breathing and circulation. Denise told another teacher to call 999.

When they reached the child's side, they were both ready to take on the challenge of dealing with the injured child. The ambulance arrived shortly after, and care was transferred to the ambulance crew. Both Denise and Sandra felt comfortable with their skills and were glad they could provide early care for the injured child.

Emergency medical care providers have long been challenged by the unique aspects of caring for ill or injured infants and children. Understanding the anatomical and physiological differences is essential to providing good patient care. It is important that First Responders understand that these patients are not little adults. They are patients with unique anatomical and functional differences that must be considered. Since the percentage of responses involving infants and children is relatively small, First Responders should practice these skills to ensure they are prepared when confronted with an ill or injured infant or child.

Special attention should be given to paediatric patients in areas such as airway management, oxygenation and ventilation, assessment, trauma and near-drowning. Unfortunately, some children are also the victims of abuse and neglect. In these instances, the First Responder must know the necessary steps to deal with these situations.

Finally, First Responders need to deal with parents who are having strong emotional responses because their child is ill or injured. In addition to the parents' emotional response, First Responders must deal with their own feelings associated with caring for an ill or injured child.

THE AIRWAY
Anatomical and physiological concerns

The most important anatomical and physiological differences in an infant or child relate to the airway. In general, the airway is smaller and more easily blocked by secretions and swelling than an adult's airway. Methods of positioning the airway of an infant or child are different to the methods for an adult. Do not hyperextend the neck because the airway is so flexible it may actually become occluded because of kinking.

The tongues of infants and children are relatively large compared to the small mandible and oropharynx. The tongue can easily cause an airway obstruction in unresponsive infants and children when they are lying on their back. A proper head-tilt, chin-lift manoeuvre or a jaw thrust without head tilt can overcome this problem. Take special care not to place pressure on the soft tissues under the jaw, as this may occlude the airway.

Infants are obligate nose breathers – that is, they do not open their mouth to breathe when their nose is occluded. Suctioning a secretion-filled nasopharynx can improve breathing problems in an infant.

Infants and children can compensate for a breathing problem for a short period of time by increasing the rate and effort of breathing. This increased work of breathing uses a tremendous amount of energy. After a short period of compensating, the child may experience rapid decompensation. This decompensation is characterised by general and muscular fatigue and is a sign of respiratory failure. Because of this, a normal respiratory rate following a fast rate may be a bad sign, especially if the child looks tired or is otherwise doing poorly. Watch for signs of alteration in mental status, including drowsiness and unusual tolerance of assessment procedures and treatment.

Opening the airway

Chapter 5 ('The airway') describes the techniques for opening an airway using the head-tilt, chin-lift manoeuvre and the jaw thrust without head tilt. Because most life-threatening problems in infants and children are related to airway difficulties, you must be knowledgeable and skilled in these techniques.

When a patient loses consciousness, the muscles relax and the tongue may fall back and occlude the airway. Because these structures are attached to the lower jaw, the airway can be opened by lifting up on the lower jaw. This can be accomplished with the head-tilt, chin-lift manoeuvre or, when trauma is suspected, by the jaw thrust without head tilt. When performing a head tilt, be careful not to hyperextend the neck. Hyperextension may occlude the small, flexible airway of infants and young children. Extend the head or the neck only until the bottom of the nose points straight up. This is referred to as the 'sniffing position' for infants and children (**Fig. 12.1**). Placing a folded towel under the shoulder may assist in maintaining an open airway.

When you suspect trauma, use the jaw thrust without head tilt. With the jaw thrust, maintain the head in a neutral position, and lift the chin up and out by applying pressure to the angle of the posterior jaw (**Fig. 12.2**). Be sure to maintain stabilisation of the spine while using this technique.

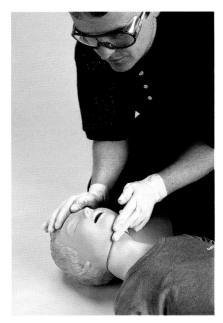

Fig. 12.1 When performing a head tilt on an infant or child, be careful not to hyperextend the neck. Use the sniffing position in children. Place a folded towel under the shoulders of infants to assist in maintaining an open airway.

Infants and children

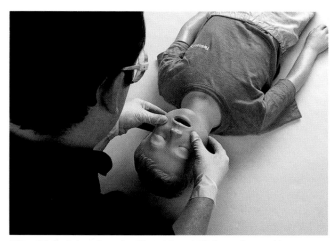

Fig. 12.2 A jaw thrust without head tilt is performed in children using the same technique as for adults.

Suctioning

Suction may be needed to clear the airway of secretions, blood or vomit. In infants, take care not to stimulate the back of the throat with the suction catheter – such stimulation can dramatically slow the infant's heart rate or cause a gag reflex or vomiting.

Suction the infant or child's airway only as deeply as you can see. In general, use a soft flexible catheter for infants and children. Measure the distance from the corner of the patient's mouth to the angle of the jaw. Place your finger on the catheter at this measurement, and do not insert the catheter any further than this. To ensure that the patient does not become hypoxic, limit the suctioning to 10–15 seconds. Rinse the catheter and suction tubing as necessary. When using a suction device on an infant or child, the vacuum should be limited to 80–120 mmHg.

It is important to consider the need for nasal suctioning. In infants, nasal secretions can cause significant upper airway obstruction. A mucus extractor can be used.

If the infant or child has an airway obstruction, follow the guidelines for foreign body airway obstruction as outlined in Chapter 5 ('The airway').

Using airway adjuncts

Oropharyngeal airways are useful in maintaining an open airway in infants and children when the head-tilt, chin-lift manoeuvre or the jaw thrust are ineffective. Airway adjuncts are not used for initial ventilation efforts.

Oropharyngeal airway

An oral airway should be used following the head-tilt, chin-lift manoeuvre only if the patient is unresponsive and has no gag reflex. If the oral airway is used in a patient who has a gag reflex, the patient may gag and vomit. This can seriously threaten the airway. The preferred method of inserting an oral airway in an infant or child is to use a tongue depressor to insert the airway without rotating. This will reduce the potential for damage to the soft palate. **Fig. 12.3** illustrates the technique for inserting an oral airway.

Nasal airways are not recommended for use by First Responders in infants or children.

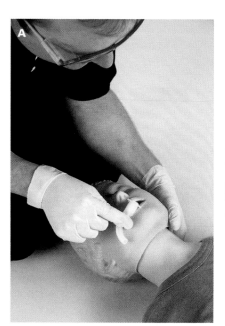

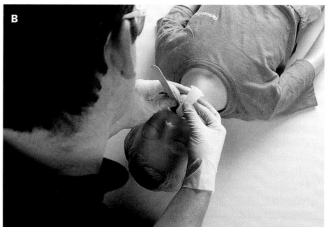

Fig. 12.3 Inserting the oral airway in infants and children. Observe universal precautions. **(a)** Select the proper sized airway by measuring from the centre of the patient's front teeth to the angle of the jaw. Position yourself at the top of the patient's head. Open the patient's mouth and use a tongue depressor to move the tongue forwards by pushing down against the base of the tongue while lifting upwards. **(b)** Insert the airway right side up (with the tip facing towards the floor of the patient's mouth). Advance the airway gently until the flange comes to rest on the patient's lips. Be sure not to push into the back of the throat. Ventilate the patient as necessary.

ASSESSMENT

Once you have assessed the scene and are prepared to assess the patient, perform an initial assessment. Be sure to include the parents in your assessment and management of infants and children. If the parents are agitated, the child may become agitated. If the parents are calm, this may help calm the child. In many cases, you can begin your assessment from a distance. Mental status, respiratory distress and many signs of shock can be assessed long before you touch the patient. Use your experience and clinical judgement to determine the assessment order that is most appropriate. Always try to assess painful areas last.

In general, begin the assessment from a distance. Observe the child's surroundings and, if the patient is injured, note the mechanism of injury. Form a general impression of whether the child is well or sick based on overall appearance. Look at the patient as you enter the room. Is he or she interacting appropriately with the people and items in the environment? Does he or she recognise the parents? Infants begin to recognise their parents at about 2 months of age. Failure to recognise parents is an ominous sign. Is the infant or child quiet and uninterested, or is the infant or child playing with a favourite toy? Is the patient appropriately distressed or scared, or is he or she unusually quiet?

Assess the mental status. Alterations in mental status should be recognised. For example, a child who is uninterested in any activity or person may be experiencing an alteration in mental status. In some cases, mental status changes may be indicated simply from the parent's statement that "There is something wrong". Mental status is characterised and documented as:

A = alert;
V = responds to voice;
P = responds to pain; and
U = unresponsive.

For newborn babies and infants, 'responds to voice' can be interpreted as 'turns to parent's voice', since young children may not obey commands under normal circumstances. Try to make eye contact with the child. Observe the child's general response to you, as well as the body tone and position.

If necessary, open the airway. Look, listen and feel for the presence of breathing. Assess the rate and effort of breathing. Increased breathing effort may be recognised by nasal flaring, the use of accessory muscles, retractions or airway noises. Airway noises include stridor, crowing and grunting; they are explained later in this chapter. Any noise made when breathing indicates a respiratory problem. Evaluate the quality of the cry or speech. If necessary, provide artificial ventilation. Look for equal expansion of both sides of the chest. As part of your respiratory assessment, assess skin colour. Look for skin that is pale, blue or mottled.

Assess circulation using the brachial and femoral pulses in infants (**Fig. 12.4**). In addition to heart rate, assess for quality of the pulse and equality of the pulses on both sides of the body. Any difference in the quality of the two pulses may be an indicator of inadequate perfusion. Assess the patient's skin colour, temperature and condition.

Based on the findings from the initial assessment, you can determine a patient priority. Infants and children with altered mental status, respiratory distress or poor perfusion should be considered priority patients.

How you perform the First Responder physical examination depends on the situation and the patient's age. In general, this examination is often best done in a trunk-to-toe-to-head approach. The components remain the same as for an adult. Even though you start with the trunk you should still assess for deformities, open wounds, tenderness and swelling. This approach provides valuable information about the patient while developing the infants or child's trust and confidence.

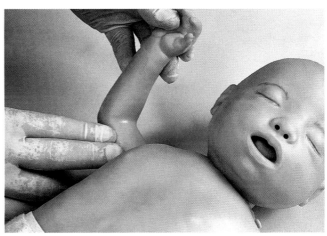

Fig. 12.4 Assessing the brachial pulse in the infant.

Review Questions

The Airway and Assessment

1. Compared to adults, the airways of infants and children are _____ and more easily _____ by secretions and swelling.

2. To open the airway of an injured child, the First Responder should perform the _____.

3. When assessing infants and younger children, the First Responder should start with the _____ of the body and finish with the _____.

4. Suctioning in the infant and child should be limited to:
   A. 5–10 seconds
   B. 10–15 seconds
   C. 15–20 seconds

5. The oral airway must be inserted by using a _____ without _____.

1. Narrower, obstructed; 2. Jaw thrust; 3. Trunk, head; 4. B; 5. Tongue depressor, rotation

COMMON MEDICAL PROBLEMS IN INFANTS AND CHILDREN

This section reviews common medical emergencies. A solid understanding of the nature of illness and the signs and symptoms related to various illnesses will help prepare you to deal with paediatric medical emergencies in the field.

Airway obstruction

Airway obstructions in infants or children are often caused by foreign bodies such as toys or food (**Fig. 12.5**). It is important to recognise the difference between partial and complete airway obstruction. If you interfere with a child's attempt to clear a partial airway obstruction you could cause a complete obstruction.

Partial obstruction

Partial airway obstructions are characterised by noisy respirations, sometimes with stridor (an abnormal, high-pitched inspiratory sound) or crowing (a harsh noise heard on inspiration). The child may be coughing. Retractions may be seen on inhalation.

In general, if the nail beds and the mucous membranes are pink, that signals good peripheral perfusion. This is because even though there is a partial obstruction, there is adequate air exchange. During your assessment of mental status, these infants and children will often be awake and agitated. If there is cyanosis or altered mental status, there may be a complete obstruction.

Emergency care

To assist an infant or child with a partial airway obstruction, first pay attention to positioning. Allow the child to maintain a position of comfort – assist a younger child to sit up, but do not allow the patient to lie supine, as this may worsen the obstruction. Many children will be more comfortable sitting in their

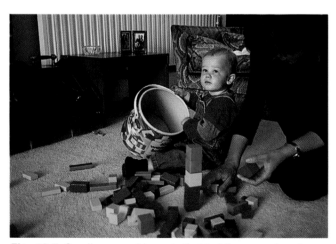

Fig. 12.5 Small, removable parts that toddlers can place in their mouths, such as small building blocks, can cause airway obstruction.

parent's lap. The patient should be transported to a hospital for further evaluation. Be aware that transporting a child sitting in a parent's lap may compromise your ability to assure their safety through proper restraints. Never buckle a lap belt over both parent and child. For safety you may need to separate the parent and child; if so, keep the parent restrained close to and within the child's field of vision.

Make every effort to keep the child comfortable; do not agitate the child. Agitation will increase the work of breathing and further complicate the situation. Perform only a limited examination. Avoid assessing blood pressure because this may upset the child. If there is a deterioration in colour or mental status, it is most likely that a complete obstruction has occurred.

Complete obstruction

Complete airway obstruction is a life-threatening emergency. Any partial airway obstruction with altered mental status or cyanosis should be treated as a complete obstruction. These obstructions require immediate intervention.

Patients with complete airway obstruction have no effective crying and cannot speak. Cyanosis is often present. When complete obstruction follows partial airway obstruction, the infant's or child's efforts to clear the airway by coughing become ineffective. Increased respiratory effort is seen. The patient may lose responsiveness or have an altered mental status.

Clear the airway using the foreign body airway procedures described in Chapter 5 ('The airway'). Attempt artificial ventilation using the mouth-to-mask technique.

Respiratory emergencies

The rapid recognition and treatment of respiratory emergencies in infants and children is equivalent in priority to the recognition of shockable rhythms, early cardiopulmonary resuscitation (CPR) and early defibrillation in adults. More than 80% of all cases of cardiac arrest in infants and children start as respiratory arrest. The two best ways of preventing unexpected death in children are the prevention of injuries and the recognition of and early intervention in respiratory emergencies.

Respiratory distress

Respiratory distress is a clinical condition in which the infant or child begins to experience an increase in the work of breathing. Infants and children increase the work of breathing at the expense of other physiological functions. Signs and symptoms of respiratory distress include a rapid respiratory rate (greater than 60 breaths per minute in infants, 30–40 breaths per minute in children), nasal flaring, retractions, stridor, use of accessory muscles, lethargy, apathy and grunting. See-saw respirations may often be present. See-saw respirations are the pronounced use of the abdomen to assist in breathing. The chest is pulled in and the abdomen is thrust out.

Nasal flaring occurs as the infant tries to get more air by increasing the size of the airway by expanding the nostrils. Retractions are contractions of muscles to increase the ability to expand and contract the chest cavity. Retractions appear as the sucking in of the muscles between the ribs (intercostal muscles), the neck muscles (supraclavicular muscles) and the muscles below the margin of the rib (subcostal muscles). Retractions occur as the effort of breathing increases (**Fig. 12.6**). Grunting is an expiratory sound made when the patient attempts to trap air to keep the alveoli open. **Box 12.1** lists the signs and symptoms of respiratory distress.

Respiratory failure

If uncorrected, respiratory distress can progress to respiratory failure. In this clinical condition, the patient is continuing to work hard to breathe, and the patient's condition begins to deteriorate. As the work of breathing increases, the infant or child will become tired and no longer able to compensate for respiratory distress. Respiratory failure is seen in the combination of the signs and symptoms of respiratory distress with decreased peripheral perfusion, cyanosis and mental status changes. **Box 12.2** lists the signs and symptoms of respiratory failure.

If respiratory failure is not treated, the patient will become too tired to breathe. A complete failure of the respiratory system will occur. As the infant or child fatigues or shows signs of decompensation, the First Responder must begin more aggressive interventions.

Role of the First Responder

Begin with a scene assessment and initial patient assessment. Complete a physical examination as needed.

Regardless of the origin of the clinical condition presented, the goal is to restore effective respiratory function. The easiest way to correct this problem is first to recognise the seriousness of the condition. Act quickly and calmly to avoid upsetting the child or the parents.

In cases of respiratory failure, the patient is focused on breathing. When the patient focuses on breathing, he or she will not resist your interventions. The child should be allowed to remain in a position of comfort. Make sure an ambulance is on the way and notify the crew of the patient's condition.

If the respiratory failure progresses, you will need to ventilate the child. This is done with the child in a supine position. If the child is able to struggle against being placed in this position and your assistance with ventilation, the child does not need to be ventilated. In all cases of respiratory arrest, your goal is to prevent cardiac arrest. Immediately begin to ventilate the child at one breath every 3 seconds. Airway management and ventilation are the highest priority for these patients. Patients in respiratory arrest should be transported rapidly to a facility capable of dealing with this emergency. Perform an ongoing assessment if the

Box 12.1	**Signs and Symptoms of Respiratory Distress**

Respiratory distress is indicated by any of the following:
- Increased rate of breathing
- Nasal flaring
- Intercostal, supraclavicular and subcostal retractions
- Mottled skin colour or cyanosis
- Stridor
- Grunting
- Altered mental status (combative, decreased mental status, unresponsive)

Box 12.2	**Signs and Symptoms of Respiratory Failure**

Respiratory failure/arrest is the presence of any of the findings of respiratory distress along with any of the following:
- Breathing rate less than 10 per minute in a child
- Breathing rate of less than 20 per minute in an infant
- Limp muscle tone
- Unresponsive
- Slow or absent heart rate
- Weak or absent distal pulses
- Cyanosis

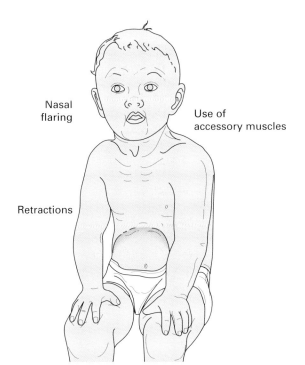

Nasal flaring

Use of accessory muscles

Retractions

Fig. 12.6 Nasal flaring, retractions, accessory muscle use and positioning are signs of respiratory distress in infants and children.

Infants and children

ambulance has not yet arrived. Carefully monitor the patient's respiratory efforts and heart rate. Ensure the receiving hospital has been forewarned about receiving a critically ill infant or child.

Circulatory failure

Shock is the failure of the cardiovascular system to supply adequate oxygenated blood to the vital organs. If uncorrected, it can rapidly lead to death. Attention to assessment findings helps you identify this condition. Shock in infants and children rarely results from a cardiac problem. Common causes include dehydration from vomiting or diarrhoea or both, trauma, blood loss and infection.

When assessing the infant or child, be alert for the following circulatory signs and symptoms. As the body attempts to compensate, respirations become rapid, and the skin becomes pale, mottled, cool and clammy. The pulse becomes rapid, and distal pulses may be absent or weak compared to central pulses. You may see mental status changes ranging from agitation and disorientation to unresponsiveness.

Role of the First Responder

The goal in the management of shock is to transport the patient to a facility capable of establishing vascular access and rapidly administering fluid. In some pre-hospital care systems this may be done by providers of advanced life support (ALS); in other systems this requires transport to a hospital by ambulance personnel. Your actions at the scene must be rapid and organised. After completing the scene assessment, perform an initial patient assessment. During the initial assessment, ensure a patent airway. Be prepared to provide artificial ventilation. Manage bleeding if present. Keep the patient warm. Carefully monitor the patient's pulse, and begin chest compressions if necessary.

Fits

Fits represent a nervous system malfunction and are among the most common complaints that pre-hospital care providers see in infants and children. Some infants and children have chronic fits; others have fits because of acute illness or injury. There are many types and causes of fits; these include chronic medical conditions, rapid rise in body temperature, infections, poisoning, low blood sugar, head injury or other trauma, decreased levels of oxygen and unknown causes. Inadequate breathing and altered mental status may occur following a fit.

The role of the First Responder is to support the patient's vital functions and prevent the patient from injuring himself or herself. Do not worry about determining the cause of the fit. Be alert for violent muscle contractions called convulsions. Keep in mind that not all fits have this violent muscle contraction. Fits may be brief or prolonged. Fits must be considered a serious emergency; however, fits themselves are rarely life threatening.

When gathering a history concerning fits be sure to include the following questions:
1. Has the child had previous fits?
2. Does the child take anti-epileptic medications?
3. Is it possible that the child ingested any other medications?

If the answer to either of the last two questions is yes, the First Responder should determine whether the medication was taken as prescribed and also whether or not the present fit is similar to previous fits.

Role of the First Responder

Following the completion of the scene assessment, the initial patient assessment and the physical examination (as needed), protect the patient from the environment. Move any objects that the patient might come into contact with during the fit. Ask bystanders, with the exception of the parents, to leave the area. Ensure a patent airway. Never restrain a fitting patient or put anything in the mouth. Patients who are fitting will often have significant oral secretions, so have suction available. If the patient is cyanosed, assure an adequate airway and begin ventilation if possible. Observe and describe the fitting activity to the ambulance personnel who will be transporting the patient to the hospital.

Following the fit, place the patient in the recovery position if there is no possibility of spinal trauma. If there is a partial airway obstruction, correct the head position, check for a foreign body, give high-flow oxygen and consider inserting an airway. Although brief fits are usually not harmful, there may be a dangerous underlying condition. If a fit lasts for more than 5–10 minutes, a specific medication may be required. Comfort, calm and reassure the patient and family that an ambulance is on the way.

Altered mental status

Another common medical condition that First Responders may encounter in an infant or child is altered mental status. There are many common causes of altered mental status; no single cause predominates in infants and children. Altered mental status may be caused by low blood sugar, poisoning, fitting, infection, head trauma, decreased oxygen levels and shock (hypoperfusion). Altered mental status in infants and young children may be characterised by lack of an appropriate response to the environment or persons, lack of interest in items in the environment and failure to recognise the parents. As with adults, the AVPU acronym can be used to assess and communicate the level of responsiveness in infants and children.

Role of the First Responder

Support the patient. Do not worry about trying to determine a specific cause of the altered mental status, except by obtaining a patient history. Maintain an open airway. Place the patient in the recovery position if there is no possibility of spinal trauma. Have suction available. If the patient is cyanosed, ensure a patent airway and provide artificial ventilation. Comfort and reassure the child's parents that an ambulance is on the way. Complete ongoing assessments as needed.

Sudden infant death syndrome (SIDS)

Sudden infant death syndrome (SIDS) is the sudden death of an infant who is generally less than 1 year old. Infants who have died from SIDS are often discovered early in the morning. The death is not apparently related to anything in the infant's history and remains unexplained even after a thorough autopsy. SIDS is the leading cause of death in infants under 1 year of age.

Role of the First Responder

Unless the baby is stiff, try to resuscitate the infant. Follow good, basic life-support procedures and alert the responding pre-hospital care personnel of the infant's condition. Be especially observant of scene details and document them well.

The death of a child is very difficult for parents and health professionals. Parents experience intense feelings of guilt, anger, denial and disbelief. The initial reaction may range from hysteria to complete silence. It is essential to allow members of the family to express their grief. Be careful to avoid comments that might suggest blame to the parents. Be prepared to provide emotional support to the parents. Some medical and law enforcement agencies provide bereavement teams to help families deal with their emotional trauma. Check to see if any agencies in your area provide this service.

This is an extremely emotional event for the First Responder. Do not hesitate to consider the need for critical incident stress debriefings, and, if necessary, request them for yourself and for others involved (see Chapter 2, 'The well-being of the First Responder'). Communicating these feelings with one another can greatly reduce the stress.

TRAUMA

Trauma is a leading cause of death in children and adolescents. Blunt trauma is most common, although unfortunately, in our society, penetrating trauma is on the rise. The injury patterns seen in infants and children are different to those seen in adults. Because the child is smaller, the traumatic forces are more generalised and may spread throughout the body rather than dissipating over a small area. Often more than one body system is involved. With the small size and the closeness of internal organs, more energy is transmitted to more organs. The bones of a child are less calcified and are more resilient. This makes the musculoskeletal system less likely to absorb the impact of trauma. In addition, there may be more significant internal damage without serious outward signs.

Children are often injured in road traffic accidents. If the infant or child has not been restrained in an infant

or child car safety seat, or if the seat is secured improperly, there are often head and neck injuries. When the infant or child is improperly restrained there are often abdominal and lower spine injuries. Air bags may cause facial trauma or asphyxiation. Children may be injured as pedestrians or bicycle riders who are struck by vehicles, resulting in head, spinal and abdominal trauma. Children may also be injured in falls from a height, as a result of burns, or from sports injuries. The following sections describe certain common injuries and their appropriate emergency medical care.

Head injury

The head is proportionally larger in infants and children than it is in adults. Head injury is the most common cause of death in paediatric trauma patients. Unfortunately, many severe injuries result in death regardless of the treatment given.

Vomiting is common in head injuries and, therefore, the airway must be protected. The most common cause of decreased oxygenation in unresponsive head injury patients is the tongue obstructing the airway. For this reason, the jaw-thrust technique is critically important. Respiratory arrest is commonly seen after severe head injuries and it may occur during transport.

Chest injury

Suspect chest injury based on the mechanism of injury. Children have soft, pliable ribs. When the child is injured in the chest, the resilience of the chest wall allows the forces to be transferred to the heart, lungs and blood vessels. There may be significant internal injuries without obvious external signs. If abrasions or contusions are present on the chest, they signal an increased risk of internal chest injury.

Abdominal injury

The abdomen is a common site of injury to infants and children. Often the injury is not obvious. Always suspect internal injuries when evaluating trauma patients. Always consider abdominal injury in a deteriorating trauma patient without external signs of trauma or blood loss. The abdomen may collect a lot of blood that cannot be seen, and the abdomen may be distended.

Injury to an extremity

Infants and children are not exempt from injuries to the extremities. In cases of injury to an extremity, provide manual stabilisation, as in injuries to adult patients.

For all trauma patients, begin with a scene assessment and an initial patient assessment. Note the mechanism of injury. Complete a physical examination, looking for specific injuries. Have your partner hold the child's head in a neutral position and do not move the patient. Make sure the patient has an open airway and is breathing adequately. If you need to open the airway, use the jaw thrust without head tilt. Have suction ready. If there are injuries to the extremities, stabilise them in the position you find them until they can be splinted. Complete ongoing assessments until transporting ambulance personnel arrive.

REACTIONS TO ILL AND INJURED INFANTS AND CHILDREN

Many First Responders feel anxiety when dispatched to a call involving an ill or injured child. This anxiety often comes from a lack of experience in treating children or from a fear of failure. First Responders who have children of their own often experience

Review Questions

Trauma

1. Which of the following areas is most often injured in infants and children?
   A. Head
   B. Chest
   C. Abdomen
   D. Extremities

2. When assessing an injured infant or child with deteriorating perfusion, the First Responder should suspect hidden injuries in the _____?
   A. Head
   B. Chest
   C. Abdomen
   D. Extremities

1. A; 2. C

stress from identifying the patient with their own child. Cases of child abuse or neglect are especially difficult, as is dealing with a child who is seriously injured or dies. Chapter 2 ('The well-being of the First Responder') describes measures you can take to manage the stress resulting from these situations. A debriefing after the event can help you think about your emotions.

Remember that you have skills that you can apply to children. Much of what you have learned about adults applies to children, but you need to remember the differences.

If you rarely see infants and children in your emergency medical services practice, staying prepared is important. Often a local paediatrician can assist you in refining your skills. Observe normal children of all ages. Finally, consider every patient encounter with an infant or child as a learning experience.

Remember that most of the children you see are not gravely ill or injured and you will be able to help them. Allow yourself to enjoy the time you spend with your smallest patients.

CHAPTER SUMMARY
The airway

Anatomical and physiological concerns related to the airway are the most important. In general, airways are smaller and more easily obstructed. Positioning the airway is different in children – take care not to hyperextend the neck as this may occlude the airway. The tongue is relatively large in infants and young children and occupies a proportionally larger amount of space. Proper positioning is important in these patients.

Airway adjuncts may be used to assist in maintaining an open airway. Insert an oral airway using a tongue depressor.

Assessment

Assessment of the infant or child begins from a distance. Use your general impression to decide if the child is sick or well. In general, use a trunk-to-toe-to-head approach in infants and young children. Assess the airway, breathing and circulation of the child.

Common medical problems in infants and children

The first priority when dealing with ill infants and children is airway and breathing. The leading cause of death in infants and children is an uncorrected respiratory problem. Follow the proper sequence for relieving a foreign body airway obstruction.

Respiratory failure is the next step in the progression of respiratory distress. Respiratory failure is characterised by an increased or decreased respiratory rate, cyanosis, decreased muscle tone and mental status changes. Infants and children in respiratory failure should undergo airway positioning as a top priority. Ventilation may be absent or just inadequate. Ensure airway patency and provide ventilation.

Other medical emergencies in infants and children include altered mental status, shock and seizures. In general, the First Responder will provide care that supports the vital functions. Ensure an open airway, have suction available and support ventilation. Make sure an ambulance is on the way and notify the crew of the patient's condition.

Trauma

Trauma is a leading cause of death in children and adolescents. The pattern of injury will be different to what it is in adults. Because of the smaller size, multiple organ systems may be involved. Management of injuries is similar to that for adults; however, it is important to have appropriately sized equipment. Vehicular trauma, burns and falls are the most common causes of childhood trauma. Head injuries are common. Chest injury should be suspected based on the mechanism of injury. It is possible for an infant or child to have a significant chest injury without obvious external signs. Abdominal injuries are common and are often hidden. The First Responder must suspect abdominal injury in any trauma patient who is deteriorating without obvious external injury.

Reactions to illness and injured children

Realise that most of your First Responder skills for adults also apply to infants and children. Take time to gain additional experience and knowledge related to infants and children. Use every opportunity to provide care to an infant or child as a learning experience.

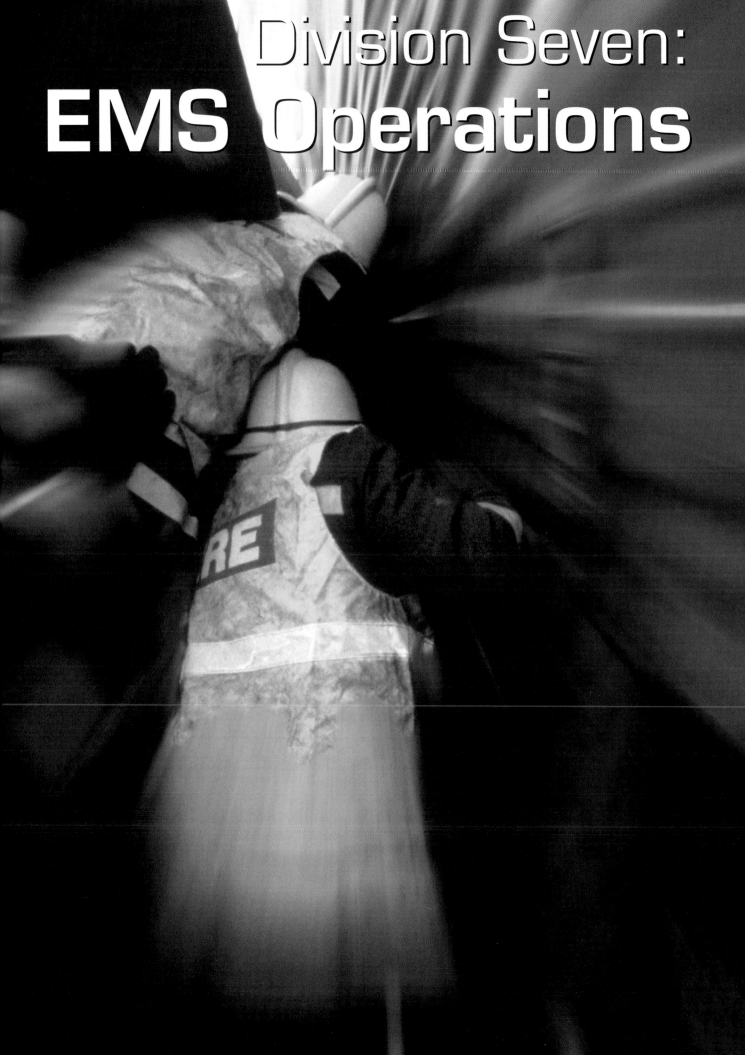

Division Seven:
EMS Operations

Chapter

EMS operations

I   Phases of an EMS response
   A   Preparation for the call
   B   Mobilisation
   C   On the way to the scene
   E   Arrival at the scene
   E   Transferring the patient to the
       ambulance
   G   Post-run

II   Air medical transport
   A   Selection of landing sites
   B   Landing site preparation
   C   Safety

III   Fundamentals of extrication
   A   Principles of extrication
   B   Team approach system
   C   Extrication techniques
   D   Supplementary restraint systems
       (SRS)

IV   Hazardous materials
   A   Safety
   B   Radiation

V   Mass casualty situations
   A   Basic triage
   B   Procedures

Key terms

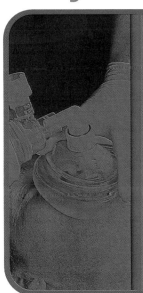

Extrication
   The process of removing a patient
   from entanglement in a motor
   vehicle or other situation in a safe
   and appropriate manner.

Hazardous material
   Any substance or material that can
   pose an unreasonable risk to
   safety, health, property or the
   environment.

Incident management system
   A system for co-ordinating
   procedures to assist in the control,
   direction and co-ordination of
   emergency response resources.

Placard
   An information sign with symbols
   and numbers to assist in
   identifying the hazardous material
   or class of material.

Triage
   A method of categorising patients
   into treatment or transport
   priorities.

Objectives

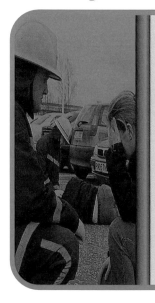

On completion of this chapter you will be able to meet the following objectives:

1. List the phases of an EMS response.
2. Define the role of the First Responder in an extrication situation.
3. Identify the need for personal and crew safety at operational incidents.
4. Understand the principles of the team approach system as it relates to the extrication of casualties.
5. List the various methods of gaining access to the casualty, and understand the principles of controlled and immediate release.

6. State the safety rules that apply when air medical transport is being used.
7. State the role a First Responder until appropriately trained personnel arrive at the scene of a hazardous material incident.
8. Understand the principle role of a First Responder in the mass casualty situation.

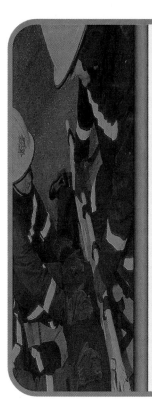

First response

THE SHIFT WAS ABOUT TO BEGIN for Jane and Roy, fire-fighters and First Responders. They arrived at their station in South Newcastle a few minutes early to prepare for their working day. In the past, they had sometimes begun a shift without adequate time to check the equipment, but this time they planned ahead. Roy began the inventory of the medical equipment, and checked that there were adequate supplies for an emergency call and that the battery-operated equipment was functioning properly. At the same time, Jane inspected the mechanics of the vehicle. She completed the daily checklist, recording fluid levels, checking tyre pressures and ensuring that all lights and warning devices were functioning properly.

With the vehicle check complete, Jane and Roy stored their personal protective equipment and checked to see that the street maps were available. They reported to control that they were 'on the run' and available. As they headed to the kitchen for a glass of orange juice, the radio interrupted, 'Respond to 81 Elm Street ... First Responder assignment; unknown problem; patient is unresponsive, unknown if breathing. Call-back in progress.' As they returned to the vehicle, they were confident they were prepared for the call.

Just as competent patient care skills are critical, non-medical operational skills are equally important. As a First Responder, you need a solid understanding of the skills required for all phases of an EMS response, as well as an understanding of your roles and responsibilities in each phase. As you read this chapter, please remember that it is intended only as an overview of First Responder operations. You should seek additional training programmes from your own service.

PHASES OF AN EMS RESPONSE

A typical medical response consists of nine stages or phases:

- preparation for the call;
- mobilisation;
- on the way to the scene;
- arrival at the scene;
- transferring the patient to the ambulance;
- on the way to the receiving facility;
- arrival at the receiving facility;
- on the way to the station; and
- the post-run phase.

First Responders are not normally involved in all these phases, but they may be involved in most of them at normal incidents.

Preparation for the call

Preparation for the call refers to the phase before a response, during which you prepare to respond. This is the phase that allows you to check that all equipment is functional, that the emergency vehicle is completely stocked (**Fig. 13.1**) and mechanically sound (**Fig. 13.2**), and that you are mentally and physically prepared to respond to an emergency call.

As a First Responder, you have a responsibility to yourself, your family, your partner and your patients to be mentally and physically fit to respond to any

emergency call. This includes eating a proper diet and taking exercise as described in Chapter 2 ('The well-being of the First Responder'). In addition to being in good physical and mental health, you must be prepared to respond through the skills and knowledge that you learned in your initial First Responder programme, and you must maintain these skills by taking part in continuing training programmes.

Continuity training is extremely important in emergency medical services, and you should attend as many additional sessions as possible. Discussing operations and patient care experiences with other emergency personnel is also beneficial. Pre-hospital emergency care is a dynamic field that continually evolves as medical advances occur. You must remain flexible and open to new ideas and procedures as you progress in your career.

The emergency vehicle must also be ready for any call, and it must always be stocked with medical and non-medical supplies. Your brigade and local protocols dictates what specific equipment is required in the vehicle (**Fig. 13.3**). Most services stock the typical emergency vehicle with a wide range of basic medical supplies (**Box 13.1**).

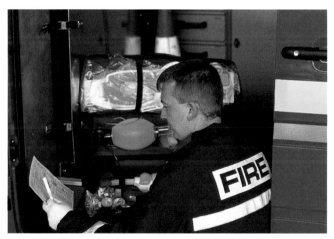

Fig. 13.1 Check all medical supplies and equipment in the emergency vehicle to make sure it is completely stocked.

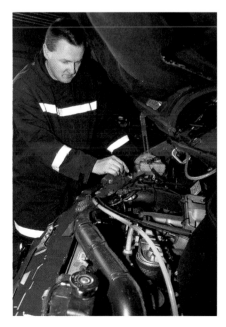

Fig. 13.2 Check all of the vehicle's mechanical systems.

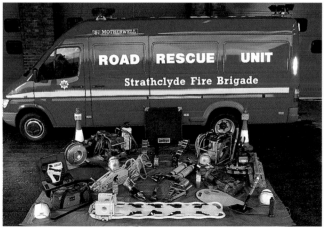

Fig. 13.3 The emergency vehicle should be well stocked with a variety of equipment and supplies for all emergencies.

| Box 13.1 | **Emergency Vehicle Equipment** |

- Basic supplies
- Airways
- Suction equipment
- Artificial ventilation devices
- Basic wound-care supplies

Besides medical supplies, certain non-medical supplies are required for the safe and efficient operation of a First Responder unit. Many services require certain specific safety and protective equipment to be in the emergency vehicle. This equipment includes gloves, masks and protective eye wear. First Responders should also have the appropriate gear to respond to a rescue situation.

Other beneficial non-medical supplies and equipment include local street maps, pre-planned routes, binoculars and patient care reports. As a First Responder, you should be familiar with your response area, and you should have a basic knowledge of traffic routes, one-way streets and alternative routes.

Mobilisation

Mobilisation is a critical phase of an emergency response. The majority of calls received at control centres are via the '999' system. The control centre is staffed 24 hours a day with personnel who may be able to provide medical instructions to the caller before the response unit arrives. This system allows a family member, friend or bystander to begin emergency medical care while help is on the way. In addition, many control centres have pre-planned response policies, including criteria-based dispatch (see Chapter 1, 'Introduction to EMS Systems') that allow the dispatcher to use a computer-assisted dispatch program or cardex system to determine which units should be dispatched and to give these units a mode of response based on the information that has been received about the patient.

When the controller notifies you of a response, you need to receive specific information. This information depends on your particular control centre and the caller providing the information. Usually you are informed of the location and the nature of the incident. In some systems, the controller provides the caller's name, location and call-back number. Additional information may be available at the time of mobilisation or become available while you are on the way to the scene, such as the number of patients, the severity of any injuries and any other special problems or complications at the scene, including hazards and safety issues.

On the way to the scene

To respond to the request for help, you must reach the scene safely. Use common sense, but also consciously remind yourself not to run to the vehicle (or later, at the scene) because of the risk of injury. You should notify the control centre that you are responding to the call. Record the essential information from control and keep this information available for review as you respond.

As an added safety measure to keep you, the crew and other passengers safe, everyone in the vehicle should always wear seat belts. This protection may save your life (**Fig. 13.4**).

As the driver of an emergency vehicle, you are responsible for knowing and following all road traffic regulations and local protocols regarding the use of emergency warning devices.

While travelling to the incident, you may obtain additional information from the control to help in your scene assessment. This is also a good time to assign personnel to specific duties and consider whether any special equipment is likely to be needed. You can also use this time to decide what equipment to take with you on initially leaving the vehicle and to prepare it. Planning in advance now may save time at the scene.

Before beginning patient care, you must consider your arrival at the scene carefully. The first step is to position the vehicle. Position the vehicle first for safety and secondly for ease of departure from the scene. Safety considerations include parking uphill or upwind from any hazardous substance, and at least 30 m from any wreckage. The incident will dictate whether to park the vehicle in front of or beyond the incident.

Apply the parking brake and turn on the necessary warning lights to alert other vehicles of your presence. At night, avoid blinding other drivers who will arrive at the scene after you by turning off the headlights, unless they are needed to illuminate the scene.

Arrival at the scene

Notify control of your arrival at the scene. Remember to assess the scene before approaching; this is an opportunity to protect yourself from harm. If there is a potential for violence or if the scene is unsafe, wait for police assistance before approaching. Consider the need

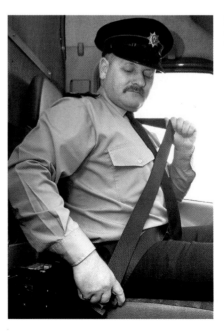

Fig. 13.4 Always wear your seatbelt in the vehicle.

for personal protective equipment (see Chapter 2, 'The well being of the First Responder'), and assess the scene for hazards. Is the vehicle parked in a safe location? Is it safe to approach the patient? Does the patient need to be moved immediately because of any hazards?

Next, note the mechanism of injury at every incident scene – this will provide you as the First Responder with a guide to possible injuries. Questioning patients and witnesses will also provide valuable information. If there are more patients than you and your crew can handle, request additional help and begin triage. The principles of triage are discussed later in this chapter. If there is only one patient, begin your initial assessment with a general impression. If the patient has sustained trauma, provide in-line spinal immobilisation.

All actions at the scene should be rapid, organised and efficient, and you should ensure that a casualty-centred approach is adopted.

Transferring the patient to the ambulance

Using the principles you learned in Chapter 5, 'Lifting and moving patients', assist the EMS personnel when they transfer the patient to the vehicle for transport. After performing all critical interventions, ensure that all dressings and bandages or splints, if used, are secure. Cover the patient to preserve body heat and to provide protection from the weather, and secure the patient to the appropriate lifting and moving device. You may sometimes be required to accompany the patient in the ambulance, for instance to assist with two-rescuer cardiopulmonary resuscitation.

Post-run

If the vehicle needs fuelling or other mechanical work, this should be handled at this phase. All paperwork from the call should be filed as required by your service. Restock any supplies that were used, and clean and disinfect the equipment. Follow your service procedure for disinfecting equipment. When you are

finished with these tasks, notify control that you are available for further calls.

AIR MEDICAL TRANSPORT

Air medical transportation should be considered when the patient's condition warrants it because of the speed of response and transfer to the appropriate hospital that is possible with air transport, or because specialist medical treatment can be given if there is a doctor on board the aircraft.

There is an obvious need for First Responders to be fully familiar with the exact services that the local air medical transport unit can offer. This includes not only a knowledge of the type and size of aircraft, but also whether the service simply provides helicopter transport, or whether it is an air ambulance or a trauma response service with doctors or paramedics on board.

The key general points to note are:

1. It is important to have knowledge of the 'call-out' procedures for the aircraft, the hours of operation (if not 24 hours a day) and the response times, as well as being familiar with the methods of communicating with the aircraft by radio or otherwise.
2. Ideally one agency, normally the ambulance service, should be responsible for tasking the aircraft if the incident or accident warrants its use.
3. Tasking (i.e. mobilising) information must be clear and concise. It should include:
   - the exact location of the accident or incident;
   - details of the type of accident or incident;
   - time of the accident or incident; and
   - any specific requirements, such as rendezvous points, details of other aircraft tasked or requested, and any peculiar or unusual equipment required.
4. Owing to the speed of the aircraft and the fact that aircraft fly in straight lines, large distances can be covered quickly and congestion or ground obstacles can be avoided.
5. Safety on site – if the aircraft is tasked, the personnel on the ground near the prospective landing site must be aware that any crowd needs to be controlled so that the aircraft can land safely and efficiently.

Selection of landing sites

Prior to arrival of any requested air transport, a suitable landing site should be identified and, if necessary, marked out (**Fig. 13.5**). Guidance on the selection of landing sites and the necessary precautions is given below. Different types of helicopter require different-sized landing sites, and although a site may have been identified beforehand, the pilot may choose to land at a different location. It must be remembered that the pilot is always responsible for the helicopter and he or she will make the final decision.

Review Questions

Phases of an EMS Response

Match the activity in the second column with the phase in the first column:

1. Predispatch	A. Crew assignments
2. Dispatch	B. Scene assessment
3. En route to the scene	C. Lifting and moving
4. Arrival at the scene	D. Checking equipment
5. Transferring the patient to the ambulance	E. Filing paperwork
6. Post-run	F. Location of the incident

1. D; 2. F; 3. A; 4. B; 5. C; 6. E

EMS operations

Although it is possible to give a rough guide to the approximate size of landing sites, contact should be made with the local helicopter service to ascertain any local requirements to suit their needs.

The current rules and regulations for night operations are that helicopters are not permitted to land after dark, unless the landing site has been formally surveyed, has adequate lighting and has been approved for use at night.

It is useful to note that, although landing is prohibited at night, if the aircraft has landed during daylight hours, there are no restrictions on taking off after dark. Consequently, if an EMS helicopter is going to be used, early tasking is essential if it is beginning to get dark.

Officially, daylight lasts from 30 minutes before sunrise to 30 minutes after sunset.

Landing site preparation

Fundamental factors

Four fundamental factors must be considered when selecting a helicopter landing site – the size of the landing site, its surrounds, its slope and its surface.

Size – The landing site needs to be large enough to accommodate the aircraft. The type of aircraft determines the size of the site and may range from 18m×18m to 30m×30m.

Surrounds – Telephone wires, electric pylons, trees and tall buildings are hazards to be considered, A suitable site is one with a clear approach and departure route. It must be remote enough – about 50 good paces from large obstructions – for landings to be carried out safely, even in bad weather. It must also be remote enough to avoid unnecessary disturbances.

Slope – The site should preferably be level – helicopters do have landing limitations, and excessively sloping ground makes movement around the aircraft difficult and potentially fatal.

Surface – A hard surface is preferable – the concrete or tarmac of a car park, or short firm grass of a field are ideal. Soft muddy ground, loose gravel and long or recently cut grass may be unsafe.

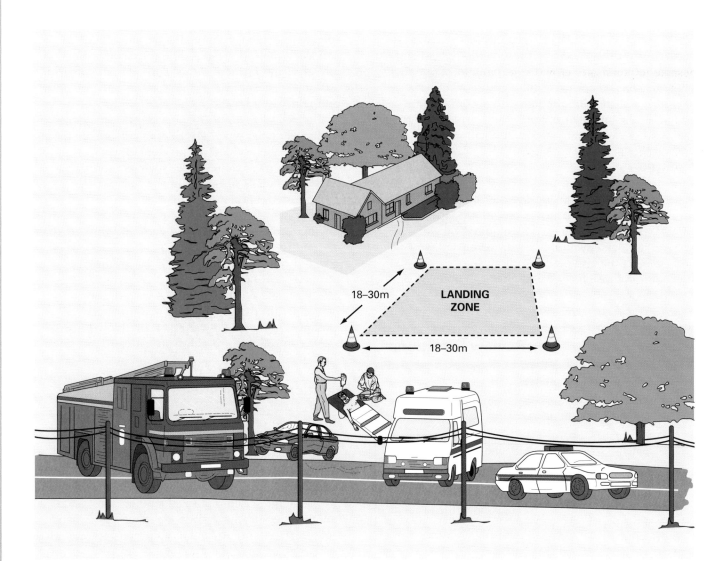

Fig. 13.5 Set up the landing zone in an area clear of obstructions such as overhead wires, trees and fences.

General principles

If a helicopter cannot land because of a sloping or soft surface, then a low hover with one main wheel or skid in contact with the ground may be carried out. Alternatively, the pilot may choose to winch to and from the site if the facility is available.

Distance from incident – The site must have reasonable access for the transport and loading of patients into the aircraft, and it should not be so close that rotor down wash will blow debris, broken glass and other loose material onto the patients or other EMS personnel. Land transport may be needed to carry patients or medical staff to and from the incident if the landing site is a long way from the site of the incident.

Damage to the aircraft from foreign objects – Helicopter engines and rotors are very vulnerable to damage from loose objects, which will cause catastrophic damage if blown into the engine intakes or rotors. The landing site should therefore be checked and cleared of any loose equipment or other objects. Ground support personnel must not wear loose articles of clothing such as caps.

Crowd control – All EMS personnel must be aware of where the landing site will be and who is co-ordinating the landing operations. The co-ordinator should not hesitate to administer crowd control and, for obvious safety reasons, keep spectators well clear of the proposed landing site. Crowd control would normally be the responsibility of the police.

The typical landing site

The typical landing site would:
- be about twice the size of the rotor diameter;
- be no more than 50–100 m from the accident site;
- not be near any overhead telephone wires or power lines, tall cranes or high buildings;
- have good access to and from the site of the accident or incident; and
- be on level, hard ground.

Alternative sites can be used if conditions are not ideal, provided that it is for the reason of saving life.

Safety

It must be remembered at all times that safety is of paramount importance when working with helicopters, not only because the tail rotor travels at very high speeds, but also because the main rotor blades are close to the ground in some helicopters.
  The basic 'do nots' are:
1. Never approach a helicopter or come under the rotor disk without the permission of either the pilot or winch operator (a 'thumbs up' is the normal sign of permission in daylight; a flashing torch is used at night).
2. Never approach a helicopter or come under the rotor disc from the 'uphill side' (**Fig. 13.6**). Although the

helicopter may have landed on a slight slope, the rotor disk remains in the horizontal plane and consequently will be closer to the ground on the 'uphill side' (**Fig. 13.7**).
3. The safest area to take up station if working in the vicinity of a helicopter is the safety zone, which is outside the main rotor disc area and between 9 o'clock and 3 o'clock. This area affords the air crew the best view of people approaching the aircraft and vice versa (see **Fig. 13.6**).

The basic 'dos' are:
1. Always walk (never run).
2. Keep well back (about 25–30 m) during take-off and landing; the aircraft may have to turn or hover, or it may have to taxi to the most advantageous point for take-off or landing.
3. Allow the pilot or flight crew to open and close all doors, since there may be complicated locking mechanisms.
4. Advise the flight crew or pilot of any equipment or objects that you wish to carry in the aircraft before loading, as weight is a critical factor in helicopter performance.

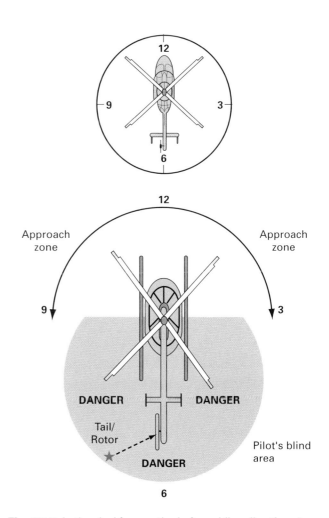

Fig. 13.6 In the clockface method of providing directions to EMS helicopters, the pilot faces the twelve o'clock position. All movement around the helicopter should be within the nine o'clock to three o'clock positions.

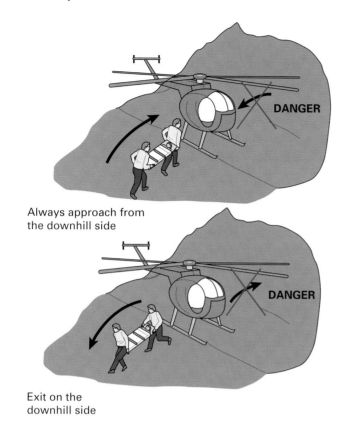

Always approach from
the downhill side

Exit on the
downhill side

Fig. 13.7 If the pilot lands on a slope, approach the aircraft from the downhill side. It is very dangerous to approach from the uphill side.

Although these are a few of the basic requirements, there can be no substitute for familiarity and co-operation with your local helicopter operator or air ambulance. They will be able to advise you of any particular requirements and operating procedures that they have developed. You should update them on your own particular operating procedures, as a good working relationship will improve the service.

Finally, safety can never be ignored because helicopters are potentially dangerous and should always be treated with respect to avoid accidents. This is especially true when the aircraft is running – aircraft noise can make people forget basic rules.

FUNDAMENTALS OF EXTRICATION

Entrapment can be described as any situation where a person cannot remove himself or be removed without the help of the emergency services because of his medical condition or environment. The continual increase in road traffic accidents (RTAs) has resulted in growing demands on the fire service to extricate casualties from vehicles (**Fig. 13.8**).

Every year the fire service carries out thousands of rescues at RTAs throughout the UK. The tendency is for cars to become smaller and lighter, and this workload is not expected to decrease despite the protection afforded to drivers and passengers by supplementary restraint systems (SRS) and side-impact protection.

Review Questions

Air Medical Transport
1. List the features of a typical landing site

_____
_____
_____

2. The approach zone to a helicopter should be from what area?

_____

3. What are the four fundamental factors to consider when preparing a landing site?

_____
_____
_____
_____

1. Twice the size of the rotor diameter; no more than 50–100 m from the accident site; not near any overhead telephone wires or power lines, tall cranes or high buildings; good access to and from the site of the accident or incident, on level ground; 2. Outside the rotor diameter, between the 9 o'clock and 3 o'clock position; 3. Size, surrounds, slope, surface.

The introduction of powered hydraulic equipment (**Fig. 13.9**) to both rescue tenders and front-line appliances has dramatically changed the approach of the fire service to RTAs. Furthermore, increased knowledge of RTA-related injury patterns and improved response, medical knowledge and equipment has further increased the potential for saving lives at RTAs.

Principles of extrication

First Responders, together with all other rescue personnel, should not lose sight of the reason for attending RTAs – namely to rescue casualties. All personnel must therefore adopt a 'safe, time-effective, casualty-centred' approach, with the principle of 'do no further harm to the casualty.'

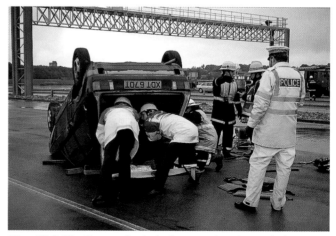

Fig. 13.8 The fire service is facing growing demands for extrication due to the increasing number of road traffic accidents.

Although the fire service is recognised as the principal rescue service, a team effort is required between the EMS rescue team and the physical rescue team if the outcome of the rescue is to be successful.

Trauma victims depend on a chain of care, which should pass smoothly through pre-hospital care to definitive care in hospital provided by accident and emergency specialists, anaesthetists, intensive care specialists and rehabilitation teams. There should be no weak links in that chain of care if the casualty is to have a truly successful outcome.

Importance of a team approach

A team approach system must be achieved to ensure the casualty arrives at definitive care as soon as possible, so enabling the casualty to have the best chance of survival (**Fig. 13.10**). The team approach system should apply to both the fire rescue operation and the combined efforts of the fire and medical rescue.

Crews should train and pre-plan for RTAs so that each member of the crew knows what the extrication plan is for a vehicle on its wheels, on its side or on its roof. Consequently, the First Responder and cutting crew can progress quickly and effectively. This pre-plan training can be extended to local ambulance crews so that all the crews involved develop into an efficient, competent rescue unit.

Research has shown that approximately 70% of all RTAs attended by emergency services involve casualties who are in the front seat of cars resting on all four wheels. A large proportion of these were trapped by the dashboard, steering wheel, driver's door, foot well or pedals

The senior fire officer can amend any pre-plan of the physical rescue if circumstances dictate. It is vital that the senior fire officer communicates, controls and supports all aspects of the physical extrication to ensure a safe, time effective, casualty-centred rescue.

Good liaison between the fire and rescue service personnel and the ambulance service needs to be established so all rescue personnel understand the condition of the casualty and the anticipated time and method of release. Rescue activities can then be tailored to meet that condition, that is either 'controlled release' or 'rapid release' can be undertaken.

It is also important that rescue personnel understand that medical rescue and physical rescue may sometimes come into conflict, such as when power tools are in operation and cannulation of the casualty is being attempted, or when medical personnel require silence and hydraulic tool power units are running. Therefore, good communication is required between all personnel on scene.

The importance of effecting RTA rescues as quickly as possible should not be misinterpreted as an encouragement to mishandle casualties.

Team approach system

Several distinct phases can be readily identified at a well-controlled RTA rescue:
- scene assessment and safety;
- initial casualty access;
- vehicle stabilisation and glass management;
- casualty stabilisation;
- creation of sufficient space to allow full access to the casualty; and
- packaging and extrication of the casualty.

Scene assessment and safety

Rescue teams should arrive at incidents with a slow, safe approach, all personnel should be correctly dressed, high-visibility jackets should be worn, as should personal protective equipment to deal with the extrication of casualties – this includes eye protection and gloves for general protection and for protection against body fluids.

Protect the incident using fend-off positions. Alight from the safe side, assess the whole incident scene for safety as soon as possible and assess the scenario. Assessing the scenario can be described as an inner and outer circle survey to appraise the situation. The

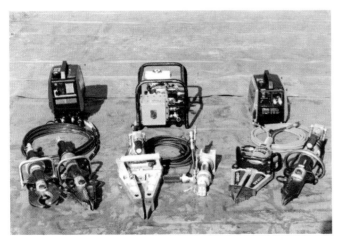

Fig. 13.9 The introduction of powered hydraulic equipment has dramatically changed the approach of the fire service to RTA extrication procedures.

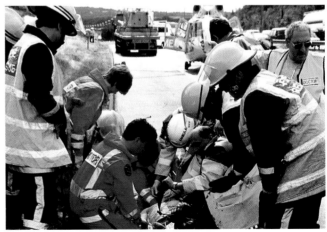

Fig. 13.10 A team approach, co-ordinated by the incident commander, facilitates definitive care of the casualty during the rescue operation and the provision of medical care.

inner circle would include any immediate hazards, the number of casualties, the degree of entrapment and so on. The outer circle would include any other vehicles or casualties outside the immediate incident.

A designated safety officer should be appointed, if the situation requires it and number of personnel allows it.

Extinguishing media should be laid out to the furthest point of the incident with an extinguisher back-up if possible.

An exclusion zone of 2 m should be adopted around the incident. This zone should be kept clear of all non-essential personnel and of equipment that is not in use. This provides a clear environment for the cutting crew and the medical crew, and for the rescue officer-in-charge to assess and plan the rescue.

Ensure that specialist rescue vehicles or specialist medical assistance is requested if the incident appears difficult or protracted.

Initial casualty access

The biggest killer at RTAs is an obstructed airway. Therefore a casualty's airway must be cleared and maintained with cervical in-line immobilisation (see Chapter 10, 'Injuries to muscles and bones') as soon as possible, by opening a door or breaking a window if necessary. Administer high-flow oxygen as soon as possible The remainder of the primary survey (AcBCs) should then be carried out.

Vehicle stabilisation and glass management

Because there is a very real possibility that casualties may have sustained spinal injuries, as a general rule crews should stabilise the vehicle before rescue personnel enter it. If there is doubt regarding the patency of the casualty's airway, immediate entry should be made with caution. Stabilisation using step chocks should provide a solid base, which will assist spinal immobilisation of the casualty; stabilisation will also help the medical team to perform intubation and cannulation when the physical rescue is taking place (**Fig. 13.11**).

Glass management should be completed early, ideally immediately after stabilisation of the vehicle. It can be dealt with in three ways:
- total removal of the front and rear windscreens if the glass is not bonded to the car body;
- controlled breakage of the side windows using glass hammers, centre punches, etc, ensuring that all casualties are informed and protected; or
- cutting of screens with a glass saw, ensuring that all casualties and personnel are protected from glass fragments and dust (**Fig. 13.12**).

Casualty stabilisation

It is imperative to gain good access to the casualty to continue to monitor vital signs, maintain cervical in-line immobilisation, administer high-flow oxygen and provide re-assurance and protection when necessary.

Creation of sufficient space to allow full access to the casualty

The early creation of adequate space is required to ensure that the time a casualty spends on the scene is reduced to a minimum. All rescue personnel should be aware of the importance of space around the casualty; therefore they should have a thorough understanding of modern space-creation techniques that are now available using powered hydraulic tools. Cutting crews should aim for an 'early first cut' and try to keep the extrication tools in continuous use in an effort to reduce entrapment times. Physical and rescue operations should be continuing simultaneously. This strategy, adopted by all team members, aims to reduce entrapment times to a minimum.

All sharp edges created during cutting operations should be covered as soon as possible using canvas covers, sheets or other appropriate material.

Liaise closely with the EMS team before releasing a casualty who has been severely trapped within the wreckage in order to ensure that the casualty's condition has been stabilised and that the EMS team is prepared for the release.

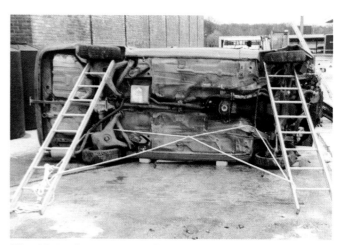

Fig. 13.11 Be sure every effort has been made to secure vehicle stability before entering. Continue to assess the vehicle's stability throughout the extrication process.

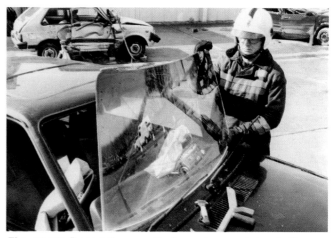

Fig. 13.12 Protect the casualty from glass, metal and other hazards during the extrication process.

Full access to the casualty should be achieved by systematic dismantling of the vehicle, unless the casualty is time critical and then an immediate release will be required in liaison with the medical team. Full access will allow for good casualty handling and better use of extrication devices. Limited access generally means poor casualty care and can compound the injuries that a casualty is suffering. Few rescuers need reminding of the consequences of mishandled spinal injuries. Always immobilize the casualty's spine before removal.

Packaging and extrication of the casualty

It is best if packaging of the casualty can take place at the same time as the physical rescue is ending – once again the aim is to reduce the time on scene. The method and route of extrication needs to be agreed early so preparations can be made by the relevant rescue personnel. The extrication should not jeopardise the good casualty care that has already been carried out during the rescue. Long spine boards and appropriate spinal care should be used where spinal injuries are suspected, and good control of the removal of the casualty to the spine board should be achieved by co-ordination of the rescue team.

Throughout the incident, ensure that the police are kept informed of anything that may assist or hinder their subsequent investigations.

Extrication techniques

The First Responder must have a thorough overview of different extrication techniques. It is essential that all rescue personnel appreciate the value of roof removal, side removal and dash rolls when attempting to create maximum space in the minimum time.

A list of space-creation techniques that rescue personnel should have an understanding of includes the following:

- full or half roof flap (forwards, backwards, side; **Fig. 13.13a &b**);
- roof removal;
- roof fold-down (**Fig. 13.13c**);
- side removal;
- boot removal;
- door removal;
- B-post rip (**Fig. 13.13d**);
- foot well removal;
- pedal removal and pull;
- cross ramming techniques (**Fig. 13.13e**);
- seat and setback removal;
- third door conversion (**Fig. 13.13f**);
- dashboard roll (**Fig. 13.13g**);
- steering wheel rim removal; and
- steering wheel relocation (**Fig. 13.13h**).

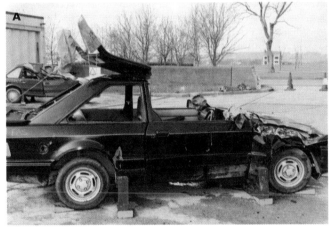

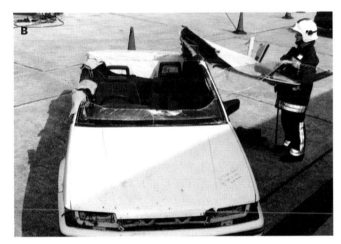

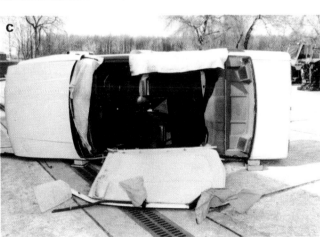

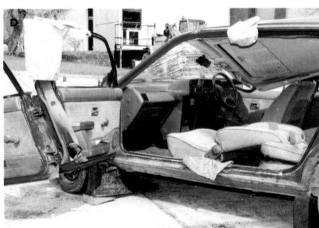

Fig. 13.13 Extrication techniques: **(a)** half roof flap; **(b)** Side roof flap; **(c)** roof fold-down; **(d)** B-post rip.

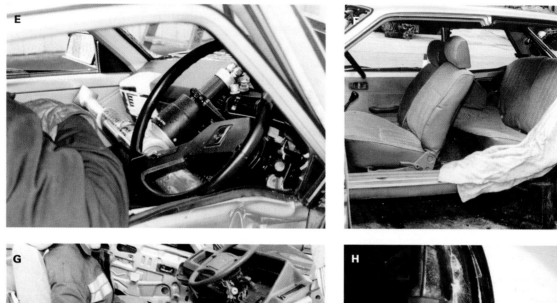

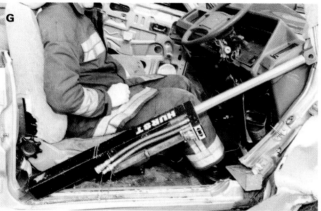

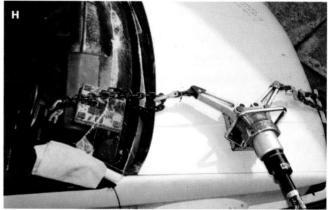

Fig. 13.13 cont. Extrication techniques: **(e)** Cross ramming; **(f)** third door conversion; **(g)** dashboard roll; **(h)** steering wheel relocation.

The casualty's medical condition will dictate the method of extrication used (that is, whether the casualty has a time-critical injury requiring rapid release (**Fig. 13.14a**) or whether time allows a controlled release (**Fig. 13.14b**)). Liaison between the senior fire officer and the senior medical officer is important, and clarity of the time available for extrication is very important. This time should be constantly re-evaluated. It is imperative that the entire rescue team is aware of the condition of the casualty and the time within which the extrication should be completed.

Supplementary restraint systems (SRS)

The past few years in the UK have seen a major increase in the number and types of airbags and other types of safety devices (such as seat belt pre-tensioners, belt grabbers) that are fitted to vehicles. Initially SRS were expensive optional extras fitted to top-of-the-range vehicles, but now airbags are standard fittings in many small family cars.

SRS present hazards to all rescue personnel in a variety of scenarios as the majority use pyrotechnic or propellant-based materials, some of which are within the scope of the Explosives Act. Hazards exist whether SRS are deployed or undeployed, or in a fire. There have been many incidents of 'post-accident airbag deployment' (PAAD) in which airbags have deployed a considerable time after the accident has occurred. Some

of these deployments have injured rescue personnel.

The design and method of operation of SRS differ from manufacturer to manufacturer and, indeed, from model to model from the same manufacturer.

Guidance from the Society of Motor Manufacturers for rescue personnel in relation to airbags

The Society of Motor Manufacturers offers guidance to rescue personnel in relation to airbags. This is summarised here.

Vehicle fires – Use normal rescue procedures and fire extinguishing methods, including water. Many airbag systems are designed to self-deploy when the internal temperature exceeds 150°C (300°F). The propellant in the airbag module will burn rapidly without fragmentation of the inflator. Airbags do not explode.

Rescue after an airbag has deployed – The following points should be noted:
1. Use normal rescue procedures immediately; do not delay medical attention.
2. Wear gloves and safety glasses or other eye protection if available.
3. Do not introduce airbag residue into your eyes or mouth or the casualty's eyes, mouth or wounds.
4. Reassure the vehicle's occupants and explain that any smoke produced from a deployed airbag module is normal and may continue for several

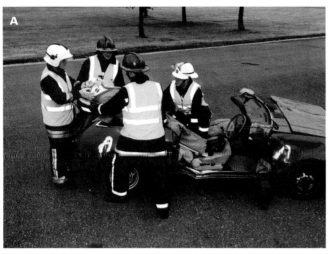

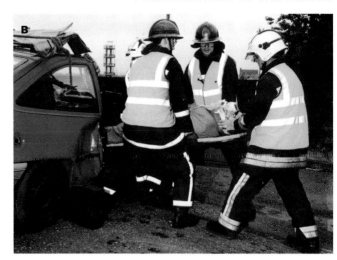

Fig 13.14 **(a)** Immediate and **(b)** controlled release.

minutes after deployment; it is not indicative of a fire. It is normal for powder to be present, but it may be alkaline and slightly irritant to skin and eyes (**Fig. 13.15**).

5. The airbag fabric, steering wheel and steering column do not get hot during deployment, but cutting away the airbag fabric during the rescue will give access to the gas generator, which may remain hot for up to 15 minutes after deployment.

6. Push deflated airbags aside for occupant removal. Airbags deflate at once after deployment. They cannot be recapped and it is not normally necessary to cover or cut away a deployed airbag during rescue operations.

7. On completion of rescue operations, brush off or remove any clothing that is coated with airbag residue. However, this should not delay the medical treatment of any casualty.

8. If gloves are not worn, wash hands after handling a deployed airbag.

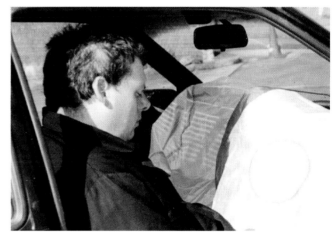

Fig. 13.15 When deployed, an airbag can create heat, smoke and residue which may irritate the skin and eyes.

Rescue after an airbag has not deployed – The following points should be noted:

1. Never cut or drill directly into an undeployed airbag module or attempt to take the unit apart. In the unlikely event of an airbag being ruptured, do not touch exposed chemicals.

2. Use normal rescue procedures immediately. Do not delay medical attention.

3. Identify whether the vehicle is fitted with any airbag modules. Look for identifying labels on the vehicle – airbags are usually marked 'SRS' (Supplementary Restraint System) or 'Airbag'. The label may be on the instrument panel, the door pillar, the steering wheel hub, the fascia on the passenger side or the back of the sun visor, or it may be under the bonnet. If in doubt presume that an airbag is present.

4. Perform the rescue from the side of the occupant and away from the potential deployment path of the bag.

5. Do not place your body or objects against any airbag module.

6. Many airbag systems are electrically activated;

therefore, as part of normal safety practices, safely disconnect or cut both battery cables. Turning the ignition off will not deactivate the airbag system. Many systems are fitted with a device that will continue to power the module for up to 20 minutes (or longer) after disconnecting the battery. Some airbag systems are mechanically operated and remain active. If in doubt treat the system as if it were active.

7. If the steering column or wiring to the steering wheel is cut, the airbag could deploy. Using an air chisel or saw may also cause deployment. Do not attempt to initiate deployment of any airbag.

Airbag dust after deployment – The fine powder or dust produced on deployment of an airbag consists primarily of talcum powder or corn starch, which act as lubricants to aid deployment. A filter retains most of the products of combustion of the inflation gas generant. However, in some cases the powder may contain small amounts of sodium carbonate (washing soda, baking soda), and traces of sodium hydroxide (caustic soda). The powder may cause slight irritation on contact with skin and eyes, but is not considered hazardous.

Treatment of contact injury due to airbag dust – If there has been eye contact, irrigate the eyes with water. If there has been skin contact, wash any affected or irritated areas with mild soap and water.

Airbags and the use of radios – There is a remote possibility that radios can activate airbags. Consequently manufacturers recommend that no radios should be used within the confines of a vehicle fitted with an airbag unless the radio is fitted to an external aerial system.

Seat belt pre-tensioners

Seat belt pre-tensioners are progressively being fitted by the majority of vehicle manufacturers in the UK. The principle is that during a frontal collision, the pre-tensioners immediately retract the seat belt by approximately 100 mm, which holds the occupant securely in the seat and therefore significantly increases the effectiveness of the seat belt. This, together with the airbag system, increases the protection of the occupants of the vehicle (**Fig. 13.16**).

Rescuers should be able to recognise the different types of seat belt pre-tensioners, know where they are likely be located and carry out extrication without cutting into the tensioners.

First Responders will need to release or cut seat belts with caution when pre-tensioners are fitted, in order to ensure that the casualty's breathing is not compromised. It is also imperative that the casualty's spine is immobilised and no excessive movement is caused.

It is likely that any cutting of pre-tensioners or associated wiring may cause the pre-tensioner to activate with a loud bang and the seat belt webbing to recoil violently. Rescuers must not presume that the disconnection of the vehicle battery will isolate airbags or seat belt pre-tensioners.

Summary of extrication techniques

More lives are lost in RTAs than in any other comparable incident, and they are the most common cause of preventable death. Victims are often young and generally healthy.

At any entrapment rescue there are higher inherent dangers to both the casualty and the rescuer than there are in most other environments. The health and safety implications for rescuers, in terms of both competence and duty of care, are therefore considerable.

There is a moral and legal obligation on all emergency personnel to ensure that the service provided to entrapped casualties is the best possible. This can only be achieved by developing a team approach and ensuring that all personnel involved in pre-hospital treatment of RTA casualties receive team training on a regular basis in addition to maintaining their own skills. First Responders, as part of a team response, will play an important role in the drive to reduce mortality rates from trauma in the UK.

HAZARDOUS MATERIALS

A hazardous material is any substance or material that can pose an unreasonable risk to health, safety or property. It will probably be hazardous to the environment too. Because there is a great chance that you will be involved in a hazardous materials incident during your emergency services career, you should receive hazardous materials ('hazmats') awareness training. This training involves learning to approach hazardous materials in the safest way for everyone involved. Check with your training officer to learn more about hazardous materials courses.

Safety

The issue of hazardous materials is an everyday concern and problem. Although some may think of hazardous materials only in terms of transport incidents such as RTAs, in reality many chemicals,

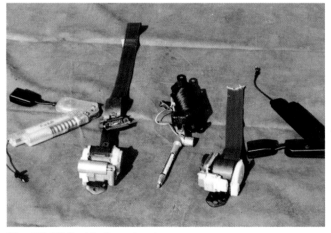

Fig. 13.16 Seat belt pre-tensioners.

Review Questions

Fundamentals of Extrication

1. List the phases of a well controlled RTA extrication.
   _____
   _____
   _____
   _____
   _____
   _____

2. What is the importance of the Team Approach system?
   _____

3. Personnel should adopt a safe, time effective casualty centred approach with the principle of _____

1. Scene assessment and safety, initial casualty access, vehicle stabilisation and glass management, patient stabilisation, space creation and full access, casualty packaging and extrication;
2. To ensure the casualty arrives at definitive care as soon as is possible enabling the casualty to have the best chance of survival;
3. 'Do no further harm to the casualty'.

pesticides and other compounds found in the home and on industrial sites may cause a hazardous materials situation. A casualty's home may have carbon monoxide leaking from the heating system, a casualty may use an oven cleaner in a poorly ventilated room or chlorine gas may leak at a local municipal swimming pool. Whenever there is a spill, leakage or fire involving chemicals, there is a potential for a hazardous materials incident (**Fig. 13.17**), and whenever First Responders, the public or the environment is at risk from these materials, there is a hazardous materials situation.

In all hazardous materials situations, your primary concern should be safety. Safety concerns include your own well-being and that of other crew members, casualties, other emergency service personnel and the local community.

Knowledge of what is involved and what to do is necessary for successful and safe management of hazardous materials situations. While on the way to the scene of a hazardous materials incident, obtain as much additional information as you can from control. There are a number of computer-based retrieval systems that are designed to assist in identifying hazardous materials. These databases list hazardous materials and the appropriate emergency procedures, and they can be a useful resource for you when dealing with the incident. Always remember the scene assessment rule – if the scene is not safe, make it safe, otherwise do not enter. In a hazardous materials scene, the expertise of a hazardous materials officer is usually required to assist in making the scene safe. Do not enter the scene unless you are protected, trained and have the skills to use the necessary equipment.

Radiation

Incidents involving radiation are rare. However, owing to the quantities of radioactive materials now used in industry and medicine and the consequent potential for an incident, emergency service personnel must be trained to deal successfully with such an incident, and they must have a knowledge of the risks involved and the standards of personal protection required. An understanding of the limitations and use of instrumentation will be required by the fire service.

Some radioactive materials are, to varying degrees, flammable or combustible, and to this extent carry a fire hazard. This hazard is, however, no greater because a material is radioactive. The most important aspect of radiation incidents is pre-planning concerning issues such as the type of material, the strength of the radiation, the location, the emergency plans of the site where the incident has occurred and liaison with the company.

Action on arrival should be to stay upwind and keep a distance of 45 m if the source of radiation is massive or unknown. Liaise with the site manager or radiation protection adviser for advice. All personnel should wear correct personal protective equipment and stay out of the restricted zone.

'Hazmats' procedures

Once you suspect that the scene may involve hazardous materials, because of information obtained either from control or from physical clues, follow these important safety guidelines as you approach the scene:

- approach the scene from an uphill and upwind direction;
- isolate the area with cordons;
- avoid contact with the material;
- be alert for unusual odours, clouds and leakage – withdraw if necessary;
- remember that some chemicals are odourless;
- do not drive any emergency vehicles through leakage or vapour clouds;
- keep all personnel and bystanders a safe distance from the scene; and
- remove casualties to a safe zone if there is no risk to the First Responder.

Approach the scene with extreme caution. Do not rush into a situation that may harm you. You cannot help others if you become a patient yourself. Until you know what the material or situation is, you cannot help. Information is the key.

Once the scene has been declared a hazardous

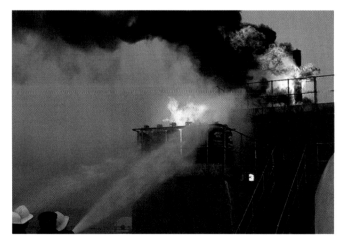

Fig. 13.17 Any spill of chemicals can become a hazardous materials incident.

Box 13.2	**Personal Protective Equipment**

- Impact-resistant protective helmet with ear protection and chin strap
- Protective eyewear. Ideally the protective eyewear has an elastic strap and vents to prevent fogging. The shield on a helmet is not considered protective eyewear
- Lightweight, puncture-resistant 'turn-out' coat
- High-visibility jacket
- Leather gloves
- Boots with steel insoles and steel toes
- Most rescuers also use lightweight, puncture-resistant turn-out trousers

materials incident, if you are trained and required to deal with decontamination issues, you should work at setting up a decontamination area in line with current procedures and advice (**Fig. 13.18**). At the site of a vehicle crash, try to determine if the vehicle is occupied and the identity of the hazardous materials. If the hazardous materials scene does not involve a vehicle, identifying the hazardous material is still important. This information may allow the hazardous materials officer to make an early termination of the incident.

Hazardous materials are often identified by a placard (**Fig. 13.19**). The placard will have a four-digit United Nations (UN) number to help you identify the material or class of material. Check the information retrieval database for any UN numbers. Shipping or transport papers are also a valuable source of information if you can safely locate and retrieve them without taking any personal risks. Shipping papers are typically located in the passenger compartment of the vehicle, with the driver. Some vehicles have a special compartment for these papers. Such papers are not usually retrievable without the use of protective equipment.

The emergency action code (EAC) should be used for first-strike emergency action. The additional personnel protection (APP) code must be sought as soon as

possible. The CHEMSAFE scheme can provide immediate on-line advice to emergency personnel at the scene of hazardous materials incidents. CHEMSAFE operates 24 hours a day, 7 days a week and it can be reached through an emergency telephone number. It is recommended that you contact CHEMSAFE as soon as possible during the incident. When you call, be prepared to provide as much information as possible regarding the incident, including the name of the substance, its UN identification number and a description of the incident. Depending on the incident, CHEMSAFE will activate one of three levels of response.

These are only some of the available resources. In general, do not rely on only one source of information when dealing with a hazardous materials incident. Other resources include poison centres, medical direction, scientific advisers and on-site specialists.

MASS CASUALTY SITUATIONS

A mass casualty situation is an incident involving more casualties than an initial emergency service response can deal with efficiently (see Chapter 6, 'Patient assessment'). In general, these situations may require the activation of all or part of a major incident plan with its added attendances.

Basic triage

In a multiple casualty situation, patient triage is a priority. Triage is a method of categorising patients into treatment and transport priorities. There are generally four priority levels. A tagging system is typically used to assist in designating the category of each of the patients. Through the use of colour-coded or numbered tags, patients are placed into one of the triage categories (**Fig. 13.20**). **Box 13.2** lists the conditions that fall into each of these categories.

Procedures

In general, the medical officer who is most knowledgeable of patient assessment and intervention and who arrives on the scene first becomes the triage

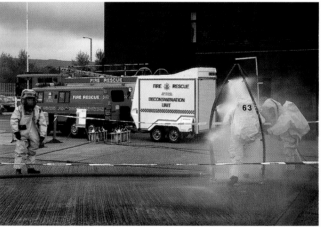

Fig. 13.18 A hazardous materials decontamination zone should be set up in line with current procedures and advice.

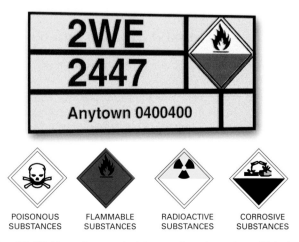

POISONOUS SUBSTANCES   FLAMMABLE SUBSTANCES   RADIOACTIVE SUBSTANCES   CORROSIVE SUBSTANCES

Fig. 13.19 Hazardous materials warning placards and labels.

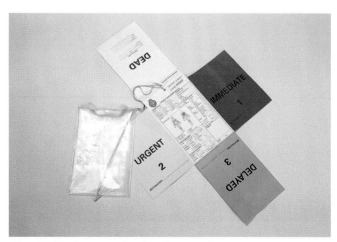

Fig. 13.20 An example of a triage card.

Box 13.2	Triage Priorities

- Priority 1 – Immediate
  Requiring life-saving interventions

- Priority 2 – Urgent
  Requiring surgery within 6 hours

- Priority 3 – Delayed
  Walking

- Priority 4 – Expectant or Dead

- arrival at the receiving facility;
- on the way to the station; and
- the post-run phase.

Your roles and responsibilities depend on the phase of the call. The first phase allows you to prepare for the call and check the vehicle for medical equipment and mechanical readiness. Mobilisation is an opportunity to gain information regarding the call. The time on the way to the scene is an opportunity for pre-planning for the actions to be taken at the scene. On arrival, you size-up the scene to ensure the well-being and safety of the crew. Remember that your actions at the scene should be organised with the goal of transport in mind. Assist other personnel with lifting and moving the patient to the ambulance. Finally, the post-run phase is a time to disinfect equipment, restock the vehicle and prepare for the next response.

officer. Additional help should be requested immediately during the assessment. The triage officer rapidly performs an initial assessment of all patients. Care is not provided during the triage sieve, except for opening the airway.

The triage officer rapidly moves from patient to patient, doing an initial assessment and using triage tags to assign patients to treatment categories. As patients are assessed and tagged they are then moved to a treatment area for further evaluation and intervention. From the treatment area, patients are moved to a transportation area for transport. Transport decisions are based on patient priority, the capabilities and capacity of the receiving hospital, and transport resources.

Once all patients have been triaged, the triage officer reports to the incident commander. Depending on the available resources, the triage officer may remain as triage officer and continue to perform triage and update patient priorities, or he or she may receive a new assignment.

The triage process forces First Responders to make difficult decisions. You may wish to practice using triage tags to be prepared when a mass casualty situation arises. The important skill in triage is to be able to prioritise patients quickly in order to give the appropriate amount of care using the available resources – in other words, to allow the greatest amount of treatment to be provided to the greatest number of patients in the circumstances.

When you report to the scene of a mass casualty incident, report to the command post and identify yourself and your level of training. Follow the directions of the incident commander.

CHAPTER SUMMARY
Phases of an EMS response

The nine phases of a typical response are:
- preparation for the call;
- mobilisation;
- on the way to the scene;
- arrival at the scene;
- transferring the patient to the ambulance;
- on the way to the receiving facility;

Air medical transport

Air medical transport is becoming the standard of care for some critically ill and injured patients. Considerations for the use of air medical transport include the mechanism of injury and the time and distance to the receiving facility. The set-up of a landing zone and communication should be delegated to persons who are not directly involved in patient care. The landing zone should be clear of debris and wires. Give the pilot as much information as possible.

Safety around the aircraft is the responsibility of everyone. Avoid running and do not smoke in or around the landing zone. The main rotor blades may dip to within nearly 1 m of the ground. The tail rotor is spinning at a speed that makes it nearly invisible. Always approach the aircraft from the twelve o'clock to three o'clock positions. Only approach the aircraft when directed by the flight crew. Never walk near the tail rotor or under the tail boom. Follow the instructions of the flight crew regarding safety around the aircraft.

Fundamentals of extrication

Extrication is the process of freeing a casualty from entanglement. This process will require physical rescue by specially trained fire-fighters. The senior fire officer should co-ordinate the efforts of everyone responsible for the physical extrication, and he or she should liaise with the medical team. Adopt a team approach system. Assess the casualty's AcBCs early and provide good-quality care to the casualty throughout the extrication. All personnel should work together to ensure that the casualty is removed in a way that minimises further injury to the casualty.

Personal safety is the number-one priority for all emergency personnel. Wear protective clothing appropriate for the situation, and take the appropriate universal precautions.

Perform a scene assessment by carrying out an inner and outer circle survey.

Stabilisation of the vehicle scene and of the casualty should be achieved as soon as possible. Glass management should ideally be achieved early and in one phase.

Early space creation, achieved by an efficient cutting team adopting a simultaneous approach, is the secret to a good extrication outcome. All rescue personnel should have a good knowledge of extrication techniques.

The casualty's condition will dictate the extrication method used. It is imperative that the seriousness of the casualty's condition is known by all rescue personnel.

SRS can be hazardous to rescue personnel. Therefore it is important to identify the presence of SRS. Ensure that none of the rescue techniques will deploy airbags or activate seat belt pre-tensioners. Ensure that all activities are carried out outside the deployment path of airbags.

Hazardous materials

Hazardous materials incidents are a common problem these days. Your primary responsibility at hazardous materials incidents is your own safety and well-being and the safety and well-being of your crew and of casualties, bystanders and the environment. Unless you are specifically trained to deal with hazardous materials situations, you must protect the scene by the use of cordons and wait for additional help to arrive. A number of resources are available to identify and provide guidance when dealing with hazardous materials. These resources include placards, transport and shipping papers, Chemdata or other information retrieval system and the CHEMSAFE scheme. You should become familiar with all of these resources. It is recommended that First Responders who are likely to be involved in hazardous materials incidents are trained and updated at regular intervals.

In a hazardous materials situation, approach the scene with extreme caution, preferably uphill and upwind. Wear suitable protection. Identify the hazard, assure safety around the scene, do whatever is possible to isolate the area and ensure the safety of the people and the environment. Move all bystanders and crew away from the scene and keep them away. Obtain additional help. Crews should not walk through leakage, or touch spilled materials. Avoid inhaling fumes, smoke or vapours.

Mass casualty situations

An incident that may require activation of the major incident plan is a mass casualty situation. These situations occur when there are more patients than the responding units can safely and effectively deal with. The first and most knowledgeable medical personnel on the scene begin triage, categorising patients according to their injury into one of four categories. This is accomplished by rapidly performing an initial assessment of each patient and indicating the priority with a triage tag. This decision-making process allows the most patients to be treated and transported using available resources.

This chapter has given you an overview of your tasks as a First Responder. You should seek additional knowledge and skills through continuing training programmes, inter-service liaison, practice drills and experience.

Division Eight:
Appendices

Appendix

Supplementary oxygen therapy

I. Oxygen

II. Oxygen delivery equipment
    A. Oxygen regulators
    B. Oxygen delivery devices

Key terms

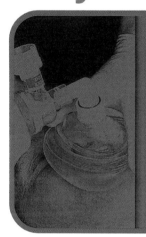

Nasal cannula
A low-concentration oxygen delivery device that should be used if the patient will not tolerate a non-rebreather mask.

Non-rebreather mask with reservoir bag
A high-concentration oxygen delivery device; the preferred method of administering oxygen in the pre-hospital setting.

Oxygen regulator
A device that attaches to an oxygen cylinder and is used to adjust the flow rate of oxygen to the patient.

Simple mask
A low-concentration oxygen mask.

Appendix A: Supplementary oxygen therapy

Objectives

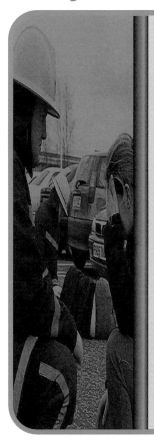

On completion of this chapter you will be able to meet the following objectives:

Cognitive objectives
1. Define the components of an oxygen delivery system.
2. Identify a non-rebreather mask and state the oxygen flow requirements needed for its use.
3. Identify a simple mask and state the oxygen flow requirements needed for its use.
4. Identify a nasal cannula and state the oxygen flow requirements needed for its use.
5. Describe the indications for using either a nasal cannula, simple mask or non-rebreather mask.

Affective objectives
6. Explain the rationale for providing adequate oxygenation through high inspired oxygen concentrations to patients who, in the past, may have received low concentrations.

Psychomotor objectives
7. Demonstrate the correct operation of oxygen cylinders and regulators.
8. Demonstrate the use of a non-rebreather mask and state the oxygen flow requirements needed for its use.
9. Demonstrate the use of a simple mask and state the oxygen flow requirements needed for its use.
10. Demonstrate the use of a nasal cannula and state the oxygen flow requirements needed for its use.
11. Demonstrate the oxygen administration for infants and children.

Oxygen is the element of life. A constant supply of oxygen is required by every cell in the body. Our bodies normally get enough oxygen from the air we breathe. In illness or injury, however, the amount of oxygen in the blood may decrease as a result of respiratory difficulty, cardiac failure or airway obstruction. In these situations, additional oxygen is necessary to decrease the risk of permanent damage to vital organs. Without exception, the ill or injured patient will benefit from supplementary oxygen.

OXYGEN

The oxygen used by most First Responders is stored in high-pressure cylinders (**Fig. A.1**). Oxygen cylinders are usually filled to a pressure of 136 bar. Because this great pressure could be explosive if a cylinder were damaged, always handle oxygen cylinders carefully. The most delicate parts of the cylinder are the valve assembly and the gauge. Oxygen cylinders should be secured during transport to prevent them from falling

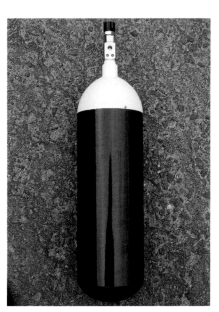

Fig. A.1 Common type of oxygen cylinder used in the UK.

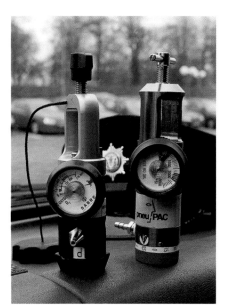

Fig. A.2 Two different types of oxygen regulator.

or rolling around. Do not smoke or allow any naked flames near oxygen. Do not use oils or grease near oxygen as this may cause an explosion.

OXYGEN DELIVERY EQUIPMENT
Oxygen regulators

To deliver oxygen to the patient at the correct pressure and flow rate, an oxygen regulator is used (**Fig. A.2**). The regulator attaches to the valve of the cylinder to control the flow of oxygen. Just as with a water tap, you control the flow rate by adjusting the regulator. **Figure A.3** shows how to attach the regulator to the cylinder.

Oxygen delivery devices

Once the flow of oxygen is regulated to the desired rate, it can be delivered to the patient. There are many types of oxygen delivery devices available for use by First Responders in pre-hospital care. These include non-rebreather masks, simple masks and nasal

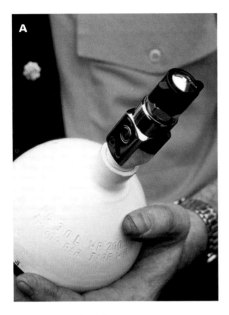
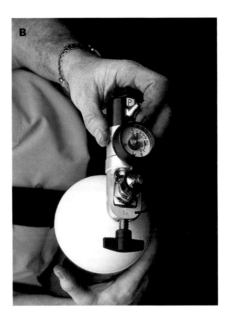
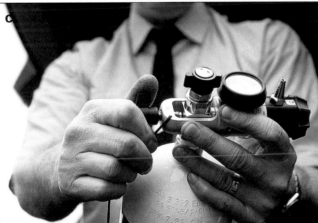
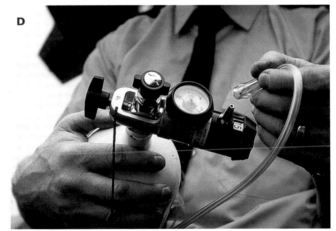
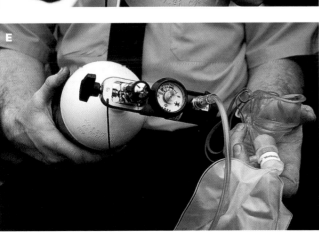

Fig. A.3 Attaching the oxygen regulator to the cylinder. (**a**) Remove the protective seal and sealing washer to reveal the the valve block and pin index system of the oxygen cylinder. Open the cylinder valve to blow off any dirt. Fit the sealing washer to the regulator. (**b**) Place the regulator over the valve and insert the pin indices into the two holes at the neck of the cylinder. (**c**) Tighten the screw of the oxygen regulator. Turn on the oxygen cylinder main valve to check for leaks. (**d**) Attach the oxygen tubing. (**e**) Inflate the reservoir bag of the non-rebreather mask with oxygen.

cannulas (**Fig. A.4**). However, the preferred mask of choice from the First Responder should generally be the non-rebreather mask with an oxygen reservoir bag.

Non-rebreather masks

The non-rebreather mask with an oxygen reservoir bag is the preferred pre-hospital method of delivering oxygen to the patient. This is a high-concentration device that can deliver up to 90% oxygen when the oxygen flow rate is set at 10–15 litres per minute. The non-rebreather mask stores oxygen in a reservoir bag. Inflate the reservoir bag with oxygen before you place the mask on the patient. This is done by attaching the tubing to the regulator, setting the flow at 10–15 litres per minute, then placing a finger over the one-way valve until the bag is completely inflated (**Fig. A.5**).

Position the mask to fit from the bridge of the nose to the chin and then adjust the straps for a comfortable fit for the patient (**Fig. A.6**). The reservoir bag should not collapse completely while the patient is breathing.

Non-rebreather masks come in adult and paediatric sizes. The proper mask should fit from the bridge of

the patient's nose to just below the bottom lip. Regardless of the mask size, the flow rate should be set at 10–15 litres per minute.

In the past, First Responders were instructed to withhold high-concentration oxygen administration for certain patients. However, this recommendation has changed for the pre-hospital setting. Any adult, child or infant who has suffered trauma or medical illness should always receive high-concentration oxygen.

Some patients become apprehensive when a mask is placed on their face. Usually, if you explain that they are receiving high concentrations of oxygen and that this will help them breathe more easily, they will calm down. Some patients are more comfortable if they hold the mask on their face, instead of having the strap around their head. Having a parent hold the mask close to a child's mouth and nose may help calm a child. If the patient will not tolerate an oxygen mask, you may need to use a nasal cannula.

Simple masks

The simple mask can deliver up to 60% oxygen with a flow rate of 8–12 litres per minute. The mask is fitted in a similar manner to the non-rebreather mask. At low oxygen flow rates atmospheric air can be drawn into the mask via the holes in the mask.

The percentage of oxygen delivered is only slightly higher than with a nasal cannula, and there is still the problem of patient apprehension caused by using a face mask.

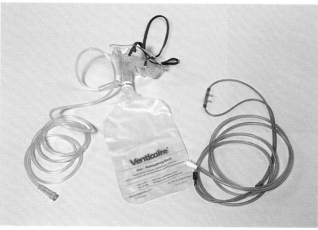

Fig. A.4 A nasal cannula (right) and a non-rebreather mask (left).

First Responder Alert

Any patient who complains of difficulty breathing (or shortness of breath), chest pain, or whose skin is bluish, pale, cool or clammy should receive oxygen by non-rebreather mask.

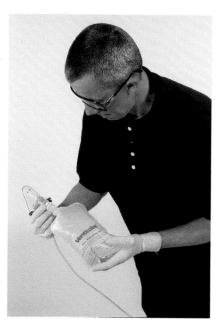

Fig. A.5 Inflate the non-rebreather mask reservoir bag with oxygen before you place the mask on the patient.

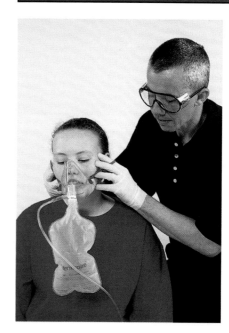

Fig. A.6 Position the mask on the patient, then adjust the straps for a comfortable fit.

Nasal cannulas

The nasal cannula is an alternative to delivering oxygen by mask. It is simply a piece of tubing that has holes through which oxygen is blown directly into the patient's nostrils. Nasal cannulas are often used for long-term oxygen therapy in a medical facility or at home. To deliver oxygen via nasal cannula, set the flow at a maximum of 2–4 litres per minute, then place the prongs into the patient's nostrils (**Fig. A.7**). Adjust the tubing for the patient's comfort. This device only delivers 25–30% oxygen at best.

In the pre-hospital setting, nasal cannulas are used only for patients who are still uncomfortable with the non-rebreather mask after you have reassured them that they are getting plenty of oxygen. The nasal cannula is a low-concentration device and is a poor alternative to the non-rebreather mask. It is, however, better than nothing if the patient absolutely will not tolerate the mask.

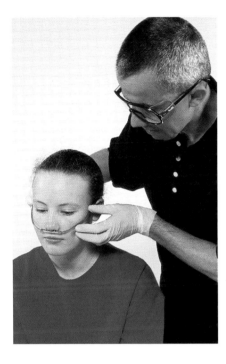

Fig. A.7 Place the prongs of the nasal cannula in the patient's nostrils, then adjust the tubing for comfort.

Review Questions

Equipment for Oxygen Delivery

1. List the steps necessary to attach a regulator to the oxygen tank.

   _____

   _____

2. The oxygen delivery device of choice for the patient having severe difficulty breathing is the _____ mask, with the oxygen regulator set at a rate of _____ l/min.

3. What should you do if the patient complains of "being smothered" by an oxygen mask?

1. Remove the protective seal and save the sealing washer. Open the tank to blow off any dirt, fit the washer to the regulator, attach the regulator onto the cylinder by inserting the pin indices into the two holes at the neck of the cylinder, turn on the main cylinder valve to check for leaks; 2. Non-rebreather mask, 10–15; 3. Explain that the patient is getting plenty of oxygen. Use a nasal cannula only if the patient cannot tolerate a mask

Appendix B

Advanced First Responder ventilation techniques

I. Advanced First Responder ventilation techniques
   A. Mouth-to-mask with supplementary oxygen technique
   B. Two-person bag–valve–mask technique
   C. Flow-restricted, oxygen-powered ventilation device technique
   D. One-person bag–valve–mask technique

II. Assessing the adequacy of artificial ventilation

Key terms

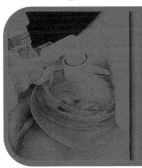

Bag–valve–mask (BVM)
A ventilation device consisting of a self-inflating bag, an oxygen reservoir, a one-way valve and a mask. The BVM is the most common ventilation device used in medicine and is most effectively used with two rescuers.

Flow-restricted, oxygen-powered ventilation device
A ventilation device that attaches directly to an oxygen regulator and delivers a constant flow of oxygen at 40 litres per minute when the trigger is depressed.

Objectives

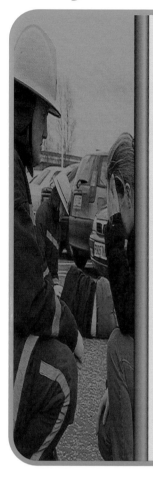

On completion of this chapter you will be able to meet the following objectives:

Cognitive objectives

1. Describe how to ventilate a patient with a resuscitation mask attached to supplemental oxygen.
2. Describe the steps in performing the skill of artificially ventilating a patient with a bag–valve–mask while using a jaw thrust.
3. List the parts of a bag–valve–mask system.
4. Describe the steps in performing the skill of artificially ventilating a patient with a bag–valve–mask for one and two rescuers.
5. Describe the signs of adequate artificial ventilation using the bag–valve–mask.
6. Describe the signs of inadequate artificial ventilation using the bag–valve–mask.
7. Describe the steps in artificially ventilating a patient with a flow-restricted, oxygen-powered ventilation device.

Psychomotor objectives

8. Demonstrate how to use a resuscitation mask with supplemental oxygen to artificially ventilate a patient.
9. Demonstrate the assembly of a bag–valve–mask unit.
10. Demonstrate the steps in performing the skill of artificially ventilating a patient with a bag–valve–mask for one and two rescuers.
11. Demonstrate the steps in performing the skill of artificially ventilating a patient with a bag–valve–mask while using the jaw thrust.
12. Demonstrate artificial ventilation of a patient with a flow-restricted, oxygen-powered ventilation device.

Sections in Chapter 5 ('The airway') describe how to ventilate a non-breathing patient by using the mouth-to-mask technique, the mouth-to-barrier device technique and mouth-to-mouth technique. While these techniques are very effective, they all use your exhaled breath to ventilate the patient. Although exhaled breath contains enough oxygen to sustain life, non-breathing patients benefit from higher percentages of oxygen.

The following techniques enable you to ventilate a patient with more oxygen than is available in your exhaled breath. Unfortunately, they all require additional equipment, which may not be available to you. If you have access to ventilation equipment, you should practise these skills frequently to ensure you are able to perform the skills quickly and effectively in an emergency.

ADVANCED FIRST RESPONDER VENTILATION TECHNIQUES

There are four ventilation techniques that you should be familiar with if you have access to the necessary equipment. You should consult your local protocols to determine which, if any, of these techniques are used. The techniques, in decreasing order of effectiveness, are:

1. Mouth-to-mask ventilation with supplemental oxygen.
2. Two-person bag–valve–mask (BVM) ventilation.
3. Flow-restricted, oxygen-powered ventilation device technique.
4. One-person BVM ventilation.

Mouth-to-mask ventilation with supplementary oxygen technique

Mouth-to-mask ventilation is the most effective method of ventilating a non-breathing patient. It is a simple technique, and because you can use two hands to create the mask seal, it provides excellent ventilation. Many masks have an inlet port on the mask (**Fig. B.1**) that enables you to attach oxygen tubing to the device. The constant flow of oxygen enriches the oxygen content of the air you are exhaling into the patient and improves the effectiveness of artificial ventilation.

Mouth-to-mask ventilation with supplementary

oxygen is performed exactly as mouth-to-mask ventilation, except that you attach oxygen tubing to the inlet port on the mask and set the regulator to flow at 10–15 litres per minute. Refer to Chapter 5 ('The airway') for a review of the mouth-to-mask ventilation technique. In normal circumstances, mouth-to-mask with supplementary oxygen will provide the patient with approximately 50% oxygen.

Two-person bag–valve–mask ventilation

The BVM is a ventilation device commonly used in medicine. The BVM consists of a self-inflating bag, a one-way valve, a mask and an oxygen reservoir (**Fig. B.2**). The adult bag has a volume of approximately 1600 ml. The bag is squeezed to ventilate the patient. Using the BVM single handed typically delivers less volume than the mouth-to-mask technique. **Box B.1** lists the features of BVMs.

The BVM is most effective when used with two rescuers. When properly performed, two-person BVM ventilations can deliver 90–100% oxygen to a non-breathing patient when attached to an oxygen source. The BVM can also be used without supplemental oxygen or a reservoir bag, but only delivers 21% oxygen. The technique is illustrated in **Figure B.3**.

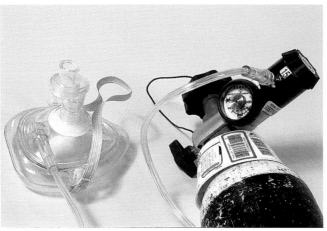

Fig. B.1 Some ventilation masks have a port to attach supplemental oxygen to enrich the rescuer's exhaled breath.

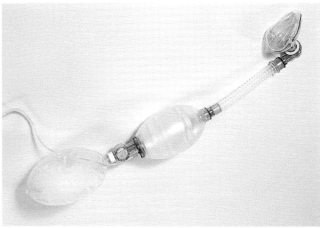

Fig. B.2 The BVM device consists of a self-inflating bag, a one-way valve, a mask and an oxygen reservoir.

A

B

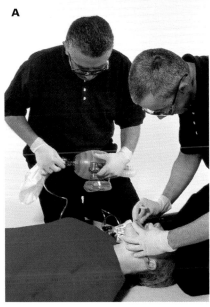
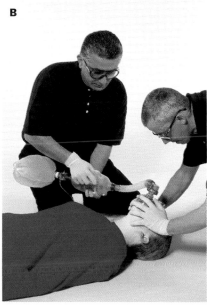

Fig. B.3 Two-person BVM technique. **(a)** The first rescuer manually opens the patient's airway from the patient's side. The second rescuer assembles and prepares the BVM (including attaching to oxygen) from a position at the top of the patient's head. The first rescuer then inserts an oral or nasal airway (if tolerated). **(b)** The first rescuer holds the bag portion of the BVM with both hands. The second rescuer seals the mask by placing the mask over the bridge of the patient's nose and then lowers the mask over the patient's mouth and upper chin. The second rescuer's thumbs are positioned over the top half of the mask and the index and middle fingers over the bottom half. If the mask has a large, round cuff surrounding a ventilation port, the port is centred over the mouth. The first rescuer squeezes the bag slowly and steadily until the chest rises. The second rescuer maintains the airway by using the ring and little fingers to bring the jaw up to the mask and evaluates the chest rise. The first rescuer continues to ventilate the patient at least once every 5 seconds for adults or every 3 seconds for infants and children. The second rescuer maintains the mask seal and open airway and continually monitors the chest rise.

Appendix B: Advanced First Responder ventilation techniques

Box B.1	**Features of the Bag–Valve–Mask**

- A self-refilling bag that is either disposable or easily cleaned and sterilised
- A port that allows a maximum oxygen inlet flow rate of 15 l/min
- Standardised 15/22 mm fittings
- An oxygen inlet and reservoir to allow for a high concentration of oxygen
- A one-way valve that prevents the rebreathing of exhaled air
- Constructed of materials that work in all environmental conditions and temperatures
- Available in infant, child and adult sizes

Flow-restricted, oxygen-powered ventilation device technique

The flow-restricted, oxygen-powered ventilation device is an alternative to BVM ventilation (**Fig. B.4**). This device provides 100% oxygen at a peak flow rate of 40 litres per minute. The valve is designed to prevent over-pressurisation of the lungs by an inspiratory pressure relief valve that opens when the pressure exceeds 60 cm of water. Most valves have an alarm that sounds when the relief valve is activated. The flow-restricted, oxygen-powered ventilation device should never be used on infants or children who weigh less than 20 kg, because it may damage the lung tissue and cause air to enter the stomach. Always refer to the manufacture's instructions and guidelines on use.

The flow-restricted, oxygen-powered ventilation devices used in the pre-hospital setting can operate in all environmental conditions. The main advantage of this technique is that it can be used single handedly by one First Responder. The flow-restricted, oxygen-powered ventilation device is preferred over the BVM

if only one First Responder is available to ventilate the patient. The technique is illustrated in **Figure B.5**.

One-person bag–valve–mask technique

Ventilation with a BVM appears to be a simple skill when practised on manikins, but on real patients it is very difficult for one First Responder to maintain an open airway, seal the mask and squeeze the bag. One-person BVM ventilation should be used only as a last resort when no other technique of ventilation is possible. One-person BVM ventilation requires a tremendous amount of practice and experience to perform properly. The technique is illustrated in **Figure B.6**.

All techniques for artificial ventilation described in this appendix require that the First Responder maintain an open airway. If the patient is not injured, the head-tilt, chin-lift manoeuvre should be used. The jaw thrust

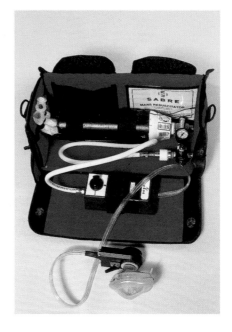

Fig. B.4 A flow-restricted, oxygen powered ventilation device may be used in place of a BVM.

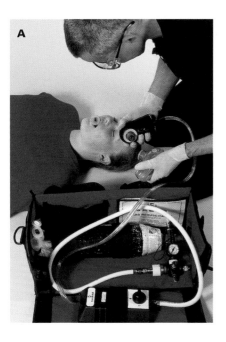
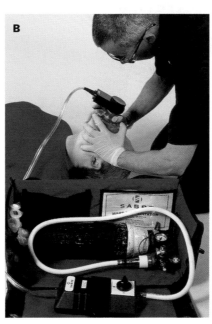

Fig. B.5 Flow-restricted, oxygen-powered ventilation device technique. Manually open the patient's airway from a position at the top of the patient's head. Insert an oral or nasal airway. **(a)** Attach the mask to the flow-restricted, oxygen-powered ventilation device. **(b)** Seal the mask by placing the apex of the mask over the bridge of the patient's nose, and then lower the mask over the mouth and upper chin. Position your thumb over the top half of the mask, and the index and middle fingers over the bottom half. Maintain the airway by using the ring and little fingers to bring the jaw up to the mask. Trigger the flow-restricted, oxygen-powered ventilation device until the chest rises. Release the trigger and allow for passive exhalation. Continue to ventilate the patient at least once every 5 seconds for adults. This device should not be used for infants or children.

without head tilt can also be used in conjunction with any of these techniques if the casualty has a potential spinal injury.

ASSESSING THE ADEQUACY OF ARTIFICIAL VENTILATION

Whenever you ventilate a patient, it is important to assess the adequacy of the artificial breathing. Especially when advanced First Responder ventilation techniques are being used, everybody attending to the patient must continually evaluate the effectiveness of the ventilation. The signs of adequate and inadequate ventilation are the same with these advanced techniques as those listed in **Boxes 5.3** and **5.4**.

If the ventilation or chest rise is inadequate, you should first check to be sure that you have adequately opened the airway. Next, check the mask seal. As you now have alternative ventilation techniques, you should consider using an alternative ventilation technique if the ventilations are not effective. Remember, not all techniques are equally effective, and one procedure may work while another has failed. If you are still having difficulty in getting an adequate chest rise after you try alternative techniques, you should consider the possibility of airway obstruction. **Box B.2** lists the steps for correcting poor chest rise during ventilation when you have additional ventilation equipment available.

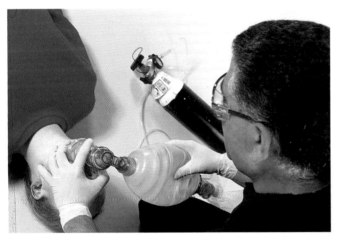

Fig. B.6 One-person BVM technique. Manually open the patient's airway from a position at the top of the patient's head. Insert an oral or nasal airway. Attach oxygen tubing to the oxygen port, and attach the mask of the BVM. Seal the mask by placing the apex of the mask over the bridge of the patient's nose, and then lower the mask over the mouth and upper chin. Make a 'C' with your index finger and thumb around the ventilation port. Maintain the airway by using the middle, ring and little fingers under the jaw to maintain the chin-lift. Squeeze the bag with your other hand slowly and steadily until the chest rises. Allow the patient to passively exhale. Evaluate the chest rise and continue to ventilate the patient at least once every 5 seconds for adults, or once every 3 seconds for infants and children.

Review Questions

Advance Ventilation Techniques

1. Place the following ventilation techniques in decreasing order of preference.
   A. One-person bag–valve-mask
   B. Flow-restricted, oxygen-powered ventilation device
   C. Mouth-to-mask
   D. Two-person bag–valve–mask

2. List at least four of the desirable features of the bag–valve–mask.
   _____
   _____
   _____
   _____

3. In the two-person bag–valve–mask technique, the EMT at the top of the head is responsible for _____ and _____.

4. The flow-restricted, oxygen-powered breathing device provides _____% oxygen at a rate of _____ l/min with a pop-off valve set at _____ cm of water.

1. C, D, B, A; 2. Self-ventilating bag, easily cleaned and sterilised, 15/22 mm fittings/oxygen inlet and reservoir, a valve that prevents rebreathing, works in all environments, available in adult, child and infant sizes; 3. Holding the mask seal, maintaining an open airway; 4. 100, 40, 60

Box B.2	**Correcting Poor Chest Rise During Ventilation when Ventilation Equipment is Available**

1. Reposition the jaw
2. Check the mask seal
3. Use an alternative technique (flow-restricted, oxygen-powered ventilation device, two-person bag–valve mask, or mouth-to-mask with supplementary oxygen)
4. Check for an airway obstruction

Appendix

Vital signs

II. Vital Signs
    A. Breathing
    B. Pulse
    C. Skin
    D. Pupils
    E. Blood Pressure

II. Vital sign reassessment

Key terms

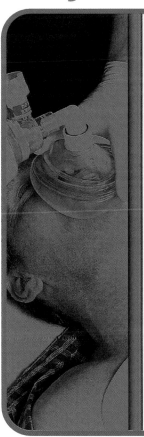

Accessory muscles
The additional muscles that a person in respiratory distress uses to facilitate breathing.

Capillary refill
The amount of time required to refill the capillary bed after applying and releasing pressure on a fingernail.

Diastolic blood pressure
The measurement of the pressure exerted against the walls of the arteries while the heart is relaxed and the chambers of the heart are being filled with blood from the great veins.

Laboured respirations
An increase in the work or effort of breathing.

Noisy respirations
Any noise coming from the patient's airway; this often indicates a respiratory problem.

Normal respirations
Respirations occurring without airway noise or effort from the patient; the usually rate in the adult is 12–20 breaths per minute.

Reactive to light
A term that describes the pupils when they constrict when exposed to a light source.

Shallow respirations
Respirations that have low volumes of air in inhalation and exhalation.

Systolic blood pressure
The measurement of the pressure exerted against the arteries during contraction of the heart.

Trending
The process of comparing sets of vital signs or other assessment information over time.

Objectives

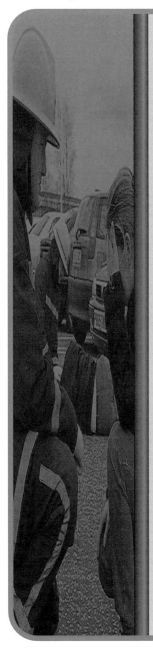

On completion of this chapter you will be able to meet the following objectives:

Cognitive objectives
1. Identify the components of vital signs.
2. Describe the methods of obtaining a breathing rate.
3. Identify the attributes that should be obtained when assessing breathing.
4. Differentiate between shallow, laboured and noisy breathing.
5. Describe the methods of obtaining a pulse rate.
6. Identify the information obtained when assessing a patient's pulse.
7. Differentiate between a strong, weak, regular and irregular pulse.
8. Describe the methods of assessing the skin colour, temperature and condition of patients.
9. Identify the normal and abnormal skin colours,
10. Differentiate between pale, blue, red and yellow skin colour.
11. Identify normal and abnormal skin temperature.
12. Differentiate between hot, cool and cold skin temperature.
13. Identify normal and abnormal skin conditions.
14. Describe the methods of assessing the pupils.
15. Identify normal and abnormal pupil size.
16. Differentiate between dilated (big) and constricted (small) pupils.
17. Differentiate between reactive and non-reactive pupils and equal and unequal pupils.
18. Describe the methods of assessing blood pressure.
19. Define systolic pressure.
20. Define diastolic pressure.
21. Explain the difference between auscultation and palpation for obtaining a blood pressure.
22. State the importance of accurately reporting and recording the baseline vital signs.

Affective objectives
24. Explain the value of performing the baseline vital signs.
25. Recognise and respond to the feelings that patients experience during assessment.
26. Defend the need for obtaining and recording an accurate set of vital signs.
27. Explain the rationale of recording additional sets of vital signs.

Psychomotor objectives
28. Demonstrate the skills involved in the assessment of breathing.
29. Demonstrate the skills associated with obtaining a pulse.
30. Demonstrate the skills associated with assessing the skin colour, temperature and condition of patients.
31. Demonstrate the skills associated with assessing the pupils.
32. Demonstrate the skills associated with obtaining blood pressure.

In some systems, First Responders function with a limited amount of equipment, and the assessment of vital signs is not within their scope of practice. In other systems, First Responders are taught to assess vital signs, and they do have the necessary equipment. If assessing vital signs is part of your responsibility as a First Responder, read the material in this appendix and practice the techniques of vital sign assessment frequently.

Listed in this appendix are the average ranges for respiratory rate, heart rate and blood pressure, listed by age. It is important that you realise that these are only average ranges. A patient's heart rate, respiratory rate or blood pressure measurement may be outside the average range and still be normal for that patient.

VITAL SIGNS

The vital signs that you will assess are:
- breathing;
- pulse;
- skin colour, temperature and condition;
- pupil size and reactivity; and
- blood pressure.

These signs are called 'vital signs' because they can reveal much about the patient's condition and the body's life-sustaining functions. The baseline vital signs are those vital signs that you measure or assess when you first encounter the patient; you can use baseline vital signs for comparison with other measurements over time as the patient's condition changes. Baseline vital signs may be assessed by any crew member as time permits. If you are working alone, assess vital signs after the First Responder physical examination.

Vital signs can provide valuable information about the patient's condition, but a single set of vital signs does not provide as much information as a comparison of the patient's vital signs over time. Trending is the process of comparing sets of vital signs or other assessment information over time.

Take care to record vital signs accurately. Record the assessment specifics as you take each vital sign, rather than trying to remember all the numbers and recording them later. Be sure to report the baseline vital signs to incoming ambulance personnel. This will give them the opportunity of comparing your findings with additional sets of vital signs assessed later in the care of the patient.

Breathing

The first vital sign to assess is the patient's breathing rate and quality. Observe the patient's breathing by assessing the rise and fall of the chest. One breath is one complete cycle of breathing in and out. Breathing is also called respiration.

Rate

You can determine the patient's respiratory rate by counting the number of breaths in 30 seconds and multiplying by two. If the patient's breathing rate is irregular, count the respirations for one full minute to obtain a more accurate rate. Because patients may subconsciously change their rate of breathing if they know you are monitoring their respirations, do not tell the patient that you are assessing the breathing rate. A good way to avoid the patient is to count respirations immediately after you assess the pulse. If you keep your hand in contact with the patient's wrist, the patient will generally think that you are still taking the pulse and will not think about breathing or subconsciously alter respirations.

Factors that affect the patient's respiratory rate include the patient's age, size and emotional state. Patients often breathe faster than normal when they are ill or injured. The average range of respiratory rates for adults is 12–20 breaths per minute. Average ranges by age are listed in **Table C.1**.

Quality

The quality of breathing is the second part of the respiratory assessment. There are four basic categories for the quality of breathing: normal, shallow, laboured and noisy.

Normal respirations – These are characterised by average chest wall motion – that is, the chest wall expands smoothly with each breath. The rhythm of normal breathing is regular and even. Normal breathing is effortless. As the patient works harder to breathe, he or she begins to use accessory muscles. Accessory muscles are the additional muscles used by a person in respiratory distress to help breathing. To decide if a patient is using accessory muscles, watch the abdominal, shoulder and neck muscles for excessive movement. Also look at the muscles between the ribs. If the patient is working hard to breathe, the accessory muscles may be being used.

Shallow respirations – These can be recognised by slight chest or abdominal wall motion and usually indicate that the patient is moving only small volumes of air into the lungs. Even when the breathing rate is within the average range, patients with shallow respirations may not be receiving enough oxygen with each respiration to support the needs of their bodies. Shallow respirations are common in cases of drug overdose (when there is depression of the respiratory centre in the brain) and in head injury.

Laboured respirations – These indicate a dramatic increase in the patient's effort to breathe. Accessory muscles are commonly used when the patient has difficulty breathing (**Fig. C.1**). The patient may be gasping for air. Nasal flaring (the widening of the nostrils during inhalation) and retractions of the supraclavicular muscles (above the clavicles) and the intercostal muscles (between the ribs) also indicate laboured respirations, especially in infants and children (**Fig. C.2**). Because children and infants normally rely heavily on their diaphragm for breathing, do not assume that the abdominal motion of their breathing automatically indicates laboured breathing.

Noisy respirations – These are abnormal respiratory sounds. Any time you hear noisy breathing, something is obstructing the flow of air. A noisy airway always indicates a respiratory problem.

Table C.1	Average Vital Sign Ranges by Age		
Age	**Pulse (beats/min)**	**Respirations (per min)**	**Blood Pressure (mmHg)**
Newborn	120–160	40–60	80/40
1 Year	80–140	30–40	82/44
3 Years	80–120	25–30	86/50
5 Years	70–115	20–25	90/52
7 Years	70–115	20–25	94/54
10 Years	70–115	15–20	100/60
15 Years	70–90	15–20	110/64
Adult	60–100	12–20	120/80

Appendix C: Vital signs

Any abnormal breathing quality is always an emergency and you need to intervene to manage the patient's airway or breathing or both. In Chapter 5 ('The airway'), Appendix A ('Supplementary oxygen therapy'), and Appendix B ('Advanced First Responder ventilation techniques') there are discussions of the techniques for maintaining an open airway, administering oxygen and ventilating the patient.

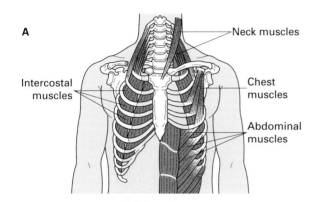

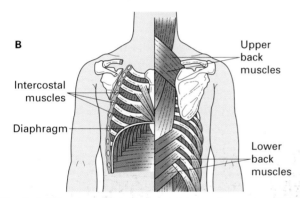

Fig. C.1 When breathing becomes laboured, accessory muscles are used to draw more air into the chest. **(a)** Anterior view. **(b)** Posterior view.

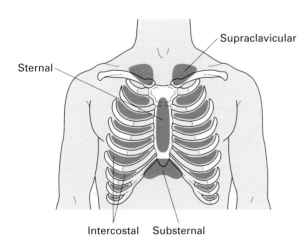

Fig. C.2 Muscle retractions indicate laboured respirations, especially in infants and children.

Pulse

The pulse is the wave of pressure in the blood generated by the pumping of the heart. You can feel the pulse wherever an artery passes over a bone near the surface of the skin. **Figure C.3** shows the location of key pulse points in the body. Assess the pulse for both rate and quality.

Rate

The pulse rate is the number of beats in 1 minute. Assess the pulse rate by counting the number of beats you feel in 30 seconds and multiplying by two. Factors such as the patient's age and physical condition, and any blood loss and anxiety, can affect the pulse rate. The average range for a resting pulse in adults is 60–100 beats per minute. An individual's normal pulse may not fall within this average range, however. For instance a well-conditioned athlete may have a resting pulse of 50, and although this pulse rate is outside the average range, it might be normal for this patient. When you measure the pulse and obtain low or high rates outside the average range, ask the patient if he or she knows what his or her normal resting pulse rate is.

Quality

The quality of the pulse is defined as its strength and regularity. The strength of the pulse can be strong or weak. The rhythm can be regular or irregular.

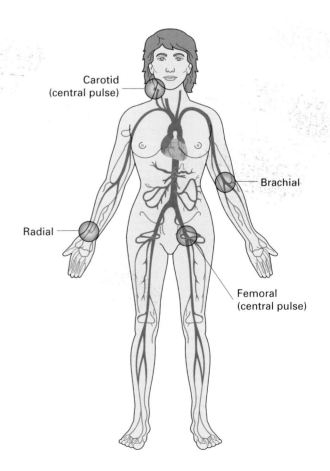

Fig. C.3 Key pulse points in the body.

The pulse should feel strong as you palpate with your fingertips. If the heart is not pumping effectively, or if there is a low volume of blood, the pulse may feel weak. A weak pulse is an early sign of shock (hypoperfusion) which may help you prioritise the patient.

The pulse should also feel regular. A regular pulse does not speed up or slow but has a constant time between beats. If there is not a constant time between beats, the pulse is irregular. An irregular pulse rate may indicate cardiovascular compromise.

Initially, assess the radial pulse in all responsive patients who are 1 year of age or older (**Fig. C.4**). The radial pulse is the pulse in the wrist on the thumb side of the forearm. Using two fingers, slide your fingertips from the centre of the patient's forearm just to the point where the wrist bends, towards the thumb side of the arm. By applying moderate pressure, you can feel the beats of the pulse. If the pulse is weak, applying more

pressure may help you feel a pulse. Too much pressure, however, may occlude the artery and you will not be able to feel the pulse. If you cannot feel a radial pulse in one arm, try the other arm.

If you are unable to feel a radial pulse in either arm, use the carotid pulse (**Fig. C.5**). The carotid pulse is felt in the neck along the carotid artery. Locate the Adam's apple in the centre of the patient's neck and slide two fingers towards one side of the neck. Never exert excessive pressure on the neck when feeling for a carotid pulse, especially with elderly patients. Excessive pressure may dislodge a clot, leading to serious effects. You should never assess the carotid pulse on both sides of the neck simultaneously because this could cause a drop in the patient's heart rate or occlude blood flow to the brain.

For patients who are under 1 year of age, assess the brachial pulse (**Fig. C.6**). The carotid pulse is normally difficult to locate in these small patients owing to the small size of the neck. The brachial pulse is on the inside of the upper arm, between the shoulder and elbow.

To assess the pulse, follow these steps:
1. Locate the radial pulse for patients who are 1 year of age or older and locate the brachial pulse for those who are under 1 year of age.
2. Count the number of beats in 30 seconds and multiply this number by two to determine the pulse rate.
3. Characterise the quality of the pulse as being strong or weak and as being regular or irregular.

Skin

The colour, temperature and condition of a patient's skin are assessed because they are good indicators of the patient's perfusion. Assess capillary refill in infants and children under 6 years of age.

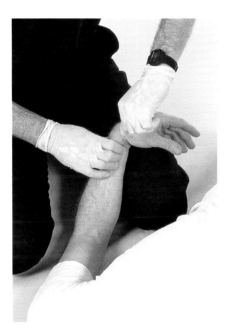

Fig. C.4 Locating the radial pulse.

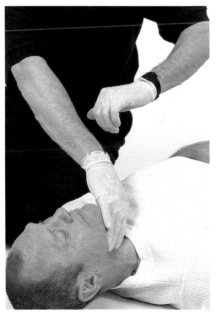

Fig. C.5 Locating the carotid pulse.

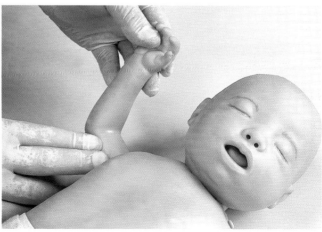

Fig. C.6 Locating the brachial pulse.

Appendix C: Vital signs

Colour

Assess skin colour in the nail beds, oral mucosa (inside the mouth) and conjunctiva (inside the lower eyelid). These places accurately reflect how much oxygen is in the blood and are easy to assess because the capillary beds run close to the surface of the skin. The normal skin colour in these areas is pink for patients of all races.

Abnormal skin colours include pale, cyanotic (blue–grey), flushed (red) and jaundiced (yellow). Poor perfusion (a lack of effective blood flow reaching all body tissues) causes pale skin colour. Cyanosis (blue–grey colour) indicates inadequate oxygenation (lack of oxygen reaching the cells) or poor perfusion. Flushed (red) skin may indicate exposure to heat or poisoning with carbon monoxide. Finally, a jaundiced or yellow skin colour may be an indication that the patient's liver is not functioning properly.

Temperature

Assess skin temperature by placing your forearm against the patient's skin (**Fig. C.7**). Assess the skin temperature in more than one location and compare findings. The patient's extremities are more susceptible to environmental changes in temperature than the trunk, so assess the temperature of the skin on the abdomen or back. Normally the skin is warm. Hot skin indicates a fever or exposure to heat. Cool skin indicates poor perfusion or exposure to cold. If the skin is cold, the patient has been exposed to extreme cold.

Condition

The condition of the skin is normally dry – but not so dry that it is cracked. Wet, moist or extremely dry skin conditions are abnormal. Extremely dry skin may be a sign of dehydration.

The term clammy is used to describe cool and moist skin. Clammy skin is a sign of shock (hypoperfusion). For more information on shock, see Chapter 9 ('Bleeding and soft tissue injuries').

Capillary refill

Capillary refill is the time it takes for the capillary beds to fill after being blanched (**Fig. C.8**). Capillary refill is a reliable indicator of hypoperfusion in children.

To assess capillary refill, press on the nail beds, release the pressure and determine the time it takes for the nail bed to return to its initial colour. A capillary refill time of less than 2 seconds is normal. Any capillary refill time longer than 2 seconds is abnormal and indicates poor perfusion.

Pupils

The pupils are the dark centres of the eye. They react to changes in the amount of light reaching the eye by constricting (getting smaller) or dilating (getting bigger). The pupils should constrict when exposed to light and dilate when protected from light. Normally both eyes react in the same manner. Sometimes head injuries or neurological problems can cause the pupils not to be reactive to light ('non-reactive' pupils) or cause one pupil to react as expected and the other to be non-reactive ('unequally reactive' pupils). The pupils are normally mid-size, neither constricted nor dilated. To assess the pupils, follow these steps:

1. Look at the patient's pupils and determine how the pupils look in the ambient light. Note if the pupils are dilated, constricted or normal.
2. Using a penlight, pass the light across each pupil and note the response. Each pupil should constrict to the same extent (**Fig. C.9**).

If the area is brightly illuminated, such as in bright sunlight, a penlight may not cause the pupils to react. In this case, cover each eye from the light for a few seconds and then uncover it. Note the reaction of the pupils. Head injuries, eye injuries and drugs can all influence the size and reactivity of the pupils. Note all your assessment findings. **Figure C.10** shows constricted pupils, uneven pupils and dilated pupils.

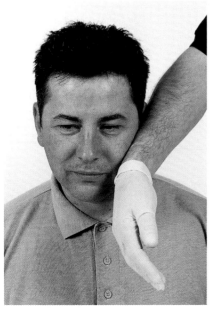

Fig. C.7 Assess the patient's skin temperature using your forearm.

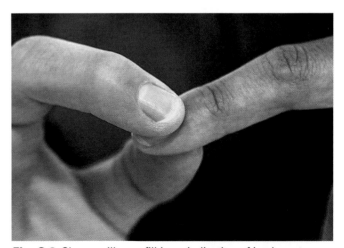

Fig. C.8 Slow capillary refill is an indication of inadequate perfusion.

Blood pressure

Blood pressure is a measurement of the force that the blood exerts against the walls of blood vessels during the contraction and relaxation phases of the heart. The systolic blood pressure is a measurement of the pressure exerted against the walls of the arteries as the wave of blood produced by the contraction of the heart passes that point in the artery. During each contraction of the heart, the pressure rises

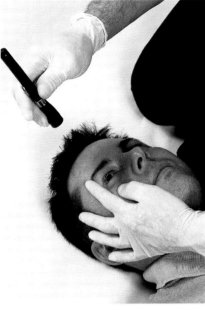

Fig. C.9 Shine a penlight across both eyes to note pupillary reaction.

momentarily as blood is pumped through the arteries. The diastolic blood pressure is the force exerted against the walls of the blood vessels as the heart relaxes and the chambers of the heart are being filled with blood from the great veins.

Blood pressure is measured in millimetres of mercury (abbreviated to 'mmHg'). Read the blood pressure with the systolic number over the diastolic number. For example, if you say, "The patient's blood pressure is 110 over 66", this means that 110 mmHg is the systolic pressure and 66 mmHg is the diastolic pressure; this is written down as '110/66 mmHg'.

It is important to understand that a single blood pressure reading is not valuable unless it is extremely high or low. Changes in successive blood pressure readings, however, may provide valuable clues about the patient's condition.

Document this information on the pre-hospital care report. Include in your verbal and written report any values outside the average range or significant changes.

There are two methods of obtaining a patient's blood pressure. Auscultation is the preferred method for assessing blood pressure. This method uses a blood pressure cuff and stethoscope. **Figure C.11** describes how to perform this technique.

Palpation is an alternative method of measuring systolic blood pressure only. You measure the systolic blood pressure by feeling for return of the pulse as the cuff deflates. You can use the palpation method in

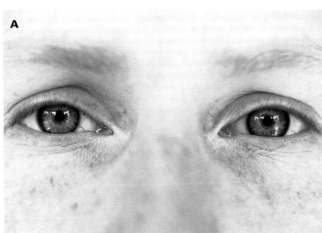

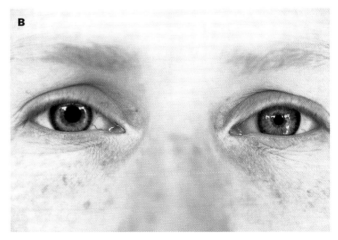

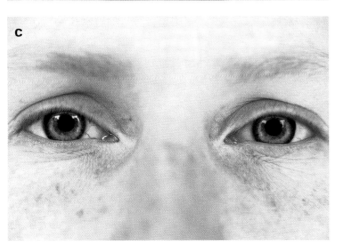

Fig. C.10 The assessment of pupils. Normal pupils are equal and reactive, neither dilated nor constricted. **(a)** Constricted pupils. **(b)** Uneven pupils. **(c)** Dilated pupils.

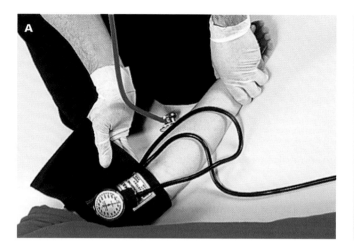

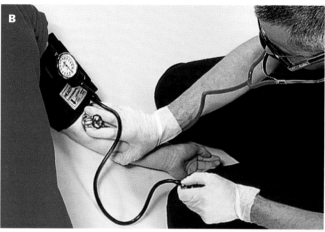

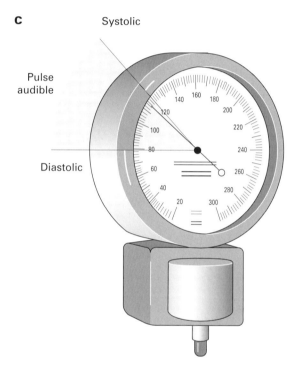

C

Systolic

Pulse
audible

Diastolic

Fig. C.11 Measuring blood pressure by auscultation. Choose a cuff of the appropriate size. Many cuffs have range finders to assist in finding the appropriate size. Apply the cuff so that the centre of the bladder is over the brachial artery. The index line should fall between the two range lines when wrapped around the arms. If a range finder is not present, the width of the cuff should go halfway around the arm. A cuff that is too large will produce a falsely low reading, while a cuff that is too small will produce a falsely high reading. Palpate the brachial pulse. **(a)** Place the blood pressure cuff around the patient's upper arm. The lower edge of the cuff should be about 2.5 cm above the point where you palpated the brachial pulse. **(b)** Place the head of the stethoscope over the location of the brachial pulse, closer to the wrist than the blood pressure cuff. Close the valve on the blood pressure cuff and inflate it until the pulse disappears, then inflate an additional 30 mmHg. Slowly release the pressure in the cuff while listening with the stethoscope. **(c)** Note the number when you hear the first beat. This is the systolic pressure. Note the number when you hear the beat disappear or become muffled. This is the diastolic pressure. Record both pressures.

situations when you cannot hear stethoscope sounds well because the patient's pulse is too weak or because the environment is too noisy. **Figure C.12** describes how to perform this technique.

Measure the blood pressure in all patients who are over 3 years of age, provided you have appropriately sized blood pressure cuffs for different age groups. The average ranges of blood pressure for adults and children are listed in **Table C.1**. Remember that these are only average ranges and that a blood pressure outside these ranges can still be normal for that individual. Ask patients if they know the usual range of their blood pressure.

VITAL SIGN REASSESSMENT

For stable patients, reassess the vital signs every 15 minutes. Stable patients are alert and oriented, with vital signs within the average ranges and with no signs that their condition is worsening. Reassess the vital signs of unstable patients every 5 minutes as you

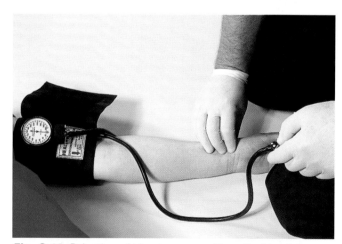

Fig. C.12 Palpation of blood pressure. Place the blood pressure cuff on the patient's upper arm as for auscultation. Find the patient's radial or brachial pulse distal to the cuff. Inflate the cuff until the radial pulse can no longer be felt, then inflate an additional 30 mmHg. Slowly release the pressure in the cuff. Note the pressure when the pulse appears. This number is the systolic pressure. The diastolic pressure cannot be measured with this method.

monitor their condition constantly (**Fig. C.13**). Patients are unstable when they have mental status changes, vital signs outside average limits or a worsening condition. Also assess vital signs before and after every intervention.

Remember that your general assessment of the patient comes before vital sign assessment. The initial assessment and First Responder physical examination provide more important information than the vital signs. Notice if the patient appears sick, is in respiratory distress, or is unresponsive. These are better assessments of status than vital signs.

It is also important to remember that the vital sign numbers provided in this chapter are only average ranges. For any individual, a blood pressure, pulse or respiratory rate not within the average limits may still be appropriate for that individual. Changes in vital signs allow us to track changes in the patient's condition.

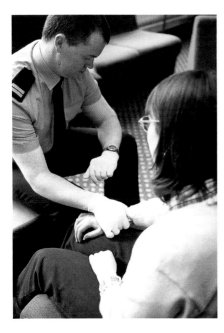

Fig. C.13 Repeat the vital sign assessment every 5 minutes for the unstable patient.

Review Questions

Vital Sign Reassessment

1. List three characteristics of a stable patient.

   _____
   _____
   _____

2. Reassess stable patients every _____ minutes, unstable patients every _____ minutes.

---

1. A stable patient is alert and orientated, with vital signs within the average ranges, with no signs that their condition is worsening; 2. 15, 5

APPENDIX SUMMARY

Vital signs

A patient's vital signs include: breathing rate and quality; pulse rate and quality; skin colour, temperature and condition; pupils; and blood pressure. Skin colours include pink (normal), pale, cyanotic, flushed and jaundiced. Skin should be warm and dry. Abnormal skin temperatures include hot, cool and cold; abnormal skin conditions include wet, moist and excessively dry. Pupils should be equal in size and reactive to light. Measure the blood pressure in patients who are over 3 years of age. Changes in vital signs can reveal changes in the patient's condition.

Vital sign reassessment

Evaluate the vital signs of unstable patients every 5 minutes and every 15 minutes for stable patients. Stable patients are alert and oriented, with vital signs within the average ranges and with no signs that their condition is worsening. Unstable patients have mental status changes, vital signs outside average limits or a worsening condition.

Appendix

Automated external defibrillation

I. **The Automated external defibrillator**
   A. Overview of the automated external defibrillator
   B. Advantages of the automated external defibrillator
   C. Operation of the automated external defibrillator
   D. Post-resuscitation care

II. **Maintenance of the automated external defibrillator**

III. **Automated external defibrillator skills**

Key terms

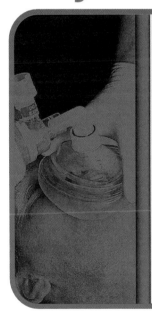

Automated external defibrillator (AED)
A machine used by basic-level rescuers to provide an electrical shock to a patient who is not breathing and who is pulseless; these machines are either automatic or semi-automatic.

Defibrillation
The delivery of an electrical shock to the patient's heart to stop a chaotic heart rhythm.

Joule
A unit of energy used to measure the amount of electricity delivered during defibrillation.

Ventricular fibrillation (VF)
A chaotic heart rhythm in which the patient has no pulse and the heart is simply 'quivering' inside the chest; the heart is not pumping so no pulse is produced.

Ventricular tachycardia (VT)
An abnormal heart rhythm in which three or more beats in a row are generated by the ventricles at a rate of 140 beats per minute or more; there may or may not be a detectable pulse, and if there is no pulse, this is referred to as 'pulseless VT'.

Objectives

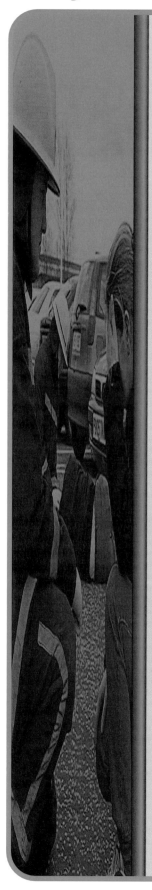

On completion of this chapter you will be able to meet the following objectives:

Cognitive objectives

1. List the indications for automated external defibrillation.
2. List the contraindications for automated external defibrillation.
3. Define the role of the First Responder in the emergency cardiac care system.
4. Explain the impact of age and weight on defibrillation.
5. Discuss the fundamentals of early defibrillation.
6. Explain the rationale for early defibrillation.
7. Explain that not all chest pain results in cardiac arrest and the First Responder does not always need to attach an AED.
8. Explain the importance of pre-hospital advanced life support (ALS) intervention if it is available.
9. Explain the importance of urgent transport to a facility with ALS if it is not available in the pre-hospital setting.
10. Discuss the various types of AEDs.
11. Discuss the procedures that must be taken into consideration for standard operations of the various types of AEDs.
12. State the reasons for assuring that the patient is pulseless and is not breathing when using the AED.
13. Discuss the circumstances that may result in inappropriate shocks.
14. Explain the considerations for interruption of cardiopulmonary resuscitation (CPR) when using the AED.
15. Discuss the advantages and disadvantages of AEDs.
16. Summarise the speed of operation of automated external defibrillation.
17. Discuss the use of remote defibrillation through adhesive pads.
18. Discuss the special consideration for rhythm monitoring.
19. List the steps in the operation of the AED.
20. Discuss the standard of care that should be used to provide care to a patient with persistent ventricular fibrillation and no available ALS.
21. Discuss the standard of care that should be used to provide care to a patient with recurrent ventricular fibrillation and no available ALS.
22. Differentiate between single-rescuer and multi-rescuer care with an AED.
23. Explain the reason for pulses not being checked between shocks with an AED.
24. Discuss the importance of co-ordinating ALS-trained providers with personnel using AEDs.
25. Discuss the importance of post-resuscitation care.
26. List the components of post-resuscitation care.
27. Explain the importance of frequent practice with the AED.
28. Discuss the need to complete the 'Automated Defibrillator: Operator's Shift Checklist'.
29. Discuss the goal of quality improvement in automated external defibrillation.
30. Define the function of all controls on an AED, and describe event documentation and defibrillator battery maintenance.

Affective objectives

31. Defend the reasons for obtaining initial training in automated external defibrillation and the importance of continuing education.
32. Defend the reason for maintenance of AEDs.

Psychomotor objectives

33. Demonstrate the application and operation of the AED.
34. Demonstrate the maintenance of an AED.
35. Demonstrate the assessment and documentation of patient response to automated external defibrillation.
36. Demonstrate the skills necessary to complete the 'Automated Defibrillator: Operator's Shift Checklist'.

Cardiac emergencies are the most prominent type of emergency in the UK. Each year, the use of the automated external defibrillator (AED) saves many lives. There is increasing use of AEDs by First Responders in the UK.

The AED is a machine used by basic-level providers to analyse the patient's cardiac rhythm and deliver an electrical shock that stops the heart's chaotic rhythm. This electrical shock is called defibrillation. For the adult patient in cardiac arrest, defibrillation is the highest priority and ideally should be done before CPR is started. Defibrillation is the primary intervention that makes the greatest difference to the survival of patients in cardiac arrest. Early defibrillation is a vital link in the chain of survival and is an important life-saving technique.

THE AUTOMATED EXTERNAL DEFIBRILLATOR

The steps of defibrillation include the recognition and treatment of a heart rhythm that produces no pulse. Basic-level providers are generally not trained in the recognition of cardiac rhythms, and therefore, in the past, they were not able to defibrillate. Since defibrillation is the intervention that has most impact on the survival of adult patients in cardiac arrest, the use of an AED will allow more providers to deliver this life-saving intervention.

The longer a person is in cardiac arrest, the less likely it becomes that defibrillation will be successful. Therefore, the availability of the AED for use by First Responders is beneficial.

Overview of the automated external defibrillator

The AED was developed in the early 1980s and has gained widespread application. Health-care providers have been using defibrillation for decades as the primary treatment of life-threatening electrical disturbances in the heart. By combining computer technology with the defibrillator, much of the need for human decision-making has been removed, and hence the possibility for error has been reduced. The use of an AED can be learned in a short time. In the future, these machines may be available in every shopping centre, airport and hotel, and their use taught in advanced CPR courses.

The AED works when two conductive patches are placed on the patient's chest and the machine is turned on. The AED then uses computer circuitry to analyse the patient's cardiac rhythm, and to deliver a shock if appropriate. To administer a shock, the AED's computer must detect a life-threatening electrical disturbance in the heart, which is generally a condition known as 'ventricular fibrillation'.

Ventricular fibrillation – Ventricular fibrillation (VF) is a chaotic dysrhythmia in which the patient has no pulse or respiration, and the heart is simply 'quivering' inside the chest (**Fig. D.1**). There is electrical activity in this rhythm but it does not cause a mechanical pumping action of the heart to produce a pulse.

Ventricular tachycardia – The AED will shock other rhythms, but these are seldom present on arrival of EMS. One of them, pulseless ventricular tachycardia (VT), occurs when there are three or more consecutive beats (originating in the ventricles) at a rate of 140 beats or more per minute (**Fig. D.2**). This rhythm occurs frequently at the onset of cardiac arrest but there is generally a rapid deterioration to ventricular fibrillation.

An AED can shock both rhythms, but the key is that the patient must be pulseless and not breathing before you attach the machine to the patient.

There are two types of AEDs – fully automatic and semi-automatic (**Fig. D.3**). With a fully automatic external defibrillator, the rescuer simply has to attach two defibrillator patches to the patient's chest, connect the lead wires and turn on the AED. With a semi-automatic external defibrillator the rescuer must attach the patches and leads to the patient's chest, turn on the AED and press a button to analyse the rhythm. The AED's computer-synthesised voice then advises you what steps to take based on its analysis of the patient's cardiac rhythm. Shocks, if advised, are delivered manually by pressing a button. Both types of AEDs are designed to deliver up to three shocks in a row.

If your AED does not have a screen that shows the patient's rhythm, you will probably never know or see the rhythm. In any case, your primary concerns are to assess the absence or presence of a carotid pulse and to follow the directions of the AED. Remember that the machine cannot detect pulses, only electrical activity within the heart. The electrical activity may or may not be producing a pulse.

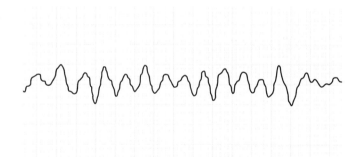

Fig. D.1 Ventricular fibrillation.

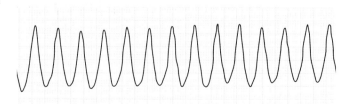

Fig. D.2 Ventricular tachycardia.

Appendix D: Automated external defibrillation

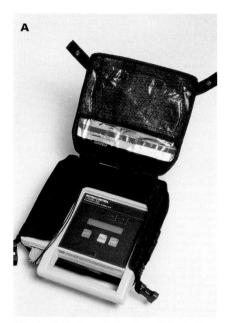
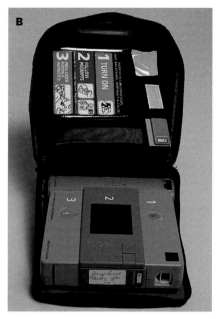
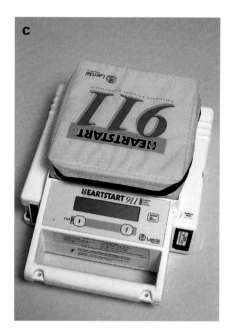

Fig. D.3 Automated external defibrillators.

These machines are very accurate in detecting both shockable rhythms and rhythms that do not need shocks. A correct and accurate analysis by the AED depends on properly charged defibrillator batteries and proper maintenance of the defibrillator. The few documented cases of inappropriate shocks occurring can be attributed to human error (such as using the device on a patient with a pulse or activating it in a moving vehicle) or mechanical error (such as low batteries).

You should stop CPR when the AED is analysing the patient's heart rhythm or when delivering shocks. During the delivery of a shock, anyone touching either the patient or anything attached to the patient may also receive a shock. It is dangerous to be close to the patient when the AED is used because contact with an object that is touching the patient can transmit the high-voltage shock.

Do not touch the patient when the rhythm is being analysed because movement may cause discrepancies in the analysis of the rhythm. You should stop CPR and artificial ventilations, and if the patient is in a vehicle, it should be stopped.

Defibrillation is a higher priority than CPR. Therefore it is beneficial to the patient to stop CPR to use the AED. CPR may be stopped for up to 90 seconds when three consecutive shocks are delivered. Resume CPR only after the first three shocks are delivered, or when the AED indicates a 'no-shock' situation.

Advantages of the automated external defibrillator

There are many advantages in the use of the AED. The biggest advantage is that the basic-level providers who are not trained to read cardiac rhythms can still deliver an electrical shock to the patient's heart.

The speed of the operation is very fast – usually the first shock can be delivered to the patient within 1 minute of arrival at the patient's side. Remote defibrillators use adhesive pads, making it a 'hands-off' process. Traditional defibrillators use paddles that the rescuer must hold on the patient's chest, placing the rescuer close to the patient when the shock is delivered. The electrodes are large and easy to place. Some models have an optional rhythm-monitoring capability that can be used when personnel with a knowledge of the interpretation of cardiac rhythms arrive on scene.

The defibrillator will automatically select the energy level of the shock to be delivered, measured in joules (often abbreviated to J). The AED can increase the energy level of each successive shock. The machine will shock the patient the first and second times at 200 joules and the third time at 360 joules.

AEDs that use biphasic wave-forms to deliver the electrical energy to the patient use lower energy levels of 130–150 joules. The biphasic AED will still deliver the shocks in stacks of three.

Operation of the automated external defibrillator

When caring for a patient, always take appropriate universal precautions. On your arrival at the scene, perform the initial assessment, and if appropriate use the AED.

Figure D.4 illustrates the steps for AED using a common type of semi-automatic external defibrillator, and **Figure D.5** illustrates a standardised algorithm for AED use.

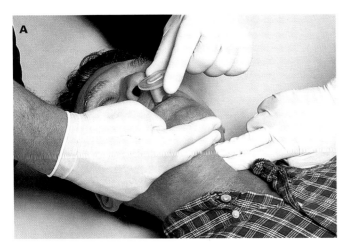

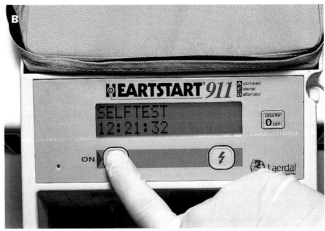

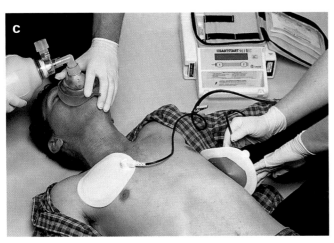

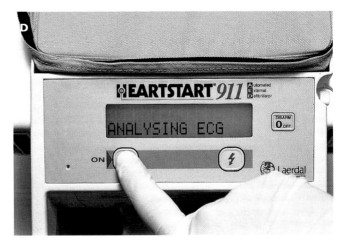

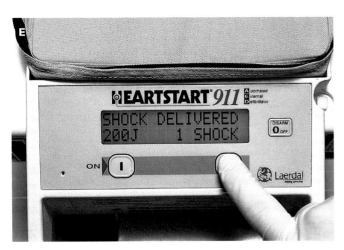

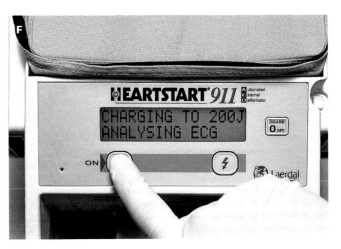

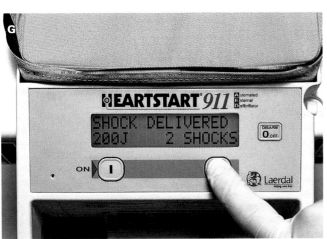

Fig. D.4 Use of the semi-automatic external defibrillator. Follow universal precautions. **(a)** Perform the initial AcBC assessment and confirm that the patient is in cardiac arrest. Stop CPR if it is in progress and verify that the patient is unresponsive, not breathing and pulseless. Resume CPR. If you are the only rescuer present, proceed with the use of the AED. **(b)** Turn on the AED's power. If the machine has a tape recorder, turn it on. **(c)** Attach the device to the patient. One electrode is placed to the right of the upper portion of the sternum below the clavicle. The other electrode is placed over the ribs to the left of the nipple with the centre in the midaxillary line. Most electrodes include diagrams showing correct placement. **(d)** Stop CPR, clear everyone away from the patient and initiate analysis of the rhythm. **(e)** If the machine advises a shock, deliver the first shock (generally 200 J); if not, go to step **k**. **(f)** Reanalyse the rhythm. **(g)** If the machine advises another shock, deliver a second shock (at 200 J); if not, go to step **k**.

Appendix D: Automated external defibrillation

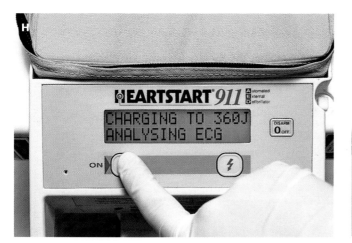

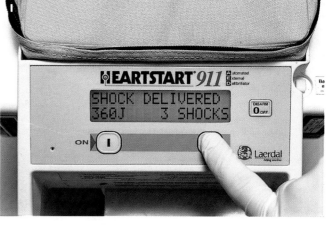

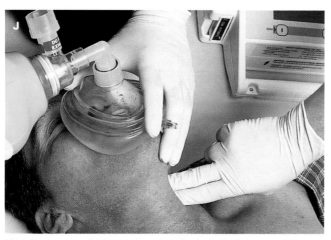

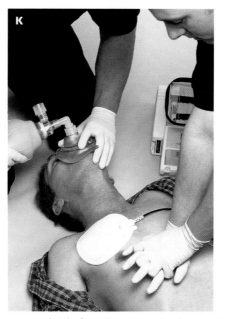

Fig. D.4 cont. **(h)** Reanalyse the rhythm. **(i)** If the machine advises another shock, deliver a third shock (at 360 J); if not, go to step **k**. **(j)** Check the patient's pulse. If the patient has a pulse, check breathing. If the patient is breathing adequately, place the patient in the recovery position and monitor the airway and pulse and have the patient transported as soon as possible. If the patient has a pulse and is not breathing adequately, provide artificial ventilations and have the patient transported as soon as possible. If the patient does not have a pulse, resume CPR for 1 minute. At the direction of the AED, deliver one more cycle of up to three stacked shocks (at 360 J), and reassess the pulse. If there is no pulse, continue the stacked shocks. If an ambulance has arrived, consult with medical direction and continue with stacked shocks or have the patient transported. Have the patient transported as soon as possible. **(k)** If the machine advises 'no shock', check the patient's pulse. If there is a pulse, check breathing and treat appropriately for adequate or inadequate breathing and have the patient transported. If there is no pulse, perform CPR for 1 minute and then recheck the pulse. Reanalyse the rhythm if there is still no pulse. If 'no shock' is again advised and there is still no pulse, resume CPR for 1 minute. Analyse the rhythm for a third time. If shock is advised, deliver up to two sets of three stacked shocks separated by 1 minute of CPR, consult the medical direction physician and have the patient transported. If 'no shock' is advised for a third time and the patient does not have a pulse, resume CPR and have the patient transported as soon as possible.

First Responder Alert

Attach the AED only to patients who are in cardiac arrest – unresponsive with no pulse and not breathing – to avoid delivering inappropriate shocks to patients who have a pulse. Shocking a patient with a pulse may put that patient into ventricular fibrillation or into other unshockable rhythms.

To use the fully automatic external defibrillator, follow the same procedure. Once the AED power is turned on, the machine will analyse and shock with no action by the rescuer. After three shocks, check the pulse and continue with the appropriate treatment. The machine will state 'clear the patient' before delivering shocks, or will state 'no shock indicated' when appropriate.

Not all patients in cardiac arrest will benefit from defibrillation. If the AED does not detect a shockable rhythm, it advises 'no shock indicated'. Make sure the patient has no pulse and then begin CPR. After 1 minute of CPR, use the AED to analyse the rhythm again.

Automated External Defibrillation (AED) Algorithm for the First Responder

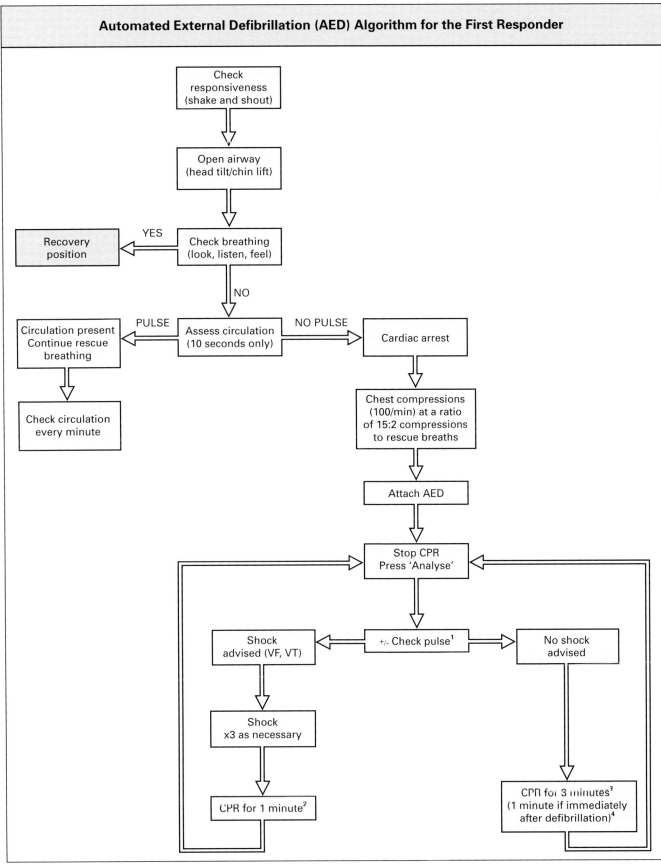

Fig. D.5 Algorithm for AED use. Use appropriate universal precautions. If CPR was started before your arrival, stop CPR to confirm lack of breathing and pulse. If you are the only rescuer, proceed to the use of the AED. **1)** When a shock is indicated, no pulse checks should be performed during the first three shocks, as the priority is rapid defibrillation. **2)** After the first three shocks, uninterrupted CPR should be given for 1 minute. **3)** If no shock is indicated, uninterrupted CPR should be given for 3 minutes. Press analyse only after 3 minutes; if this confirms no shock indicated check pulse. **4)** When no shock is indicated for the first time after an episode of VF, the period of CPR before the next analysis is only 1 minute. Continue the AED algorithm until ALS is available. In cases of persisting VF/VT, the course of actions is dictated by local policy. (Derived from Handley AJ, *et al. Resuscitation* 1998; **37**: 71.)

Appendix D: Automated external defibrillation

Because it is vital for the patient to receive defibrillation as soon as possible, pulse checks are not performed after the first and second shocks or after the fourth and fifth shocks. After the third shock, the defibrillator has reached the maximum energy level required. A pulse check should be performed after the third shock and again after the sixth shock. Follow standard operating procedures in all cases (**Box D.1**).

The AED generally is not used for patients younger than 12 years of age or patients weighing less than 41 kg. The airway and artificial ventilation are of prime importance in these patients. In young children, cardiac arrest usually results from respiratory compromise, not from cardiac problems. Patients weighing less than 41 kg may receive too high an electrical charge for their size, resulting in damage to the heart.

Do not remove the AED, even after a successful resuscitation. Ventricular fibrillation may recur even after successful shocks. If you are with a patient who has been resuscitated but is unresponsive, check pulses every 30 seconds. If at anytime the patient becomes pulseless, analyse the rhythm. Deliver up to three stacked shocks if indicated and continue the resuscitation according to your local protocol.

If you are with a responsive patient having chest pain who becomes unresponsive, stops breathing and becomes pulseless, attach the AED, analyse the rhythm, deliver up to three shocks if indicated and continue the resuscitation according to your local protocol. Not all patients who are experiencing chest pain progress to cardiac arrest. Follow the steps in Chapter 7 ('Circulation') for the care for a patient who is responsive and has a pulse. The AED should only be attached to patients who are unresponsive and do not have a pulse – do not attach the AED to a patient who is responsive or who has a pulse.

If a situation arises in which you are the only rescuer with an AED, take universal precautions and perform an initial assessment to verify that the patient is not breathing and has no pulse. Turn on the AED power, attach the device to the patient, initiate analysis of the rhythm and deliver a shock if necessary. Follow the local protocol for the remainder of the treatment. Defibrillation should always be the first step before CPR. Do not leave the patient in order to call for assistance until the 'no shock indicated' command has been given, the pulse has returned, three shocks have been delivered or help has arrived.

Always follow the local protocol for the use of the AED. Each organisation has guidelines for continuing education and the use of the AED. Use of the defibrillator does not require advanced life support (ALS) personnel to be at the scene, although they should be notified as soon as possible. It is vital that EMS personnel are contacted and arrive as soon as possible.

For safety reasons, do not use the defibrillator near water or in the heavy rain. The defibrillator is an electrical device. If the patient is lying in water or on ice and you are standing in the water beside the patient, the electrical shock will travel from the patient to you through the water. Move the patient to a dry area and remove any wet clothes from the patient. You should also ensure that the patient is not touching any metal, because the electrical discharge from the defibrillator would travel through the patient and through the metal to anyone touching it.

Post-resuscitation care

If the patient does not regain a pulse after the AED algorithm has been completed, follow local protocol regarding whether or not to continue with the use of the defibrillator. It is vital that care is maintained after resuscitation of the patient. The patient's airway, breathing and circulation must be monitored continuously so that the cardiac arrest does not re-occur. Do not remove the defibrillator from the patient if he or she has been resuscitated. The paramedic personnel may remove it when they transport the patient. Do not forget to administer high-flow oxygen via a non-rebreather mask with reservoir bag.

Document all findings in your report and inform the ALS personnel of all interventions. Be sure to document each step performed, any changes in patient condition and any responses to interventions. Document all vital signs before and after use of the AED. Document all interactions with bystanders and any information obtained regarding the patient. The pre-hospital care report is a vital part of the emergency medical care.

Box D.1	Standard AED Operating Procedures

- If no other EMS personnel are on scene, the First Responders should continue CPR and use of the AED until they arrive
- One First Responder operates the defibrillator while the other performs CPR
- After opening the airway and confirming the patient is in cardiac arrest, defibrillation comes first. Do not delay the analysis of the rhythm or defibrillation. The first shock should be delivered within 60 seconds of arrival at the patient's side
- All contact with the patient must be avoided during analysis of the rhythm and delivery of shocks. Never analyse the rhythm in a moving vehicle
- State "clear the patient" before delivering shocks, and verify that everyone is clear
- No defibrillator can function correctly without properly working batteries. Check the batteries at the beginning of each shift, and carry extra batteries
- Be familiar with the specific AED used by your service
- If you are alone when approaching a cardiac arrest patient, use the AED after assessing the AcBCs, instead of initiating CPR

Automated Defibrillators: Operator's Shift Checklist

Date _____ Shift _____ Location _____

Make/Model No. _____ Serial No. or Facility ID No. _____

At the beginning of each shift, inspect the unit. Indicate whether all requirements have been met. Note any corrective actions taken. Sign the form

	OK as found	Corrective Actions/ remarks
1. Defibrillator Unit Clean, no spills, clear of objects on top, casing intact		
2. Cables, connectors a. Inspect for cracks, broken wire, or damage b. Connectors engage securely and are not damaged*		
3. Supplies a. Two sets of pads in sealed packages, within expiration date* b. Hand towel c. Scissors d. Razor e. Alcohol wipes* f. Monitoring electrodes* g. Spare charged battery* h. Adequate ECG paper* i. Manual override module, key or card* j. Cassette tape, memory module, and/or event card plus spares*		
4. Power supply a. Battery-powered units (1) Verify fully charged battery in place (2) Spare charged battery available (3) Follow appropriate battery rotation schedule as per manufacturer's recommendations b. AC/battery backup units (1) Plugged into live outlet to maintain battery charge (2) Test on battery power and reconnect to line power		
5. Indicators*/ECG Display a. Remove cassette tape, memory module and/or event card* b. Power-on display c. Self-test OK d. Monitor display functional* e. 'Service' message display off* f. Battery charging; low battery light off* g. Correct time displayed; set with control room		
6. ECG recorder* a. Adequate ECG paper b. Recorder prints		
7. Charge/Display Cycle a. Disconnect AC plug – battery backup units* b. Attach to simulator c. Detects, charges and delivers shock for VF d. Responds correctly to non-shockable rhythms e. Manual override functional* f. Detach from simulator g. Replace cassette tape, module and/or memory card*		
8. Pacemaker* a. Pacer output cable intact b. Pacer pads present (set of two) c. Inspect per manufacturer's operational guidelines		
Major problem(s) Identified (Out of Service)		

* Applicable only if the unit has this supply or capability

Signature _____

Fig. D.6 Example of an AED operator checklist.

MAINTENANCE OF THE AUTOMATED EXTERNAL DEFIBRILLATOR

Defibrillators require regular maintenance. There should be a maintenance schedule for each unit. A checklist, the 'Automated Defibrillator: Operator's Shift Checklist', must be completed on a daily basis (**Fig. D.6**). The most common cause of defibrillator failure is improper device maintenance, usually battery failure. Battery replacement schedules should be maintained for each unit. Many AEDs now use lithium batteries, which have a specified life and do not need to be recharged. Many AEDs will carry out an automatic self-check at a predetermined frequency. This, however, does not remove the requirement for carrying out other checks on the equipment.

AUTOMATED EXTERNAL DEFIBRILLATOR SKILLS

You must maintain your AED skills. The AED is not a frequently used device in most systems. Therefore, the skills may be easily forgotten if they are not practised. It is recommended that a skill review is undertaken every 90 days to reassess competency. Every event in which an AED is used should be reviewed by a physician or a designated representative. Reviews of events using the AED may be accomplished by a written report and a review of the voice–electrocardiogram tape recording made by the AED machine or the solid-state memory modules and magnetic tape recordings stored in the device. Quality improvement involves both the personnel who use the AEDs and the organisation in which the AEDs are used.

Organisations using AEDs should have all the necessary links in the chain of survival, medical supervision, an audit or quality-improvement programme in place, and mandatory continuing education with skill competency reviews for AED providers.

APPENDIX SUMMARY

The automated external defibrillator

The automated external defibrillator (AED) allows basic-level providers who are not trained in rhythm recognition to deliver an electrical shock to a patient in cardiac arrest. The AED uses computer circuitry to analyse the patient's heart rhythm, and, if appropriate, to deliver a shock. AEDs can be fully automatic or semi-automatic. The AED allows for early defibrillation, a vital link in the chain of survival.

If the patient does not regain a pulse after using the AED, follow your local protocol for transport, CPR and further defibrillation. If the patient does regain a pulse, place him or her in the recovery position, administer high-flow oxygen and monitor the airway and breathing until paramedic personnel arrive.

Maintenance of the automated external defibrillator

AED failures are often caused by improper maintenance. The AED should be checked daily. Check the batteries and complete the 'Automated Defibrillator: Operator's Shift Checklist'.

Automated external defibrillator skills

You must refresh your skills with the AED periodically. A review every 90 days is recommended by many organisations. Following an event in which an AED is used, the medical director or a designated representative will review the case for quality improvement.

Appendix

E

Principles and techniques of splinting

I. **Injuries to bones and joints**
    A. Signs and symptoms of bone and joint injury
    B. Emergency care for casualties with bone or joint injuries

II. **Splinting**
    A. Reasons for splinting
    B. Principles of splinting
    C. Splinting equipment and techniques
    D. Risks of splinting

Key terms

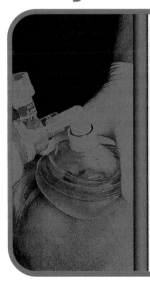

Distal
A directional term meaning further away from the trunk (more peripheral).

Pneumatic splint
A device that uses air or vacuum to stabilise an injury.

Position of function
The relaxed position of the hand or foot in which there is minimal movement or stretching of muscle.

Proximal
A directional term meaning closer to the trunk (more central).

Rigid splint
A type of immobilisation device that does not conform to the body.

Sling and swathe
Bandaging used to immobilise a shoulder or arm injury.

Splint
A device used to immobilise a musculoskeletal injury.

Objectives

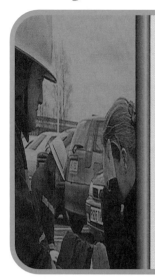

On completion of this chapter you will be able to meet the following objectives:

Cognitive objectives
1. State the reasons for splinting.
2. List the general rules of splinting.
3. List the complications of splinting.
4. List the emergency medical care for a patient with a painful, swollen, deformed extremity.

Affective objectives
5. Explain the rationale for splinting at the scene versus load and go.

6. Explain the rationale for immobilisation of the painful, swollen, deformed extremity.

Psychomotor objectives
7. Demonstrate the emergency medical care of a patient with a painful, swollen, deformed extremity.

The specialised emergency medical care of a casualty with a painful, swollen or deformed extremity includes applying a splint to immobilise the injury and prevent further damage. This appendix describes various types of splints, and it discusses the principles of splinting and some techniques for splinting.

Musculoskeletal injuries are among the most common injuries you will encounter. Usually, these injuries are not life threatening, although they are often painful. Prompt identification and treatment of musculoskeletal injuries is crucial to reduce pain, prevent further injury and minimise permanent damage.

Splinting an extremity is within the scope of practice for some First Responders. If splinting is not within your scope of practice, you should care for injuries as described in Chapter 10 ('Injuries to muscles and bones').

INJURIES TO BONES AND JOINTS

Signs and symptoms of bone and joint injury

Various signs and symptoms are characteristic of bone or joint injuries. The area of injury may have some deformity or angulation and it may be painful to move and tender to the touch. If the bone ends are separated, some crepitation (grating) may be heard or felt during the examination. Crepitation is caused by bone ends rubbing together. Do not purposely seek this sign, and do not try to repeat it if you note it during the assessment. Bone ends rubbing together may produce further injury.

The area of injury may be swollen, appearing larger than the same area on the other side of the body, and it may be discoloured. If the injury is open, bone ends may be protruding through the skin and exposed to the outside environment. With a joint injury, the joint may be locked in position and immovable. **Box E.1** summarises the signs and symptoms of a bone or joint injury.

Emergency care for casualties with bone and joint injuries

As described in Chapter 10, emergency medical care for bone and joint injuries consists of both basic techniques and specialised techniques. First, always take appropriate universal precautions before examining the casualty. Even a closed injury that is not bleeding may become an open injury because of movement or pressure.

Establish a clear airway and ensure the adequacy of breathing. Assess the casualty's circulation and look for major bleeding. Any major bleeding or life-threatening situations should be controlled. Always care for life-threatening injuries before focusing on a painful, swollen, deformed extremity. Do not waste time caring for an extremity if the casualty is not breathing adequately or has other threats to life!

Splint the injury appropriately to prevent movement of bone ends or fragments (described later in this appendix), and prepare the casualty for transport. After splinting the injury, a cold pack may be applied to the injured area to reduce swelling and pain. An injured extremity should be elevated to reduce blood flow to that area unless there are other injuries that could cause complications if this were done.

Box E.1	**Signs and Symptoms of a Bone or Joint Injury**

- Deformity or angulation
- Pain and tenderness
- Crepitation (grating)
- Swelling
- Bruising (discolouration)
- Exposed bone ends (open injury)
- Joints locked into position

Review Questions

Injuries to Bones and Joints

1. Emergency medical care includes the application of a _____ and _____ to reduce swelling and pain.

2. Injuries to the arm should always be splinted, even if the patient has more serious injuries. True or False?

3. List three signs and symptoms of a musculoskeletal injury:

_____

_____

_____

1. Cold pack, splint; 2. False; 3. Deformity or angulation, pain and tenderness, crepitation, swelling, bruising, exposed bone ends, joints locked into position

SPLINTING

The specialised emergency medical care provided for a painful, swollen, deformed extremity includes applying a splint to immobilise the injury and prevent further damage. A splint is a device used to immobilise a musculoskeletal injury. This appendix describes some types of splints and how they are used.

Reasons for splinting

Splinting a painful, swollen, deformed extremity prevents movement of bone fragments, bone ends or injured joints. The splint minimises damage to muscles, nerves and blood vessels caused by broken bones. Immobilisation helps to prevent a closed injury from becoming an open injury. It also minimises the restriction of blood flow resulting from bone ends compressing blood vessels, and it limits the bleeding caused by tissue damage from the bone ends. Splinting reduces pain by limiting the movement of bone ends. Paralysis resulting from spinal damage is also minimised. **Box E.2** summarises the reasons for splinting.

Box E.2	**Reasons for Splinting**

- Prevent movement of bone fragment, bone ends or injured joints
- Minimise damage to muscle, nerves and blood vessels
- Minimise the chance of converting a closed injury to an injury
- Minimise the restriction of blood flow resulting from bone ends compressing blood vessels
- Minimise bleeding from damaged tissue caused by bone ends
- Minimise pain associated with movement of bone ends
- Minimise chance of paralysis of extremities due to spinal damage

Principles of splinting

Before splinting, always assess the casualty as a whole first. After performing a primary assessment, physical examination and treating any life-threatening injuries, you should care for the injured extremity. Evaluate the pulse at the end of the injured extremity, the motor function (the ability to move the extremity) and sensation (the ability to feel) distal to the injury. Assessing distal to the injury means assessing further away from the trunk than the injury. For example, if the injury is to the knee, you should assess the pulse, motor function and sensation in the lower leg or foot. If the injury is to the wrist, you should assess the fingers. Assess the pulse, motor function and sensation both before and after applying a splint, and record the findings. A splint that is placed improperly or secured too tightly may impede circulation. If there is a change in circulation, loosen the splint and reassess. If the circulation does not return, you may need to remove the splint and apply it again.

The bones and joints above and below an injury site must be immobilised with the splint to minimise muscle movement near the injury. Before splinting, cut away loose clothing to expose the area and make the splint more effective. Open injuries should be dressed and bandaged before application of the splint.

If there is a severe deformity or the extremity is cyanotic or lacks a pulse, the injury should be aligned with gentle traction under analgesia (such as Entonox inhalation) before splinting, in an attempt to regain circulation. (Entonox is a half-and-half mixture of oxygen and nitrous oxide. It is contained in blue and white cylinders.) If resistance is felt, splint the extremity in the position in which you find it. If no pulse returns in the injured extremity, rapid transport is indicated to prevent possible loss of the extremity. If any bones are protruding through the skin, do not try to reposition them, although they may retract when the splint is applied. Splints should be padded to prevent pressure and discomfort to the casualty.

When splinting a hand or foot, immobilise it in the position of function. This is the most comfortable position for the hand or foot and requires the least amount of muscle use or stretching. The position of function is a natural resting position. For the hand, place a roll of gauze in the palm to support the hand; for the foot, support the sole (**Figs E.1** and **E.2**).

First Responder Alert

Always care for life-threatening injuries before focusing on a painful, swollen, deformed extremity. Do not waste time caring for an extremity if the patient is not breathing adequately or has other threats to life!

Appendix E: Principles and techniques of splinting

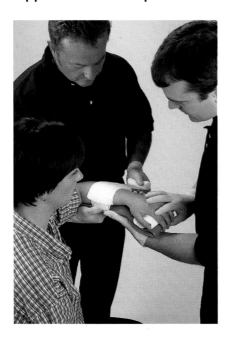

Fig. E.1 For a hand injury, place a roll of gauze in the palm to support and immobilise the hand in the position of function.

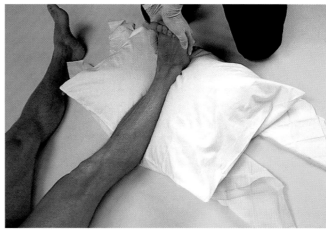

Fig. E.2 For a foot injury, support the sole and immobilise in the position of function.

If you are in doubt whether to splint an injury, you should splint it – it is better to err on the side of caution. It is acceptable to splint an injury that does not need it, but it is unacceptable to fail to splint an injury that does need it. Without an X-ray, it is impossible to differentiate between a broken ankle and a sprained or strained ankle; therefore, you should assume the ankle is broken. Do not waste time trying to identify the actual injury. See **Principle E.1** for the principles of splinting.

If the casualty is showing the signs and symptoms of shock, place the casualty in neutral alignment and transport using total body immobilisation, including spinal board and cervical collar. Do not waste time splinting each injury separately.

Splinting equipment and techniques

Many types of splints are used to immobilise various musculoskeletal injuries. For all types of splints, remember the general principles previously described.

Rigid splints
Rigid splints can be used to support a painful, swollen and deformed extremity and immobilise the joints or bones above and below the injury. Common examples are padded-board splints, cardboard splints and box splints. **Figure E.3** illustrates one technique for using rigid splints.

Pneumatic splints
Pneumatic splints are flexible splints that use air to maintain rigidity. Air splints are an example of a pneumatic splint. Vacuum splints are also pneumatic splints; they work by removing the air in the splint, so that it becomes rigid and immobilises the injured extremity (**Figs. E.4** and **E.5**).

The vacuum splint is applied to the injured area and then suction applied until it is snug. The advantages of the vacuum splint include the fact that it places uniform pressure on bleeding areas, and that it is

Principle E.1	**Principles of Splinting**

1. Assess pulse, motor function and sensation distal to the injury before and after splinting, and record your findings
2. Immobilise the joint above and below the musculoskeletal injury. If the joint is injured, immobilise the bone above and below the injury
3. Remove or cut away clothing before splinting
4. Cover open wounds with sterile dressings before splinting
5. Splint the injury in the position found, unless there is severe deformity or the extremity is cyanotic or lacks a pulse. If these conditions are found, attempt to align the extremity with gentle traction before splinting
6. Do not intentionally replace protruding bones, but note them in your report
7. Pad the splint to prevent pressure and discomfort to the patient
8. Splint the injury before moving the patient unless there are life-threatening situations present
9. If in doubt whether an injury is present, apply a splint
10. If the patient has the signs and symptoms of shock, use full-body immobilisation, align the patient in the normal anatomical position on a spinal board and assist in the transport as soon as possible

comfortable for the casualty. The disadvantage is that air may leak into the splint if damaged.

When using a pneumatic splint, cover all wounds with clean dressings before applying the splint. Using an air splint requires two rescuers, one to support the extremity and one to apply the splint. As when applying any splint, check the patient's pulse, motor function and sensation distal to the injury before and after application.

Improvised splints

Improvised splints, such as pillows, may be used to support joint injuries and are commonly used for ankle injuries. The pillow is wrapped completely around the ankle and secured. The toes are left visible so that assessment may be made of the pulse, motor function and sensation (**Fig. E.6**). Cardboard splints are also useful for joint injuries, because they may be cut to form an angle and then secured in place.

The sling and swathe

The sling and swathe is a common splinting technique used for a shoulder injury. The arm is placed into the sling and the swathe is wrapped around the arm and the body so that the arm and shoulder cannot move (**Fig. E.7**). The sling and swathe may be used along with other types of splints for arm injuries (**Figs E.8** and **E.9**).

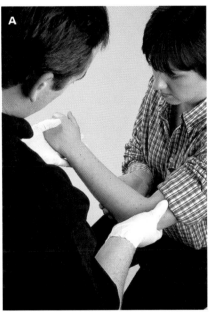 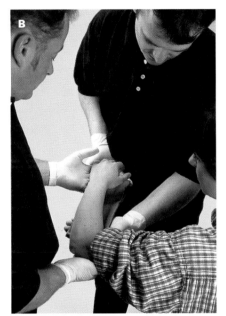 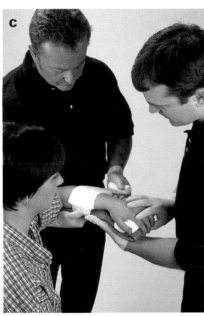

Fig. E.3 Splinting a long bone with a rigid splint. Use appropriate personal protective equipment for universal precautions. **(a)** Check the casualty's pulse, motor function and sensation distal to the injury. **(b)** Provide manual stabilisation and support the injured extremity, maintaining gentle traction if indicated while applying the rigid splint. Measure the rigid splint to the extremity. **(c)** Pad the open spaces between the splint and the extremity with roller gauze tied snugly. Tie the knots over the splint, not the skin, for comfort. Immobilise the joints above and below the injury site. Secure and immobilise the hand or foot in the position of function. Secure the entire injured extremity to the body. Repeat the assessment of pulse, motor function and sensation distal to the injury.

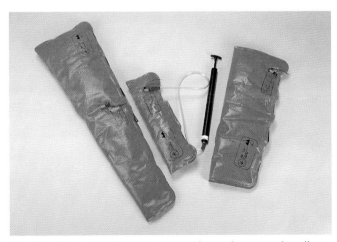

Fig. E.4 Vacuum splints are commonly used pneumatic splints.

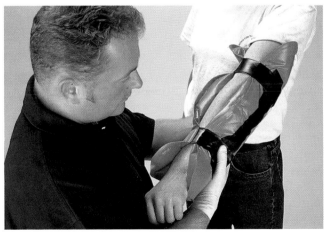

Fig. E.5 An injured arm immobilised by a vacuum splint.

Appendix E: Principles and techniques of splinting

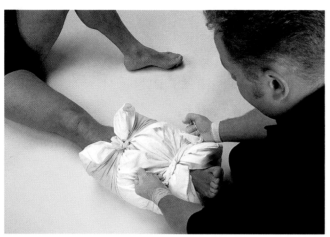

Fig. E.6 An improvised pillow splint can provide support for an injured ankle or foot.

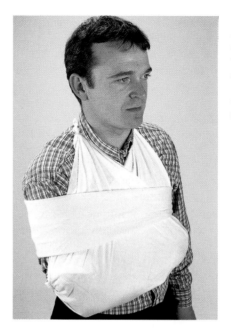

Fig. E.7 A sling and swathe is a common splinting technique for a shoulder injury to prevent movement of the arm and shoulder.

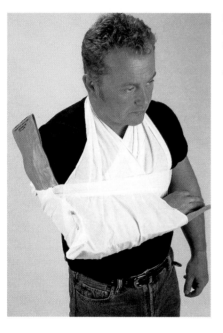

Fig. E.8 A deformed humerus can be immobilised using a sling and swathe.

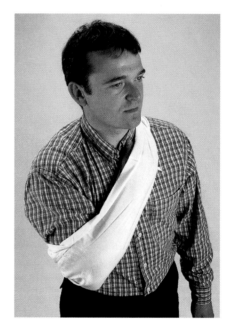

Fig. E.9 Immobilisation of an injured elbow using a high-arm sling.

Always use properly sized splints. Some devices come in infant and child sizes. Familiarise yourself with the equipment used by your local EMS agency.

Risks of splinting

Using splints improperly can lead to complications. If splints are used incorrectly, they may cause more harm than benefit. A splint can compress nerves, tissues and blood vessels; therefore, the pressure of the splint should be monitored continuously together with the pulse, motor function and sensation of the injured extremity. A splint applied too tightly on an extremity can reduce distal circulation. An improperly applied splint can increase bleeding and tissue damage associated with the injury, cause permanent nerve damage or disability, convert a closed injury to an open injury or increase the pain caused by excessive movement.

Splinting an injury takes time. If you are not able to complete splinting of a critically injured casualty before the ambulance arrives, do not delay treating or transporting in order to complete splinting. Splinting may be done on the way to the hospital or not at all if the casualty has life-threatening injuries. When moving the casualty, take extreme care to keep the injury stable.

APPENDIX SUMMARY
Injuries to bones and joints

Emergency medical care for musculoskeletal injuries includes universal precautions, airway assessment, control of major bleeding and care for life-threatening situations. The injured area may be elevated to reduce blood flow to that area, and cold packs may be applied to reduce swelling. Splints can be used to restrict movement and prevent further damage to the injured tissue. Never delay transport of a critical casualty to splint an extremity.

Splinting

Splinting a painful, swollen, deformed extremity minimises movement and pain, and helps prevent further damage. Always follow appropriate splinting principles.

When splinting, assess the pulse, motor function and sensation distal to the injury before and after splinting, and record your findings. Immobilise the joints or bones above and below the injury. Remove or cut away clothing before splinting, and cover any open wounds with sterile dressings. Splint the injury in the position found unless there is impaired distal circulation or sensation, or the casualty has a life-threatening condition. Types of splints include rigid or non-formable splints, pneumatic splints and improvised splints.

Because a splint might compress nerves, tissues and blood vessels, the pressure of the splint should be checked continually together with the pulse, motor function and sensation distal to the injury. Excessive movement may cause or aggravate damage to tissues, nerves, vessels or muscle. Never delay treating or transporting a critically ill casualty with life-threatening injuries in order to splint.

Review Questions

Splinting

1. Always check pulse, motor function and _____ distal to the injury before and after applying splints.

2. The injury should be splinted before transport even when the patient is not breathing. True or False?

3. Splinting an injury properly should _____ (increase, decrease) the pain associated with the injury.

4. If the pulse distal to the injury is absent, _____ _____ should be applied gently to the extremity.

1. Sensation; 2. False; 3. Decrease; 4. Manual traction

Glossary

Abortion
The medical term for any delivery or removal of a human foetus before it can live on its own.

Abrasion
An open injury involving the outermost layer(s) of skin.

AcBC A mnemonic for the initial protocol to be adopted by the First Responder when performing the primary assessment; it stands for 'Airway with cervical spinal control, Breathing and Circulation'.

Accessory muscles
Muscles in the neck, chest, and abdomen used to assist breathing. The use of accessory muscles indicates difficulty in breathing.

Advanced life support (ALS)
Cardiopulmonary resuscitation using various medical and paramedical procedures, including intravenous drug administration, and using specialised artificial ventilation equipment.

Agonal respirations
Weak and ineffective chest wall movements immediately before or after cardiac arrest.

Airway
The respiratory system structures through which air passes.

Altered mental status
An ailment resulting in a patient's increased or decreased awareness, which can range from hyperactivity to unconsciousness.

Ambulance Paramedic
An emergency provider with training above the level of Ambulance Technician to include advanced airway management, intravenous (IV) cannulation, drug therapy and defibrillation.

Ambulance Technician
An emergency care provider, cardiac trained, who may administer low risk drugs and gases and may carry out defibrillation.

Amniotic sac
The membrane forming a closed, fluid-filled sac around a developing foetus.

AMPLE history
A mnemonic used in the secondary assessment; it stands for the history of allergies, medications, pertinent history, last oral intake and events leading to illness or injury.

Amputation
The detachment of an extremity or part of an extremity.

Atria The two upper chambers of the heart, which function to receive blood and pump it to the ventricles.

Automated external defibrillator (AED)
A machine used by basic-level rescuers to provide an electrical shock to a patient who is not breathing and who is pulseless; they are either automatic or semi-automatic.

Bag–valve–mask (BVM)
A ventilation device consisting of a self-inflating bag, an oxygen reservoir, a one-way valve, and a mask. The BVM is the most common ventilation device used in medicine and is most effectively used with two rescuers.

Bandage
A non-sterile cloth used to cover a dressing and secure it in place.

Barrier devices
Typically a piece of plastic that is designed to create a barrier between the patient's and rescuer's mouth during ventilation.

Basic life support (BLS)
Maintaining an airway and supporting breathing and the circulation without the use of equipment other than a simple airway device or protective shield.

Behaviour
The manner in which a person acts or performs.

Birth canal
The lower part of the uterus and the vagina.

Bleeding
The loss of blood, either externally or internally, because of a wound, injury, or illness.

Bloody show
The expulsion of the mucus plug as the cervix dilates; the show is sometimes mixed with blood and it often occurs at the beginning of labour.

Body mechanics
The principles of effective use of the muscles and joints of your body when lifting and moving casualties.

Burn An injury to surface body tissue and, in some cases, underlying tissue caused by a significant change in heat to the affected area.

Burnout
A condition characterised by physical and emotional exhaustion resulting in chronic unrelieved job-related stress and ill health.

Capillary refill

The amount of time required to refill the capillary bed after applying and releasing pressure on a fingernail.

Cardiac muscle

The muscle found only in the heart.

Cardiopulmonary resuscitation (CPR)

The process of one or two rescuers providing artificial ventilations and external chest compressions to a patient that is pulseless and not breathing.

Casualty

A term used to describe a person requiring treatment, specifically as a result of trauma.

Cervix

The neck of the uterus.

Chain of survival

The term for the optimum process that should be followed for saving a life. The chain consists of: early access, early BLS, early defibrillation and early ALS.

Chief complaint

The patient's description of the medical problem.

Child Generally, a young person over the age of 1 year.

Child neglect

The act of not giving attention to a child's essential needs.

Closed injury

An injury that does not produce a break in the continuity of the skin.

Contusion

A wound caused by the rupturing of blood cells under the skin surface, often resulting in a bruise; the skin is not broken.

Convulsions

Jerky, violent muscle contractions.

Criteria-based dispatch

A system by which an Ambulance Control Operator, who has received special training, uses a computerised dispatch program or cardex system to prioritise calls according to information received, and may provide pre-arrival instructions to emergency callers or others over the telephone before arrival of the EMS.

Critical Incident Stress Debriefing (CISD)

A debriefing process conducted by either a team of peer counsellors or specially trained health professionals, in order to help emergency workers deal with their emotions and feelings after a critical incident.

Critical incident

Any situation that causes an emergency worker to experience strong emotional reactions and that interferes with their ability to function, either immediately or at sometime in the future.

Crowing

A harsh noise heard on inspiration.

Crowning

The stage in which the head (or other presenting part) of the baby is seen at the vaginal opening.

Defibrillation

The delivery of an electrical shock to the patient's heart to stop a chaotic heart rhythm.

Diaphragm

The large, dome-shaped muscle that separates the thoracic and abdominal cavities; the main muscle used in breathing.

Diastolic blood pressure

The measurement of the pressure exerted against the walls of the arteries while the heart is relaxed and the chambers of the heart are being filled with blood from the great veins.

Direct injury

The result of force applied to a part of the body.

Distal

A directional term meaning further away from the trunk (more peripheral).

DOTS

An acronym for the information that is identified when the First Responder performs the secondary assessment; it stands for deformities, open injuries, tenderness and swelling.

Dressing

A sterile cloth used to cover open injuries in order to protect them from further infection, stem fluid loss, and assist healing.

Drowning

Death due to suffocation by immersion in water.

Emergency Medical Services (EMS) System

A system of many agencies, personnel and institutions involved in planning, providing and monitoring emergency care.

Emergency move

A casualty move used when there is an immediate danger to the casualty or crew members if the casualty is not moved, or when life-saving care cannot be given because of the casualty's location or position.

Epiglottis

A leaf-like flap that prevents food and liquid from entering the windpipe during swallowing.

Evisceration

An open injury in which the internal organs are protruding.

Extrication

The process of removing a patient from entanglement in a motor vehicle or other situation in a safe and appropriate manner.

Finger sweep

Placing a gloved finger deep into the patient's mouth to remove solids or semi-solid obstructions.

First Responder physical examination

A hands-on evaluation performed by the First Responder to obtain information about the illness or injury.

First Responder

An EMS provider who utilises a minimum amount of equipment to perform initial assessment and intervention and who is trained to assist other EMS providers, e.g. a suitably trained fire-fighter, First Aider or member of the public.

Fitting

A type of impaired consciousness that may be characterised by convulsions or other sudden changes in responsiveness.

Flow-restricted, oxygen-powered ventilation device

A ventilation device that attaches directly to an oxygen regulator and delivers a constant flow of oxygen at 40 litres per minute when the trigger is depressed.

Foetus

An unborn, developing baby.

Gag reflex

A reflex that causes the patient to retch when the back of the throat is stimulated; this reflex helps the unresponsive patient protect the airway.

General impression

The First Responder's immediate assessment of the environment and the patient's chief complaint, accomplished in the first few seconds of contact with the patient.

Grunting

A sound made when a patient in respiratory distress attempts to trap air to keep the alveoli open.

Gunshot wound

A wound caused by a bullet or similar projectile entering the body.

Hazardous material

A substance that poses a threat or unreasonable risk to life, health, property or the environment if not properly controlled during manufacture, processing, packaging, handling, storage, transportation, use, or disposal.

Heimlich manoeuvre

Abdominal thrusts used to relieve a foreign body airway obstruction (FBAO).

Hormones

Chemicals that regulate the body's activities and functions.

Hyperthermia

A rise in the body temperature.

Hypothermia

A drop in the body temperature.

Impaired consciousness

A form of altered mental status in which there is a sudden or gradual decrease in a patient's level of responsiveness.

Incident management system

A system for co-ordinating procedures to assist in the control, direction and co-ordination of emergency response resources.

Incision

A clean cut that bleeds freely, caused by a sharp edge.

Indirect injury

The injury affecting an area that results from a force applied to another part of the body.

Infant

Generally, a child under the age of 1 year.

Involuntary muscle

Smooth muscle found in the digestive tract, blood vessels, and bronchi. Involuntary muscle is not under the individual's conscious control.

Joule A unit of energy used to measure the amount of electricity delivered during defibrillation.

Laboured respirations

An increase in the work or effort of breathing.

Laceration

A wound that usually occurs from the tearing or ripping of tissue.

Laryngectomy

A surgical procedure in which the larynx is removed.

Larynx

The voice box; contains the vocal cords that vibrate during speech.

Manual handling

An activity involving the movement or support of a load by hand or other bodily force.

Mechanism of injury

The event or force that caused the casualty's wounds.

Medical Direction

The process (usually by medically trained personnel) of ensuring that the care given to casualties is medically appropriate; also called medical control ('MEDCON'). This may include direct communication between medically trained personnel and care providers in the field.

Miscarriage

Spontaneous delivery of a human foetus before it is able to live on its own.

Mucus extractor

A device that is used to provide suction to the mouth and nose of infants and infants.

Nasal cannula

A low-concentration oxygen delivery device that should be used if the patient will not tolerate a non-rebreather mask.

Nasal flaring

An attempt by the infant in respiratory distress to increase the size of the airway by expanding the nostrils.

Nasopharyngeal airway

A flexible tube of rubber or plastic that is inserted into the patient's nostril to provide an air passage.

Nasopharynx

The region of the pharynx that lies directly behind the nose.

Nature of illness

The event or condition leading to the patient's medical complaint.

Near-drowning

Initial survival following immersion in water.

Noisy respirations

Any noise coming from the patient's airway; this often indicates a respiratory problem.

Non-rebreather mask with reservoir bag

A high-concentration oxygen delivery device; the preferred method of administering oxygen in the pre-hospital setting.

Non-urgent move

A casualty move used when there are no present or anticipated threats to the patient's life and care can be adequately and safely administered.

Normal respirations

Respirations occurring without airway noise or effort from the patient; the usually rate in the adult is 12–20 breaths per minute.

Occlusive dressing

A airtight dressing, such as a petroleum gauze, that is placed over a wound and sealed.

Open injury

An injury that produces a break in the continuity of the skin.

Oropharyngeal airway

A curved piece of plastic that goes into the patient's mouth and lifts the tongue away from the back of the throat.

Oropharynx

The region of the pharynx that lies just below the nasopharynx and extends to the level of the epiglottis.

Oxygen regulator

A device that attaches to an oxygen cylinder and is used to adjust the flow rate of oxygen to the patient.

Patient

A general term used to describe a person requiring treatment.

Perfusion

The process of circulating blood to the organs, delivering oxygen and removing waste products.

Perineum

The area of skin between the vagina and anus.

Pharynx

Part of the airway behind the mouth and nose, divided into two regions, the nasopharynx and the oropharynx, commonly referred to as the throat.

Placard

An information sign with symbols and numbers to assist in identifying the hazardous material or class of material.

Placenta

The foetal and maternal organ through which the foetus absorbs oxygen and nutrients and excretes wastes; it is attached to the foetus via the umbilical cord.

Pneumatic splint

A device that uses air or vacuum to stabilise an injury.

Position of function

The relaxed position of the hand or foot in which there is minimal movement or stretching of muscle.

Presenting part

The part of the foetus that appears at the vaginal opening first.

Primary assessment

The first step in the evaluation of every medical patient and trauma casualty used to identify immediate threats to life.

Proximal

A directional term meaning closer to the trunk (more central).

Pulse points

A location where an artery passes close to the skin and over a bone, where the pressure wave of the heart contraction can be felt.

Puncture wound

A wound caused by a pointed object piercing the skin; though apparently small it often conceals underlying damage.

Quality Improvement

A system for continually evaluating and making necessary adjustments to the care provided within an EMS system.

Reactive to light

A term that describes the pupils when they constrict when exposed to a light source.

Recovery position

Position in which the casualty is placed on his or her side, used to maintain an open airway by preventing the tongue from blocking the rear aspect of the mouth and allowing gravity to assist in draining secretions.

Rescue board

A flat, rigid board of plastic, wood or aluminium, used to immobolise the entire spine; 'long-spinal board' or 'backboard' are synonymous terms.

Rescue breathing

The artificial ventilations provided to a non-breathing patient by a rescuer during CPR.

Respiratory distress

A clinical condition in which the infant or child begins to increase the work of breathing.

Respiratory failure

A clinical condition in which the patient is continuing to work hard to breathe, the effort of breathing is increased, and the patient's condition begins to deteriorate.

Resuscitation masks

Small, lightweight masks that can be used when ventilating a patient.

Retractions

The use of accessory muscles to increase the work of breathing, which appears as the sucking in of the muscles between the ribs and at the neck.

Rigid splint

A type of immobilisation device that does not conform to the body.

Scene assessment

The evaluation of the entire environment for safety, the mechanism of injury or the nature of illness, the number of casualties, and the need for additional help.

Secondary assessment.

The final step in the process of assessing the casualty; it involves repeating the primary assessment and then continues until patient care is transferred to the arriving EMS personnel.

Shallow respirations

Respirations that have low volumes of air in inhalation and exhalation.

Shock

Inadequate oxygenation of the body tissues and inadequate organ perfusion caused by an abnormality in the cardiovascular system.

Simple mask

A low-concentration oxygen mask.

Sling and swathe

Bandaging used to immobilise a shoulder or arm injury.

Splint

A device used to immobilise a musculoskeletal injury.

Strategic Medical Direction

Any direction provided by medically qualified personnel that does not involve speaking with providers in the field, including but not limited to, systems design, protocol development, education and quality improvement.

Stress

Bodily or mental tension caused by physical or emotional factors; can also involve a person's response to events that are threatening or challenging.

Stridor

An abnormal high-pitched inspiratory sound, often indicating airway obstruction.

Suction catheter

A flexible or rigid tip placed on the end of suction tubing. The suction catheter goes into the patient's mouth.

Suction

Using negative pressure to remove liquids or semi-liquids from the airway.

Sudden infant death syndrome (SIDS)

The sudden, unexplained death of an infant, generally between the ages of 1 month and 1 year, for which there is no discernible cause on autopsy.

Systolic blood pressure

The measurement of the pressure exerted against the arteries during contraction of the heart.

Trachea

The windpipe.

Tracheal stoma

A permanent artificial opening into the trachea.

Trending

The process of comparing sets of vital signs or other assessment information over time.

Triage

A method of categorising patients into treatment or transport priorities.

Twisting injury

The result of a force applied to the body in a twisting motion.

Umbilical cord

The cord that connects the placenta to the foetus.

Universal distress signal

Both hands clutching at the neck; a sign of upper airway obstruction.

Universal precautions

Measures taken to prevent First Responders from coming into contact with a patient's blood, body fluids, or airborne pathogens via secretions.

Uterus

The female reproductive organ in which a baby grows and develops.

Vagina

The canal that leads from the uterus to the external opening in females.

Ventricles

The two lower chambers of the heart, which pump blood out of the heart.

Ventricular fibrillation (VF)

A chaotic heart rhythm in which the patient has no pulse and the heart is simply 'quivering' inside the chest; the heart is not pumping so no pulse is produced.

Ventricular tachycardia (VT)

An abnormal heart rhythm in which three or more beats in a row are generated by the ventricles at a rate of 140 beats per minute or more; there may or may not be a detectable pulse, and if there is no pulse, this is referred to as pulseless VT

Voluntary muscle

Muscle that is attached to bone. Voluntary muscle is under the individual's direct control.

Wheeze

A high-pitched whistling sound caused by narrowed air passages, which can indicate an airway obstruction.

Xiphoid Process

The bony protrusion that extends from the lower portion of the sternum.

Further Reading

Advanced Life Support Group. *Major Incident Medical Management and Support. The Practical Approach.* BMJ Publications, 1995.

British Red Cross and St John's Ambulance. *First Aid Manual of the Voluntary Aid Societies,* 7e. Dorling Kindersley Ltd, 1997.

Caroline N. *Emergency Care in the Streets,* 4e. Little Brown and Co., 1991.

Colquhoun MC, Handley AJ & Evans TR. *ABC of Resuscitation,* 3rd Edn. BMJ Publications, 1995.

Greater Manchester County Fire Service and the Advanced Life Support Group. *Firefighter's Manual of Trauma Care.* The Institution of Fire Engineers, 1996.

Greaves J, Hodgetts T & Porter K. *Emergency Care: A Textbook for Paramedics.* WB Saunders, 1997.

Huckstep RL. *A Simple Guide to Trauma.* Churchill-Livingstone, 1995.

Manual of Firemanship. Practice Firemanship 2. Book 12. Her Majesty's Stationery Office, 1995.

McSwain NE, Paturas JL & Weitz E (Eds) *PHTLS: Basic and Advanced Pre-hospital Trauma Life Support,* 3rd Edn. Mosby Inc., 1994.

Robinson C & Redmond T. *Management of Major Trauma.* Oxford University Press, 1991.

Skinner D, Driscoll P and Earlam R. *ABC of Major Trauma,* 2nd Edn. BMJ Publications, 1996.

The Manual Handling Operations Regulations. Resuscitation Council Guidelines, 1992.

Watson L. *Advanced Vehicle Entrapment Rescue.* Greenwave Publishers, 1994.

Index

Abbreviations; CPR, cardiopulmonary
    resuscitation; Emergency medical
    services; RTA, road traffic
    accident.

ABC, *see* AcBC
Abdominal injury
    infants/children, 184
    open, 141
Abdominal palpation, 92-93
Abdominal thrusts (Heimlich
    manoeuvre), 71-72
    children, 74
    definition, 52
Abortion, spontaneous (miscarriage),
    165, 169
Abrasions, 139
    definition, 131
AcBC (Airway with cervical spinal
    control, breathing and
    circulation), *see also* Airway;
    Breathing; Circulatory system;
    Spinal column
    in adult CPR, 106-107
    definition, 52, 80, 101, 131, 151
    in head injury, 159
    in infant/child CPR, 110-111
    in spinal injury, 157
Acceptance by dying patient, 13
Access
    to casualty, space creation
        allowing, 198-199, 199, 206
    to EMS system, 6
        in cardiac emergencies, early,
        105
Accessory muscles, *see* Respiratory
    muscles
Additional help, need for, 86
Advanced life support, 105
    definition, 101
    early, 105
Advanced safety precautions, 20
Age and vital signs, 223
Agonal respirations, 52
Air
    in artificial ventilation
        forced into stomach, 70
        volume delivered, 65
    exchange, *see* Exchange, air/gas
Air medical transport (helicopter/air
    ambulance), 193-196, 205-206
    landing site, 193-195, 205
        preparation, 194
        selection, 193 194
Airbags, 200-202
Airway, 55-63, *see also* AcBC
    adjuncts, 57
        infants/children, 178
    anatomy/physiology, 24, 55, 177
    burn cases, 145, 146
    clearing (of compromised
        airway), 60-63, 75
    in CPR
        adult, 106
        infant/child, 110-111, 112
    elderly persons, 97
    fitting and, 122

head injury and, 159
impaired consciousness, 121
infant/child, *see* Child; Infant
inspection (in general), 56-57
near-drowning, 125
obstruction
    by foreign body, *see* Foreign
    body
    by tongue, *see* Tongue
    open, maintaining (in general),
    60-63, 75, 218-219
    opening (in general), 55-60, 75, 89
        infant/child, 177, 179
    primary assessment, 89
    RTA victim, 198
    special situations in management,
    69-70, 76
    spinal injury and, 158
    in triage, 87
Alcohol and hypothermia, 123
Alertness, assessment, 88, *see also* AVPU
    head injury, 160
Alimentary tract, 33-34
Allergies, 95, *see also* Anaphylactic shock
Ambulance
    air, *see* Air medical transport
    transferring patient to, 193
Ambulance crew
    ambulance paramedic, definition,
    3, 6
    ambulance technician, definition,
    3, 6
    reporting to, 8, 91, 96
Amniotic sac, 167
    definition, 165, 167
AMPLE history, 80, 94-95
Amputations, 141
    definition, 131
Anaphylactic shock, 134
Anger, dying patient, 13
Anxiety in dealing with ill or injured
    infants/children, 184
Aorta, 27, 103
Arm, *see* Upper extremities
Arteries, 27, 103-104
    bleeding from, 136
Artificial ventilation, *see* Ventilation
Assessment
    patient, 7, 79-77, *see also specific
    aspects and conditions*
    child/infant, *see* Children;
    Infants
        primary, *see* Primary
        assessment
        at RTA, 198
        secondary, *see* Secondary
        assessment
    scene, *see* Scene
Atria, definition/function, 23, 27, 103
Auscultation, blood pressure, 227
Automated external defibrillator, *see*
    Defibrillator
AVPU, 88-89
    head injury, 160-161
    infants/children, 179
    in primary assessment, 88-89

Baby, newborn, initial care, 171, 171-172
Back blows
    children, 74
    infants, 73
Back injury in first responder, 37
Backboards, *see* Rescue boards
Bag-valve-mask, 217, 218-219
    definition, 215
    one-person, 218-219
    two-person, 217
Bandages, 146-148, 149
    definition, 131
Bargaining, dying patient, 13
Barrier devices for ventilation, 20, 67
    definition, 52
Basic life support, 105
    in cardiac emergencies, early, 105
    definition, 101
Behavioural emergencies, 127-130, 130
Birth canal, definition, 165
Blast injuries, 142, 149
Bleeding/haemorrhage, 135-138, 148
    definition, 131
    evaluation (for major bleeding),
    90-91, 135-136
    external, 136-138
        management, 136-138
    internal, 138
        management, 138
        signs/symptoms, 138
    intracranial, 159
    vaginal (post-delivery), 171
Blood, 28, 104
    circulation of, 28, *see also*
    Circulatory system
    as infection risk, 19, 82, 135
    perfusion by, *see* Perfusion
Blood pressure, 221, 227-228
    age and, 223
Blood vessels, 27-28, 103-104
Bloody show, 165, 168
Blunt trauma, 85
Body fluids as infection risk, 19, 82
Body mechanics and lifting patients, 35,
    37-42, 48
Body temperature, *see* Temperature
Bomb (blast) injuries, 142, 149
Bones, 29-30, 153, *see also specific bones*
    injuries (fractures etc.), 154-157,
    161-162, 242-247
        mechanisms, 154
        signs/symptoms, 155, 242
        splinting, *see* Splints
Brachial arteries, 27, 103
    pulse, assessment, 27, 103
        infant, 111, 225
Brain injury, 159-161, 162
Breathing/respirations, 64, 89-90, 223-224
    agonal, 52
    assessment, 64, 75, 89-90,
    223-224, *see also* AcBC
        of adequacy, 64
    in adult CPR, 106-107
    children/infants, *see* Children;
    Infants
    in head injury, 159
    of presence, 64

in primary assessment, 89-90, 157
of quality, 223
in spinal injury (suspected), 157
inadequate, signs/symptoms, 65
laboured, 221, 223
muscles of, *see* Respiratory muscles
noisy, 221, 223
normal, 221, 223
rate, *see* Respiratory rate
rescue, *see* Ventilation, artificial
in respiratory failure, infant/child, 181
see-saw, 180
shallow, 221, 223
Bullet wounds, *see* Shooting injuries
Burn(s), 143-146, 149
area (extent), 144
causes, 143-144
critical, determination of, 146
depth, 143, 146, 149
location, 144
Burnout, 11, 14

Call, preparation for, 191-192
Calming/comforting/reassuring
family/friends, 96, 114
patient, 96
with behavioural emergency, 128, 129-130
with general medical complaint, 120
Capillaries, 27-28, 104
bleeding from, 136
refill, 226
definition, 221
in triage, 87
Car accidents, *see* Road traffic accidents; Vehicle
Carbon dioxide in blood, 27
Cardiopulmonary resuscitation, *see* Resuscitation
Cardiovascular system, *see* Circulatory system; Heart
Carotid arteries, 27, 103
pulse, assessment, 27, 103, 225
in adult CPR, 107
in head injury, 160
Carrying, guidelines, 37-39
Carrying chairs, 38, 46
Casualty/casualties
assessment, *see* Assessment
definition, 80
extrication, *see* Extrication
moving, *see* Moving
number of, 86, *see also* Multiple casualties
space creation allowing access to, 198-199, 199, 206
Catheter, suction, 52, 63
infants/children, 63, 178
Central nervous system, 33
Cervical collars, 43, 47
Cervical spine, *see* Spinal column
Cervix
definition, 165
dilation, 168
Chain of survival, definition, 101, 105
Chairs, carrying, 38, 46
Checklist, defibrillator, 238, 239
Chemical burns, 144, 145, *see also* Hazardous materials
CHEMSAFE, 204
Chest
injuries
infant/child, 184
penetrating, 140
palpation, 92
rise/fall in artificial ventilation,

poor
correction, 68-69, 219
reasons, 68-69
Chest compressions (in CPR), 104, 105, 108-109
adult, 108-109
hand positions for, *see* Hands
infant/child, 112-113
Chest thrusts, 72
children/infants, 73, 74
Chief complaint, 84, 119
definition, 80, 84
in head injury, 160
Childbirth, 165-173
Children, 175-185, *see also* Infants
airway, 177-178, 184
anatomy, 26, 55, 177
opening, 177, 179
airway obstruction (foreign body predominantly), 73, 74, 180
emergency care, 73, 74, 180
finger sweep, *see* Finger sweep
partial vs. complete, 180
artificial ventilation, 70
non-breathing child (=rescue breathing), 111
resuscitation masks, 67
assessment, 179, 185
breathing, *see below*
circulation, *see below*
pulse, *see below*
breathing, assessment, 90, 179, 223
in CPR, 111, 112
circulation, assessment, 179, 182
in CPR, 111, 112
common medical problems, 180-183
CPR, 110-113, 114
defibrillation contraindicated in, 237
definition, 175
physical examination, 93-94
pulse, assessment, 90, 179
in CPR, 111
respiratory system, 26, 55, 177
suctioning, 63, 178
trauma, 183-184, 185
Chin lift, *see* Head-tilt, chin lift
Circulatory system/the circulation, 26-28, 101-114, *see also* AcBC
anatomy and function/physiology, 26-28, 34, 103-104, 114
assessment
in adult CPR, 107
child/infant, *see* Children; Infants
in head injury, 159
primary, 90-91
failure, *see* Shock
Clammy skin, 226
Clothing, protective, *see* Protective clothing/equipment
Cold injuries, 122-125
generalised, *see* Hypothermia
local (freezing; cold burns), 124-125, 144, 146
Collarbone injury, 155
Colour, skin, 91, 226
Comforting, *see* Calming/comforting/reassuring
Communication/liaison (EMS team), extrication and, 197, 199, *see also* Information
Compressions, chest, *see* Chest
Consciousness, *see also* Mental status, altered; Responsiveness
impaired, 120
definition, 117, 120
management, 121

questioning related to spinal injury, 157, 159
Contact injury, airbag dust, 202
Continuity training, 191
Contusion wounds, 139
definition, 131
Convulsions, *see* Fits
Cot death (SIDS), 175, 183
Criteria based dispatch, 3
definition, 3
Critical incident
definition, 11
stress debriefing, 11, 15-17
Cross ramming, 200
Crowd control and air medical transport, 195
Crowing, 175
Crowning, 169, 170
definition, 165
Crush injuries (and crush syndrome), 141-142, 149
Cutting operations, 198, 199
airbags and, 202
Cyanosis, 226

Dash board roll, 200
Death
patient coping with imminent, 13
sudden infant (syndrome), 175
Debriefing, stress, critical incident, 11, 15-17
Deceleration injury, 85-86
Decontamination area, 204
Defibrillation, 231-240
definition, 101, 105
Defibrillator, automated external, 90, 231-240
advantages, 234
algorithm for use, 237
definition, 101, 231
maintenance, 238, 240
operation, 234-238
overview, 233-234
skills, 238, 240
Defusing, 16
Delivery of baby, 169, 170-171, 173
care of mother after, 172
emergencies prior to, 169
Denial in dying, 13
Dentures and airway management, 70
Depression, dying patient, 13
Diaphragm, 25, 55
definition, 23, 52, 55
Diastolic blood pressure, 227
definition, 221
Diet and stress, 14
Digestive system, 33-34
Disability, *see* Mental/neurological status, altered
Doctor, emergency, definition, 6
Documenting of information, *see* Information
DOTS (deformities/open injuries/tenderness/swelling), 80, 91
palpation for, 92
Dressings, 146-148, 149
definition, 131
occlusive, 131, 146
Drowning, definition, 117, 125
Drug (medication) history, 95
Dust, airbag, 202
Dying patient, emotional aspects, 13

Education of pre-hospital care providers, levels, 6
Ejection from vehicle, 85
Elbow, dressing/bandaging, 147
Elderly persons
assessment, 97

hypothermia, 123
Electric shock from defibrillator,
    accidental, 238
Electrical burns, 144, 145
Emergency care/first aid
    airway obstruction in
        infants/children, 73-74, 180
    blast injuries, 142
    bone and joint injury, 242
    head injury, 160
Emergency doctor, definition, 6
Emergency medical services (EMS)
    system, 5-7, 10, 189-206
    access to, see Access
    activating, 108
    definition, 3, 5
    phases of response, 191-192, 205
Emergency move, 35, 43, 43-44
Emergency vehicle
    on way to scene, 192
    parking at scene, 192
    stocks, 191
Emotional aspects of emergency care,
    13-17, 20-21, 191, see also
    Behavioural emergencies;
    Calming/comforting/reassuring;
    Family; Patient
    in dealing with ill/injured infants
    and children, 184, 185
Endocrine system, 34, see also
    Hormones
Entrapment, see Extrication
Epiglottis, definition, 23, 24, 52, 55
Equipment
    emergency vehicle, 191-192
    moving, 45-46, 48
    protective, see Protective
    clothing/equipment
    splinting, 244
Eviscerations, 141
    definition, 131, 141
Exchange, air/gas (in lungs/tissues),
    25-26
    in foreign body airway
    obstruction
        good, 71
        poor, 71
Exclusion zone, 198
Exercise and stress, 14
Exhalation, 25, 55
Extremities
    amputation, see Amputation
    elevation to control bleeding,
        136-137
    injuries, 156-157
        immobilisation, 156-157,
            242-247
        infants/children, 184
    lower, see Lower extremities
    upper, see Upper extremities
Extrication (in RTA etc.), 18, 40-41,
    196-202, 206
    definition, 189
    devices, 43
        immobilisation, 46-47
    principles, 197
    team approach, 197-198
    techniques, 199-202, 206
Eyes
    injury, 140
    personal protection, 20

Facial trauma, airway management, 70
Falls, evaluation of injury, 84
Family, relatives and friends (of patient),
    interacting with, 94, 96, 114
    in sudden infant death syndrome,
        183
Femoral artery, 27, 104
Femur, 29

Fetus, see Foetus
Fibula, 30
Finger(s), in chest compression
    adult, 108
    infant/child, 112
Finger sweep, 60, 72
    definition, 52
    infants/children,
        contraindications, 60, 73
Fingertip pressure, 136
Fire(s), vehicle, airbags and, 200-201
Fire service, extrication and, 190, 198
First aid, emergency, see Emergency care
First Aider, certificated, 6
First responder
    definition, 3, 6
    emotional aspects of emergency
        care, see Emotional aspects
    role/responsibilities, see Role and
        responsibilities
    sexual misconduct, accusations,
        130
Fits/convulsions/seizures, 121-122, 130,
    182
    causes, 121-122
    definition, 117, 121
    infants/children, 182
Flow-restricted, oxygen-powered
    ventilation device, 218
    definition, 215
Foetus, 167
    anatomy/physiology, 167
    definition, 165
Food, last intake, 95
Forehead, dressing/bandaging, 147
Foreign body, airway obstruction, 69,
    70-74, 76
    children/infants, see Children;
        Infants
Fractures, see Bones
Freezing/cold burns, 124-125, 144, 146
Friction burns, 144
Frontal impact (RTA), 85
    seat belt pretensioners in, 202
Frostbite, 125

Gag reflex, 57
    definition, 52
    infants/children, 178
    loss, 57
Gas/air exchange, see Exchange, air/gas
Gastric distension when ventilating, 70
Gastrointestinal tract, 33-34
General impression of patient, 88
    definition, 80
Glasgow coma scale, head injury, 88-89
Glass, 198
Gloves, 19-20
Gowns, 20
Grunting, 175, 181
Gunshot injuries, see Shooting injuries

Haemorrhage, see Bleeding
Half roof flap, 199
Hand(s)
    in chest compression
        adult, 108-109
        infant/child, 112-113
    dressing/bandaging, 147
    pressure to control bleeding,
        136-137
    washing, 19
Handover report, 8, 96
Hazardous materials, 17-18, 202-204, 206,
    see also Chemical burns
    definition, 11, 17, 189
'Hazmats' procedures, 203-204
Head
    bones, 29
    emergency medical care, 160

fore-, dressing/bandaging, 147
    immobilisation, 158
    infant (at delivery), 170
    injury, 159-161, 162
        assessment, 159-160
        complications, 160
        infants/children, 183-184
        management, 159-160, 161
        signs/symptoms, 160
    palpation, 92
Head-tilt, chin lift manoeuvre, 56
    infants/children, 177
Health care system, EMS services as
    component of, 6-7
Heart
    anatomy/physiology, 27, 103
    arrest (no pulse), and cardiac
        emergencies in general
        causes, 104
        CPR in, see Resuscitation,
            cardiopulmonary
        defibrillation, see Defibrillation;
            Defibrillator
    muscle, 32, 151, 153-154
    shock caused by, 133
Heat
    exposure, 126-127
    loss in hypothermia, prevention
        of further, 123
Heimlich manoeuvre, see Abdominal
    thrusts
Helmet removal, 42
Help, additional, need for, 86
High-velocity injuries, 85, see also
    Shooting injuries
Hip injury
    dressing/bandaging, 147
    elderly, 97
History (patient), 94, 94-95, 97
    AMPLE, 80, 94-95
    head injury and, 159
    spinal injury and, 157
Hormones, 34
    definition, 23
Hydraulic equipment, 196, 198
Hyperthermia, 126-127
Hypoperfusion, see Shock
Hypothermia, 122-124
    causes, 123
        near-drowning, 125
    definition, 122
    signs/symptoms, 123
Hypovolaemic shock, 133
Hypoxia in head/brain injury, 162

Illness, see Medical problem
Immobilisation
    cervical spine, 43, 88, 158
    for extrication, 46-47
    extremities, 156-157, 242-247
Immunisation, 20
Impaled objects, 140-141
Incident management system, definition,
    189
Incision wounds, 139
    definition, 131
Infants, 175-185
    airway, 177-178, 185
        adjuncts, 178
        anatomy, 26, 55, 177
        in CPR, 110-111, 112
        opening, 177, 179
    airway obstruction (foreign body
        predominantly), 73-74, 180
        emergency care, 73-74, 180
        finger sweep, see Finger sweep
        partial vs. complete, 180
    artificial ventilation, 70
        newborn, 171
        non-breathing infant (=rescue

breathing), 111
resuscitation masks, 67
assessment, 179, 185
breathing, *see below*
circulation, *see below*
pulse, *see below*
breathing, assessment, 90, 179, 223
in CPR, 111, 112
circulation, assessment, 179, 182
in CPR, 111, 112
common medical problems, 180-183
CPR, 110-113, 114
definition, 175
mucus extractor, *see* Mucus extractor
newborn, initial care, 171, 171-172
physical examination, 93-94
pulse, assessment, 90, 179, 225
in CPR, 111
respiratory system, 26, 55, 177
suctioning, 63, 178
trauma, 183-184, 185
Infection risk
burns, 146
health care personnel, safety precautions with, 19, 82, 135
Information (and its recording/documentation), *see also* Communication
for air medical transport, 193
vital signs, 223
defibrillation, 238
on way to scene, 192
Inhalation, 25, 55
hot air, 145, 146
Injury, *see* Trauma
Intercostal muscles, 25

Jaw thrust without head tilt, 56, 218-219
infants/children, 177
Joints, 30
injury, 154-157, 160-161, 242-247
dressing/bandaging, 147
mechanisms, 154
signs/symptoms, 155, 242
splinting, *see* Splints

Knee, 30
dressing/bandaging, 147

Labour, 168-171, 173
1st stage, 168
2nd stage, 169, *see also* Delivery
3rd stage, 169
Lacerations, 139
definition, 131
Landing site, *see* Air medical transport
Laryngectomy
airway management with, 69
definition, 52
Larynx (voice box), 24, 55
definition, 52
Leg, *see* Lower extremities
Liaison, *see* Communication; Information
Lifting patients, 35, 37-42
guidelines, 37
Light, pupillary reactions, 221, 226
Limbs, *see* Extremities
Long spinal boards, *see* Rescue boards
Lower extremities, *see also* Amputation; Extremities
bones, 29-30, 153
palpation, 93
Lungs, 25-26

Major incidents, *see* Multiple casualties
Manual handling, definition, 35
Manual positioning for airway opening, 56

Manual stabilisation
extremity, 156-157
spine, *see* Spinal injury
Masks
oxygen, 209, 212
protective, 20
resuscitation, *see* Resuscitation masks
Mass casualties, *see* Multiple casualties
MEDCON, *see* Medical direction
Medical direction (MEDCON), 3, 10, *see also* Strategic medical direction
definition, 3, 8
Medical office as triage officer, 205
Medical problem/illness
chief complaint (patient's description), *see* Chief complaint
evaluation, 83-84, 94
of events leading to illness, 95
general complaint, 119-120, 130
signs/symptoms, 119-120
identification insignia, 94
infants/children, 180-183
nature of, 83-84
definition, 80
evaluation, 83-84
specific complaint, 120-127, 130
Medication history, 95
Mental/neurological status, altered, 120-121, 130, *see also* AVPU; Consciousness; Responsiveness
assessment for, 121
in head injury, 160
infants/children, 179, 182
primary, 88-89
causes, 121
hypothermia, 123
definition, 117
infants/children, 182-183
assessment for, 179, 182
management, 182-183
Miscarriage, 165, 169
Missile injuries, 85, *see also* Shooting injuries
Mobilisation phase, 192
Motor function, assessment, 93
Motor nerves, 33
Motorcycle helmet removal, 42
Mouth-to-barrier device ventilation, 67, 76, *see also* Barrier devices
Mouth-to-mask ventilation, 65-66, 75, 111, *see also* Resuscitation masks
with supplemental oxygen, 216-217
Mouth-to-mouth and nose ventilation, 111
Mouth-to-mouth ventilation, 67-68, 76, 111
Moving, 42-47, 48, 193
to ambulance, 193
emergency, 35, 43, 43-44
equipment, 45-46, 48
non-urgent, 35, 44
Mucus extractor, 63, 178
definition, 52
Multiple/mass casualties, 86-87, 204-205, 206
triage, *see* Triage
Muscles, 30-32, 153-154
cardiac, 32, 151, 153-154
respiratory/of breathing, *see* Respiratory muscles
skeletal/voluntary, 31, 151, 153
smooth/involuntary, 32, 151, 153
Musculoskeletal system, 29-32, 34, 151-162, 241-247, *see also specific components*
anatomy/physiology, 29-32, 153-154, 161
injuries, 154-162, 161-162, 241-247

mechanisms, 154
signs/symptoms, 155, 242
splinting, *see* Splints

Nasal canula, 209, 212, 213
Nasal flaring, 175, 181, 223
Nasopharyngeal airway, 57
definitions, 42, 57
Nasopharynx, 24
definition, 23, 52, 54
Near-drowning, 125-126, 130
definition, 117
Neck palpation, 92
Neglect of child, 175
Neonate (newborn baby), initial care, 171, 171-172
Nervous system, 33
Neurogenic shock, 134
Neurological status, *see* Mental/neurological status; Responsiveness
Newborn baby, initial care, 171, 171-172
Non-rebreather oxygen mask, 209, 212
Nose, *see* entries under Nasal

Obstetrics, *see* Childbirth; Pregnancy
Occlusive dressing, 131, 133
Old people, *see* Elderly persons
Oral intake, last, 95
Oropharyngeal airway, 57
definition, 52, 57
infants/children, 178
Oropharynx, 24
definition, 23, 52, 54
Oxygen
in/entry into blood, 26-27
supplementary (therapy), 209-213
ventilation techniques using, 216-218
Oxygen cylinders, 210-211
Oxygen regulators, 209, 211

Packaging of casualty, 199
Painful stimuli, responsiveness, 88, *see also* AVPU
head injury, 160
Palpation, 92-93
pulse, *see* Pulse
systolic BP measurement by, 227-228
Panic, 128
Paramedic, ambulance, definition, 3
Parents in sudden infant death syndrome, 183
Parking at incident, 192
Past medical history, 95
Patella, 30
Patient
calming/comforting/reassuring, *see* Calming/comforting/reassuring
history, *see* History
treated as whole person, 94, 96
Pelvis, 29-30
palpation, 93
Penetrating trauma, 85, 140-141, *see also* Puncture wounds
chest, 140
Perfusion
assessment, 91
decreased, *see* Shock
definition, 23, 28
Perineum, definition, 165, 167
Peripheral nervous system, 33
Personal safety, *see* Safety
Pharynx (throat), 24, 54
definition, 23, 52
Photographs of RTAs, 154
Physical examination, first responder, 91-95, 97

definition, 80
infant/child, 179
Placards, 204
definition, 189
Placenta, 167
definition, 165
delivery, 171
Pneumatic splints, 157, 244
Polaroid camera at operational incidents, 154
Positioning of casualties, 43, 44
for airway opening, 56
of infant/child with airway obstruction, 180
Post rip, 200
Post-run phase, 193
Pregnancy, 165-173
maternal/foetal anatomy and physiology, 167, 173
pre-delivery emergencies, 169
Pre-hospital care
handover report, 8, 91, 96
providers, recognised levels, 6
Presenting part of foetus, definition, 165, 169
Pressure (to control bleeding)
direct, 136
on pressure points, 137-138
Primary assessment/survey, 88-91, 97
definition, 80
head injury, 159
at RTA, 198
spinal injury (suspected), 157
Professional attributes, 8
Professional help, stress management, 15
Protective clothing/equipment, 19-20, 203
for RTAs, 18, 197-198
Psychogenic shock, 134
Psychological dimensions of emergency care, see Emotional aspects
Pulling, guidelines, 42
Pulse, 90, 224-225
age and, 223
assessment (e.g. palpation), 27, 103-104, 224-225
in adult CPR, 107, 109
children/infants, see Children; Infants
in defibrillation, 237
in head injury, 160
primary, 90
no, see Heart
points/sites, 23, 28, 104, 224
Puncture wounds, 131, 139, see also Penetrating trauma
Pupillary reactions, 221, 226
Pushing, guidelines, 42

Quality improvement, definition, 3, 10
Questions for responsive trauma patients, 157, 159

Radial artery, 27, 103-104
pulse, assessment, 27, 103-104, 225
Radiation, 203
burns, 144
Radio report to EMS personnel, 91
Reaching, guidelines for, 40
Rear impact (RTA), 85
Reassurance, see Calming/comforting/reassuring
Recording, see Information
Recovery position, 60
in adult CPR, 106
definition, 35
Relatives, see Family
Report to responding services, 91
handover report, 8, 96
Reproductive anatomy and physiology,

167, 173
Rescue boards (long spinal boards/backboards), 40-41, 46
definition, 35
elderly persons, 97
Rescue breathing, see Ventilation, artificial
Reservoir bag (non-rebreather oxygen with), 209, 212
Respirations, see Breathing
Respiratory distress (infants/children), 180-181
definition, 175
signs/symptoms, 175, 180-181
Respiratory failure (in infants/children), 181, 185
definition, 175
management, 181
signs/symptoms, 177
Respiratory muscles/muscles of breathing, 25, 55
accessory, 52, 223
definition, 52, 221
use by infants/children, 175, 181
Respiratory rate, 223
normal, 64
age and, 223
in triage, 87
Respiratory system, 24-26, 34, 54-55
components and function, 24-26, 54-55, 74-75
infants/children, 26, 55, 177
Responsibilities, see Role and responsibilities
Responsiveness, level of, see also Consciousness; Mental/neurological status
assessment of, 88-89, see also AVPU
in adult CPR, 106
in child/infant CPR, 110
in head injury, 160
assessment of breathing regarding, 64
foreign body obstruction and, 71-72, 73-74
Restraint systems, supplementary (SRS), 199-202, 206
Resuscitation, cardiopulmonary (CPR), 105-113, 114
adult, 105-109, 114
definition, 101, 105
hypothermia, 124
infants/children, 110-113, 114
near-drowning, 125, 126
one-rescuer vs. two-rescuer, 109, 113
stopping for defibrillator use, 234
Resuscitation masks, 52, 65-67, see also Bag-valve-mask; Mouth-to-mask ventilation
Retractions, 181
definition, 175
Rewarming, 123, 124
Ribs, 29
fractures, chest compression causing, 109
Rigid splints, 157, 244
Road traffic accidents, 18, 40-42, 84, 85-86, 196-202
deceleration injury, 85-86
evaluation of injury, 84
extrication from, see Extrication
head injury, 160
infants/children, 183
motorcycle helmet removal, 42
photographs, 154
safety considerations, 18
Role and responsibilities (of first responder), 5, 7-8, 10

behavioural emergencies, 128, 130
bleeding, 138
burns, 144-145
childbirth, 169, 171-172, 172
cold emergencies
generalised (hypothermia), 123
localised, 124-125
general medical complaints, 120
heat exposure, 127
infants/children
fitting, 122, 182
mental state alteration, 182-183
respiratory emergencies, 181
shock, 182
sudden infant death syndrome, 183
injuries
head, 159-161
musculoskeletal, 156-157
soft tissue, 139-140
spinal, 158
mental status alteration, 121
moving patients, 37, 48
near-drowning, 125-126
shock, 134-135
Rollover RTA, 85
Roof fold down, 200
Rule of nines (Wallace's), 144

Safety, 7, 17-20, 21
helicopters, 195-196, 205
personal, 7, 19-20, 21
defibrillators, 238
extrication, 18, 197-198, 206
infection risk, 19, 82, 135
oxygen cylinders, 210-211
scene, see Scene
Scalds, 144
Scene, 17-19, 82-87
assessment, 82-87, 97, 192-193, 197-198
on approaching scene, 192-193
bleeding and, 138
definition, 80
extrication and, 197-198
on way to, 192
polaroid photograph, 154
safety, 7, 17-19, 21, 82-83, 197-198
air medical transport and, 193
extrication and, 197-198
hazardous materials and, 203
Scoop stretcher, 45-46
Seat belt pretensioners, 202
Secondary assessment/survey, 95-96, 97
definition, 80
injuries
head, 160
spinal (suspected), 157
See-saw respirations, 180
Seizures, see Fits
Semi-automatic external defibrillator, 233, 235-236
Sensory nerves, 33
Sexual misconduct, accusation, 130
Shivering, 123
Shock (hypoperfusion), 133-135, 148
anaphylactic, 134
cardiogenic, 133
in crush injury, 141
definition, 28, 131
hypovolaemic, 133
infants/children, 182
management, 134-135
neurogenic, 134
psychogenic, 134
signs/symptoms, 134, 226
Shock (psychogenic), 134
Shooting/gunshot/bullet injuries, 85
definition, 131

evaluation, 84
Shoulder wound, dressing/bandaging, 147
Show, bloody, 165, 168
Side impact (RTA), 85
Side roof flap, 199
SIDS, 175, 183
Skeletal (voluntary) muscle, 31, 151, 153
Skeleton, 29-30, 153, see also Bones; Joints
Skin, 33, 225-226
    colour, 91, 226
    condition, 226
    temperature, 91, 226
        with cold exposure, 123, 124
Skull, 29, see also Head
    injuries, 159-161, 162
Sling and swathe, 245
    definition, 241
Slopes and helicopters, 194, 195
Smoking and stress, 14
Smooth (involuntary) muscle, 32, 151, 153
Soft tissue injuries, 138-142, 148-149
    types, 139
Space creation allowing access to casualty, 198-199, 199, 206
Spinal boards, see Rescue boards
Spinal column
    bones, 29
    injury, see Spinal injury
Spinal injury (actual/possible and implying mainly cervical spine), 44, 157-158, 162
    assessment, 157, 162
    elderly, 97
    management (other than manual stabilisation), 158, 162
    mechanisms, 157, 159
    signs/symptoms, 157-158
    stabilisation/control, 43, 88, 156, 158, see also AcBC; Immobilisation
        in adult CPR, 106
Splints, 157, 241-247
    definition, 241
    equipment/techniques, 244
    principles, 243-244
    risks with, 246
Stabilisation
    patient, 198
        manual, see Manual stabilisation
    vehicle, 198
Stairs, carrying chairs, 38, 46
Steering wheel relocation, 200
Steps, carrying down, 39
Sternum and chest compression, 108
Stocks, emergency vehicle, 191
Stomach, air forced into, when ventilating, 70
Strategic medical direction, 10
    definition, 3, 10
Stress, 11, 14-17
    debriefing, critical incident, 11, 15-17
    management, 14-17
    warning signs, 14
Stretcher
    scoop, 45-46
    wheeled, 45
Stridor
    definition, 52
    infants/children, 175
Suction, 60-63
    definition, 52
    evices, 52, 61-63, 178
    fants/children, 63, 178
    spinal trauma, 158
    fant death syndrome, 175, 183

Supplementary restraint systems (SRS), 199-202, 206
Systolic blood pressure, 227
    definition, 221

Tachycardia, ventricular, 231, 233
Team approach to extrication, 197-198
Temperature, body
    abnormal, see Hyperthermia; Hypothermia
    skin, 91, 226
Thermal burns, 143
Third door conversion, 200
Thorax, bones, 29
Throat, see Pharynx
Tibia, 30
Tongue, airway blocked by, 56
    infant/child, 26, 55, 177
Tongue depressor, 178
Toxic substances in crush injury, 141
Trachea (windpipe), 25, 55
    infant/child, 55
    stoma
        airway management with, 69
        definition, 52
Training
    continuity, 191
    hazardous materials, 203
Transfering patients, see Carrying; Lifting; Moving
Transport, see Air medical transport; Moving
Trauma/injury (first responder), back, 37
Trauma/injury (patient), 84-86, 138-147, 148-149, 154-162, 241-247, see also Contact injury; Road traffic accidents
    abdominal, see Abdominal injury
    bleeding with, see Bleeding
    closed, definition, 151, 154-155
    direct, 154
        definition, 151, 154
    elderly, 97
    head, see Head
    indirect, 154
        definition, 151, 154
    infants/children, 183-184, 185
    mechanisms, 157, 159
        evaluation, 84-85
    multiple casualties, see Multiple casualties
    musculoskeletal, see Musculoskeletal system
    open, definition, 151, 154, see also DOTS
    rib, chest compression causing, 109
    shooting, see Shooting injuries
    soft tissue, see Soft tissue injuries
    spinal, see Spinal injury
    splints causing, 246, 247
    thermal, see Cold injuries; Thermal burns
    twisting, 151, 154
    ventilation in, 68, 70, 158
Trending, 221, 223
Triage, 86-87, 204-205, 206
    definition, 189
    'sieve' (categories/priorities/tagging), 86-87, 204, 205, 206
    'sort', 86
Triage officer, 205
Twisting injury, 151, 154

Umbilical cord, 167
    definition, 165
    tying, 171
UN number, hazardous materials, 204
Unconsciousness, 120, see also

Consciousness; Mental status, altered; Responsiveness
United Nations number, hazardous materials, 204
Universal distress signal, definition, 52, 71
Universal safety precautions, 19-20, 21, 82
    definition, 11
Unresponsiveness, see Responsiveness, level of
Upper extremities, see also Amputation; Extremities
    bones, 30, 153
    palpation, 93
Uterus, 167
    definition, 165

Vaccination, 20
Vagina, definition, 165
Vehicle
    emergency, see Emergency vehicle
    involved in RTA
        fires, airbags and, 200-201
        stabilisation, 198
Veins, 28, 104
    bleeding from, 136
Ventilation, artificial, 65-69, 75-76, 106-107, 215-219
    adequacy/effectiveness, assessing, 68-69, 219
    advanced techniques, 215-219
    barrier devices, see Barrier devices
    in CPR (rescue breathing)
        adult, 106-107, 107
        child, 111
        infant, 111
        newborn, 171
        principles, 66
        rate, 65
    in special situations, 69-70
        foreign body obstruction, 72, 74
        in respiratory failure (infant/child), 181
        trauma patients, 68, 70, 158
    techniques, 65-68
Ventricles
    definition/function, 23, 27, 103
    fibrillation, 231, 233
    tachycardia, 231, 233
Verbal stimuli, responsiveness, 88, see also AVPU
    head injury, 160
Violence, 18-19, 129
    predicting potential for, 129
Vital signs, 221-229
    in head injury, 160
    reassessment, 228-229, 229
Voice box, see also Larynx

Wallace's rule of nines, 144
Warming (rewarming), 123, 124
Washing of hands, 19
Wheeled stretcher, 45
Wheeze, definition, 52
Windpipe, see Trachea
Work schedule and stress, 14-15
Wounds, see Trauma

Xiphoid process, 29, 101
    chest compression and, 108